Manual on
Control
of Infection
in Surgical
Patients

By The Committee on Control of Surgical Infections
of the Committee on Pre- and Postoperative Care

AMERICAN COLLEGE OF SURGEONS

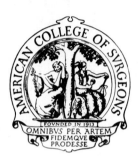

Editorial Committee

William A. Altemeier, M.D., Chairman

John F. Burke, M.D.

Basil A. Pruitt, Jr., M.D.

William R. Sandusky, M.D.

Manual on
CONTROL OF INFECTION IN SURGICAL PATIENTS

Second Edition

J.B. LIPPINCOTT COMPANY
Philadelphia

London   Mexico City   New York   St. Louis   São Paulo   Sydney

Sponsoring Editor: Sanford J. Robinson
Manuscript Editor: Rosanne Hallowell
Indexer: Kathleen Garcia
Art Director: Maria S. Karkucinski
Designer: Patrick Turner
Production Supervisor: J. Corey Gray
Compositor: Progressive Typographers
Printer/Binder: R.R. Donnelley & Sons Company

Second Edition

1   3   5   6   4   2

Library of Congress Cataloging in Publication Data
Main entry under title:

Manual on control of infection in surgical patients.

  Bibliography: p.
  Includes index.
  1. Surgery, Aseptic and antiseptic — Handbooks, manuals,
etc.   2. Nosocomial infections — Prevention — Handbooks,
manuals, etc.   3. Hospitals — Hygiene — Handbooks,
manuals, etc.   I. Altemeier, William A.   II. American
College of Surgeons. Committee on Control of Surgical Infections. [DNLM: 1. Cross infection — Prevention and control —
Congresses. 2. Surgical wound infection — Prevention and
control — Congresses. WO 185 M295 1980 – 82]
RD91.M3   1984   617'.9101   83-18695
ISBN 0-397-50575-2

The authors and publisher have exerted every effort to ensure that drug selection and dosage set forth
in this text are in accord with current recommendations and practice at the time of publication.
However, in view of ongoing research, changes in government regulations, and the constant flow of
information relating to drug therapy and drug reactions, the reader is urged to check the package
insert for each drug for any change in indications and dosage and for added warnings and precautions.
This is particularly important when the recommended agent is a new or infrequently employed drug.

NOTICE

This volume attempts to provide a useful guide to control of infection in surgical patients. The
manual does not attempt to define in exhaustive detail a particular patient's requirements for therapy,
nor to prejudge for a particular physician the therapeutic regimen he or she may deem necessary in
regard to that patient. The Committee does not claim that other methods or approaches than those
presented in this volume may not be equally successful in a specific case.

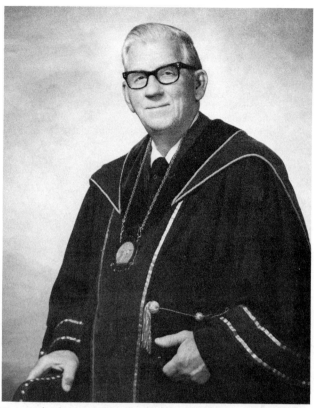

"I am indeed appreciative for the life of fulfillment I have had as an active investigator in the areas of surgical bacteriology and surgical infections, as well as a clinical surgeon and a professor and teacher. It has stimulated my interests, satisfied my inquisitiveness, enlarged my scope of knowledge and friends, and given me the privilege of providing help through knowledge and research to physicians and their patients everywhere."

(Surg Clin North Am 60:1, 1980)

William A. Altemeier, M.D., July 6, 1910 – November 23, 1983

FOREWORD

Modern surgery became a reality when Lister applied the work of Pasteur in the domain of surgery; this greatly reduced the infections that had largely blocked earlier efforts to develop surgical procedures for the internal organs. However, just as a great advance against a disease does not necessarily eliminate it, surgical infections are still a serious problem in spite of Lister's contribution and many subsequent advances (such as the development of sulfanilamide, and the development of penicillin and other antibiotics).

Surgical infections fall into two categories: spontaneous infections, including those following trauma, which come to surgeons for cure; and hospital-acquired infections, that is, those occurring as complications of surgical and other procedures performed on uninfected patients. The control of surgical infections has always been important, but it has varied in its degree of importance from time to time and from place to place. Thus, after a period during which antibiotics gave us remarkable control of staphylococcus infections, resistant strains developed, with an epidemic of serious and sometimes fatal infections occurring in the late 1950s.

More recently, the great increase in the use of inert prostheses has given the area of surgical infections a fresh importance. For instance, the indwelling plastic catheter for intravenous hyperalimentation is from time to time associated with a bloodstream infection. If prosthetic heart valves become infected, the result is all too frequently a fatal outcome. If sections of the aorta and iliac vessels are replaced with woven prostheses of Dacron or other plastic material, and infection occurs, this too may well lead to a fatal issue. And if a modern prosthetic knee or hip joint becomes infected, the work of the orthopedist can be ruined and the patient suffers greatly.

It was with this background that the Regents of the American College of Surgeons authorized the Committee on Control of Surgical Infections as a subcommittee of the Pre- and Postoperative Care Committee, and named Dr. William A. Altemeier as its chairman. Dr. Altemeier was influenced by three of the residents of William Stewart Halsted. Dr. George J. Heuer and Dr. Mont Reid successively served as Chairman of the Department of Surgery at the University of Cincinnati, where Dr. Altemeier attended medical school, and they gave the department much of its direction in the second quarter of this century. Dr. Altemeier took his surgical residency at the Henry Ford Hospital under Dr. Roy D. McClure, a third Halsted resident. All of these men emphasized careful technique to minimize tissue injury, a tradition continuously emphasized by Dr. Altemeier throughout his chairmanship of the Department of Surgery at the University of Cincinnati from 1952 to 1979. He devoted most of his career to the study of microbiology in relation to surgery, and it is a matter of record that during his service the Cincinnati General Hospital had an outstandingly low incidence of infections in clean wounds.

With characteristic energy and thoroughness, Dr. Altemeier organized four workshops on the control of surgical infections, to which came most of the active investigators in this field in the United States and other parts of the world. The first edition of the *Manual on Control of Infection in Surgical Patients* was a summary of their reports and discussions. Since the first edition appeared in 1976, the Surgical Infection Society was organized, again through the initiative, the diplomacy, and the drive of Dr. William A. Altemeier. An organization meeting was held on May 17, 1980, in Chicago. A constitution and bylaws were adopted and officers were elected. Dr. Altemeier became the first president and carried over with the other officers for a second year. Annual meetings with scientific programs were held in 1980, 1981, and 1982, and much of the new material presented at those meetings, as well as at other surgical meetings, is reflected in the second edition of this manual. It is a source of deep regret that Dr. Altemeier did not live to see the second edition in print. His death occurred November 23, 1983. The essential parts of the new edition had been completed with his participation, and the final phases of the work were finished by his co-editors.

The persistence of surgical infections, particularly nosocomial infections, is sometimes the source of much discouragement to doctors as well as patients. On the other side of the ledger, however, is the fact that we are doing operations and other procedures that would not have been undertaken before we had the antibiotics and certain other advances. In other words, surgeons have extended their range of procedure as far as modern methods for the prevention and treatment of infections have allowed.

In this sense, advances in the field of surgical infections, both in science and in the conscientious application of what we now know, have permitted many of the advances in surgery. An example of this taken from a field with which I am familiar is intravenous hyperalimentation using an indwelling central venous catheter. In my judgment, this method would have had to be given up early were it not for the fact that a large majority of the infections encountered were curable by antibiotics.

This second edition of the *Manual on Control of Infections in Surgical Patients* revises and updates the first edition and presents in highly usable form the best information available from a very distinguished group of authors. It will only benefit the patient, however, to the extent that it is understood and applied.

Jonathan E. Rhoads, M.D., F.A.C.S.

EDITORIAL COMMITTEE
of the
Manual on Control of Infection
in Surgical Patients

William A. Altemeier, M.D., F.A.C.S. (Deceased)
Christian R. Holmes Professor of Surgery, Emeritus, University of Cincinnati Medical Center, Cincinnati, Ohio

John F. Burke, M.D., F.A.C.S.
Helen Andrus Benedict Professor of Surgery, Harvard Medical School, Boston, Massachusetts

Basil A. Pruitt, Jr., M.D., F.A.C.S.
Colonel, M.C., U.S. Army; Commander and Director, U.S. Army Institute of Surgical Research, Brooke Army Medical Center, Fort Sam Houston, Texas

William R. Sandusky, M.D., F.A.C.S.
Professor of Surgery, Emeritus, University of Virginia School of Medicine, Charlottesville, Virginia

COMMITTEE ON CONTROL OF SURGICAL INFECTIONS
of the
Pre- and Postoperative Care Committee
American College of Surgeons

William A. Altemeier, M.D., F.A.C.S. (Deceased)
Christian R. Holmes Professor of Surgery Emeritus, University of Cincinnati Medical Center, Cincinnati, Ohio

John F. Burke, M.D., F.A.C.S.
Helen Andrus Benedict Professor of Surgery, Harvard Medical School, Boston, Massachusetts

George H.A. Clowes, Jr., M.D., F.A.C.S.
Professor of Surgery, Harvard Medical School, Boston, Massachusetts

William R. Cole, M.D., F.A.C.S.
Department of Surgery, Bothwell Memorial Hospital, Sedalia, Missouri

William R. Culbertson, M.D., F.A.C.S.
Professor of Surgery, University of Cincinnati Medical Center, Cincinnati, Ohio

John H. Davis, M.D., F.A.C.S.
Professor of Surgery, and Chairman, Department of Surgery, University of Vermont College of Medicine, Burlington, Vermont

Lloyd D. MacLean, M.D., F.R.C.S. (C)
Professor of Surgery, McGill University, Montreal, Quebec

Basil A. Pruitt, Jr., M.D., F.A.C.S.
Colonel, M.C., U.S. Army; Commander and Director, U.S. Army Institute of Surgical Research, Brooke Army Medical Center, Fort Sam Houston, Texas

Edwin J. Pulaski, M.D., F.A.C.S. (Deceased)
Director, Clinical Research, Baxter-Travenol Laboratories, Morton Grove, Illinois

William R. Sandusky, M.D., F.A.C.S.
Professor of Surgery Emeritus, University of Virginia Medical Center, Charlottesville, Virginia

Carl W. Walter, M.D., F.A.C.S.
Clinical Professor of Surgery Emeritus, Harvard Medical School, Boston, Massachusetts

PRE- AND POSTOPERATIVE CARE COMMITTEE
CURRENT MEMBERSHIP — 1984

†Donald S. Gann, M.D., F.A.C.S.,
Chairman *Providence, Rhode Island*

†Murray F. Brennan, M.D., F.A.C.S.,
Vice Chairman *New York, New York*

* Arthur E. Baue, M.D., F.A.C.S.
New Haven, Connecticut

John R. Border, M.D., F.A.C.S.
Buffalo, New York

Frank B. Cerra, M.D., F.A.C.S.
Minneapolis, Minnesota

* Joseph M. Civetta, M.D., F.A.C.S.
Miami, Florida

Arnold G. Coran, M.D., F.A.C.S.
Ann Arbor, Michigan

* P. William Curreri, M.D., F.A.C.S.
Mobile, Alabama

John W. Duckett, Jr., M.D., F.A.C.S.
Philadelphia, Pennsylvania

* John H. Duff, M.D., F.A.C.S.
London, Ontario

* James H. Duke, Jr., M.D., F.A.C.S.
Houston, Texas

C. McCollister Evarts, M.D., F.A.C.S.
Rochester, New York

Josef E. Fischer, M.D., F.A.C.S.
Cincinnati, Ohio

Joel B. Freeman, M.D., F.A.C.S.
Ottawa, Ontario

J. Byron Gathright, Jr., M.D., F.A.C.S.
New Orleans, Louisiana

* Ruben F. Gittes, M.D., F.A.C.S.
Boston, Massachusetts

* Lazar J. Greenfield, M.D., F.A.C.S.
Richmond, Virginia

Alden H. Harken, M.D., F.A.C.S.
Denver, Colorado

Herbert B. Hechtman, M.D., F.A.C.S.
Boston, Massachusetts

Clifford M. Herman, M.D., F.A.C.S.
Seattle, Washington

James W. Holcroft, M.D., F.A.C.S.
Sacramento, California

Joel H. Horovitz, M.D., F.A.C.S.
Dallas, Texas

Jonas T. Johnson, M.D., F.A.C.S.
Pittsburgh, Pennsylvania

* M. J. Jurkiewicz, M.D., F.A.C.S.
Atlanta, Georgia

Nicholas T. Kouchoukos, M.D., F.A.C.S.
Birmingham, Alabama

Frank R. Lewis, Jr., M.D., F.A.C.S.
San Francisco, California

Byron J. Masterson, M.D., F.A.C.S.
Louisville, Kentucky

William E. Matory, M.D., F.A.C.S.
Washington, D.C.

†Jonathan L. Meakins, M.D., F.A.C.S.
Montreal, Quebec

* William W. Monafo, Jr., M.D., F.A.C.S.
St. Louis, Missouri

* Gerald S. Moss, M.D., F.A.C.S.
Chicago, Illinois

†Richard M. Peters, M.D., F.A.C.S.
San Diego, California

Albert L. Rhoton, Jr., M.D., F.A.C.S.
Gainesville, Florida

John L. Rombeau, M.D., F.A.C.S.
Philadelphia, Pennsylvania

Robert A. Schimek, M.D., F.A.C.S.
New Orleans, Louisiana

William A. Scoville, M.D., F.A.C.S.
Baltimore, Maryland

* George F. Sheldon, M.D., F.A.C.S.
Chapel Hill, North Carolina

* Harry M. Shizgal, M.D., F.A.C.S.
Montreal, Quebec

Richard L. Simmons, M.D., F.A.C.S.
Minneapolis, Minnesota

* Jessie L. Ternberg, M.D., F.A.C.S.
St. Louis, Missouri

* Roby C. Thompson, Jr., M.D., F.A.C.S.
Minneapolis, Minnesota

* Daniel G. Vaughan, M.D., F.A.C.S.
San Jose, California

Walter W. Whisler, M.D., F.A.C.S.
Chicago, Illinois

Willis H. Williams, M.D., F.A.C.S.
Atlanta, Georgia

†Douglas W. Wilmore, M.D., F.A.C.S.
Boston, Massachusetts

Elvin G. Zook, M.D., F.A.C.S.
Springfield, Illinois

*Senior member
†Executive Committee member

PREFACE

The second edition of the *Manual on Control of Infection in Surgical Patients* is published in consideration of the wide acceptance of the first edition and its general usefulness in the United States and many other countries throughout the world. Prepared by the Editorial Committee of the Committee on Control of Infections of the Pre- and Postoperative Care Committee of the American College of Surgeons, this edition includes an authoritative update and extensive revision of the first, commensurate with the increase in available knowledge and new skills that have since been acquired.

The objectives of the manual continue to be essentially the same, with appropriate emphasis on newly introduced information and techniques:

- Its *target* is infection that can develop in the surgical patient as a postoperative, post-trauma, or hospital-acquired complication.
- Its *aim* is to provide an up-to-date readily available source of information and guide that will be useful for the prevention and control of surgical infections in hospital practice.
- Its *purpose* is to minimize infections, reduce morbidity and mortality, improve wound healing, lower costs of hospital care, avoid unnecessary deformity or disability, and reduce the incidence of permanent effects on the quality of life, both physical and psychological. In addition, it gives increased attention to the problems of getting the surgical patient well after he has acquired an infection.

The development of the first edition of the manual came about by action of the Board of Regents of the American College of Surgeons in an effort to meet the need of clinical surgeons to reduce the incidence of infection in surgical patients. The board, in conjunction with the Committee on Pre- and Postoperative Care, appointed the Committee on Control of Surgical Infections. This committee, headed by me, undertook the study of the problems underlying the continuing incidence and importance of infections in surgical patients. It became increasingly apparent that *controversy, confusion,* and frequently *lack of information* existed in many areas of the art and practice of surgery relative to infection. One of the obvious reasons for this state of affairs was the paucity of factual information available on many subjects. Thus, the Committee on Control of Surgical Infections recognized the need to establish a broad and authoritative data base from which solutions to the problems of infection could be developed.

Four symposia were then organized and held, beginning in March, 1970 and ending in November, 1972. Each concentrated attention on selected and specific areas of surgical infections. In attendance were the ten committee members, numerous invited authorities, and other special participants. The contributors and participants, all of whom were experts in various areas of surgical infections, were also selected on a geographic basis to extend the breadth of the base. Their contributions and discussions were recorded, transcribed, and studied by members of the Committee on Control of Surgical Infections. Subcommittees, assisted by consultants and other knowledgable persons, then reviewed and revised the data in a series of working sessions.

The conscientious efforts of the committee members and other contributors were then collated, refined, updated, and edited by the Editorial Committee, consisting of John F. Burke, Basil A. Pruitt, Jr., William R. Sandusky, and me. Carl W. Walter has also contributed significantly to the review and revision of many of the chapters of this manual. Beyond their input in committee deliberations, the symposia, and the overall development of this manual, several members of the Committee on Control of Infections have contributed significantly to the preparation of specific chapters. For this effort, special thanks are due to George H. A. Clowes, Jr., for Chapter 5, to William R. Sandusky for Chapter 11, to J. Wesley Alexander for Chapter 12, and to Carl W. Walter for Chapter 16. The results of the total effort formed the basis upon which the *Manual on Control of Infection in Surgical Patients* was developed.

Like the first, the second edition of the manual does not attempt to be a final text, but it is hoped that it will continue to serve as a ready, updated reference and useful guide for those who would appreciate a collated, practical account of the factors presently considered to be significant in the prevention and control of surgical infections. The Editorial Committee has continued to be conscious of the importance of cost effectiveness in these matters, but it has addressed itself primarily to the determination of the best methods known today for the prevention and control of infections in surgical patients, irrespective of cost.

The recommendations and procedures in this manual have been developed as reasonable proposals with balance between the theoretical and the practical. Disagreement with some of the recommendations is inevitable and expected as a result of conflicting ideas and lack of factual information. Indeed, there exists a difference of opinion in some cases among the members of the Committee on Control of Surgical Infections. The importance of revising this manual at this time and periodically thereafter to keep abreast of continuing advances in knowledge and technique is obvious.

The unusual time and effort spent by members of the Committee on Control of Surgical Infections, the many contributors to the symposia, and other participants are gratefully acknowledged. Our appreciation also goes to Jonathan E. Rhoads, James D. Hardy, C. Rollins Hanlon, Donald S. Gann, and Edwin W. Gerrish for their counsel and assistance.

Appreciated also have been the efforts of J. Stuart Freeman of the J.B. Lippincott Company, and of Dorothea Altemeier, Ella Turner, and other secretaries whose diligence and skill have made the final preparation possible.

It is the hope of the Editorial Committee that the second edition will continue to provide authoritative information that will serve as a guide useful to busy clinical surgeons, surgical interns and residents, operating room nurses, anesthesiologists, epidemiologists, infectious disease specialists, infection control committees and personnel, microbiologists, hospital administrators, architects, and others in their efforts to prevent and control infections in surgical patients.

William A. Altemeier, M.D., F.A.C.S.

CONTENTS

Manual on
Control
of Infection
in Surgical
Patients

1

Postoperative and hospital-acquired infections have been problems for as long as there have been hospitals, and attempts to prevent their occurrence and spread began hundreds of years ago when separate hospitals were built for patients with communicable diseases. Fever hospitals, smallpox hospitals, tuberculosis sanitoria, and "pest houses" were established in efforts to separate infected patients from other patients and from the community.

Before Pasteur's revolutionary studies in bacteriology and Lister's application of them to wounds a little more than 100 years ago, most if not all wounds became infected, and the resultant mortality of deep or extensive wounds approached the levels of 70% to 90%. Since the great majority of major wounds in the pre-Listerian era were caused by trauma, much of the stimulation for solutions to the problems of infection came during times of war and during the industrial revolution.

In such times the chief causes of death in patients with trauma were associated with putrefaction and infection, and were described as erysipelas ("St. Anthony's Fire"), hospital gangrene ("hospitalism"), sepsis, and tetanus ("lockjaw"). Such conditions forced surgeons to avoid elective amputations, and most elective surgical operations were limited in peace times to the more minor and superficial operations.

The introduction of gunpowder into Europe in the 13th century worsened this situation. For over 600 years thereafter, Europe was involved in a series of almost unending wars during which many wounds seen by surgeons were extensive, badly lacerated, and grossly contaminated. Thus, most surgeons acquired a doctrine of therapeutic despair based upon their belief that gunshot wounds were poisoned and that wound healing would not occur unless treated by some method to remove the poison.

A study of the Crimean War affords us the opportunity to observe the awesome significance of infection from 1853 to 1856. According to a report by Chenu on the health condition of the French army in Crimea and in Turkey at that time, wound

Introduction

infections played a significant role in this historical event. Of an army of about 300,000, approximately 10,000 were killed, but eight times as many or 85,375, died as the result of sickness and wounds. In other words, one-fourth of the army, composed of strong and healthy men, fell victim to various types of infections. The number of men who died as a result of wounds was 10,000, approximating the number killed. They were reportedly victims of erysipelas, scab, gangrene, general septicemia, and "hospital gangrene." The amputation cases, especially, succumbed to the latter. According to Chenu, the mortality of the wounded on whom resection of the femur was performed was tremendous. Of 1,681 individuals submitting to that operation, only 136 recovered from it. Thus, the mortality reached 92%. Amputations of the tibia had a better record, but nevertheless close to 1000 patients, or 71%, died of them. Sepsis was widespread in all the field hospitals.

Into this milieu of wounds, sepsis, and death, came Louis Pasteur and Joseph Lister. Louis Pasteur, a chemist who was studying fermentation for the French wine industry, also showed that putrefaction was a "fermentation" caused by the growth of microbes and proved that this could not arise *de novo*. Thus, the germ concept of infection gradually developed, and the dreaded changes in wounds complicating injuries were thereafter viewed with a new perspective.

It remained for Lister to identify an antimicrobial chemical that would inhibit or kill bacteria finding their way into wounds. He found that dilute carbolic acid would serve this purpose, and the principle of antisepsis was established. The introduction of antisepsis has been considered to be one of the great milestones of surgery and the reader is directed to the writings of Lister for a better understanding of the problems of that time.

Von Bergmann, assisted by Schimmelbusch, later developed his principle and practice of *aseptic* surgery in Germany; gradually and sporadically a new day dawned in the practice of surgery, offering the hope of surgery free from infection. A review of the experience of the past century, however, indicates that this hope has never been fully realized, and that this heritage has been largely taken for granted.

The introduction of modern antibiotic therapy during the second quarter of the 20th century had a revolutionary effect on the treatment of many established infections. Clinical experience and experimental bacteriological studies, however, have shown that its general use for over a third of a century has failed to decrease the overall incidence of surgical infections. This is misleading, however, since we are now able to prevent many types of infection, and we are operating on many patients whom we would not have operated on 10 or 20 years ago. As we have learned to prevent some types of infection, other types have taken their place. In addition, the widespread use and misuse of antibiotic therapy undoubtedly have increased the problems of preventing surgical infections. Too often, the widespread prophylactic use of antibiotics in surgical patients has contributed to the development of an unwarranted overdependence on their effectiveness, a de-emphasis or discredit of the importance of established surgical principles, a relaxation of the "surgical conscience," a breakdown of isolation procedures, and the establishment of a reservoir of antibiotic-resistant and virulent bacteria concentrated in the hospital environment.

These trends have been accentuated by the complexities of modern surgical practice, with the concentration of large numbers of patients with established infections admitted into hospitals, the extension of prolonged surgical operations and supportive procedures to a rapidly increasing number of high-risk patients, the increase of the number of individuals with severe trauma, and the growing use of drugs that decrease bodily resistance to infection. The extension of surgical treatment to aged and debilitated patients, and the widespread use of complicated invasive diagnostic, therapeutic, and anesthetic procedures also have favored the development of nosocomial infections. The development of noninvasive diagnostic techniques such as computerized tomography and sonography have been recent additions to medical practice which avoid or decrease other invasive technics.

It must be kept in mind, therefore, that the modern general hospital has become a complex community in which the opportunities for hospital-acquired infection are numerous and ever present. Moreover, the urgency associated with the treatment of many patients with life-threatening disease or extensive injuries, and the demands of large numbers of patients seen in a short period of time have tended to produce compromises and administrative trends not necessarily in the best interests of infection control.

A particularly important effect of general and indiscriminate antibacterial therapy in hospitals has been the progressive development of resistance to penicillin and to many of the other antibiotic agents that has been acquired by a large variety of important bacteria concentrated in the hospital environment. These virulent organisms, both gram-positive and gram-negative, have formed the "hospital reservoir" and have shown the potential of becoming pathogenic in patients weakened by disease, injury, metabolic conditions, surgery, and other debilitating factors.

There are a number of other important factors that influence the incidence of postoperative infections at the present time. In a 2½ year collaborative investigation of 15,613 consecutive operative procedures done in five American university centers, an overall infection rate of 7.4% for all types of operations was determined under close, energetic, and continuing surveillance. These centers included the University of Pennsylvania, Hahnemann Medical College, the University of California in Los Angeles, George Washington University, and the University of Cincinnati. This project was carried out with the support of the United States Public Health Service and under the aegis of the National Research Council.

The present reservoir of antibiotic-resistant bacteria in hospital environments and a continuing high infection rate, despite antibiotic prophylaxis, have resulted in the appointment of numerous committees by the American College of Surgeons, the American Medical Association, the American Hospital Association, and others to study this problem and make recommendations for its solution.

Many national and international conferences have been held in an effort to bring the various aspects of this situation into proper perspective, to disseminate existing knowledge among countries and scientific disciplines, and to stimulate research. One of the first and most highly significant meetings was the National Conference on Hospital-Acquired Staphylococcal Disease, held from September 15 to 17, 1958, in Atlanta, Georgia, under the joint sponsorship of the United States Public Health

Service and the National Research Council. An International Seminar on Hospital Infections was also held by the Council for International Organizations of Medical Sciences in London, September 24 to 28, 1962. Other important examples are the International Conference on Nosocomial Infections, which was held at the Center for Disease Control in Atlanta, August 3 to 6, 1979; the International Conference on Surgical Infections, held by the International Society of Surgery in Moscow from August 21 to 28, 1971; and the International Staphylococcus Symposium held in Aberdeen, Scotland, September 11 to 13, 1980.

These conferences and others have been helpful, but the fact remains that the problem of postoperative and hospital-acquired infections persists as a public health problem of major importance, and that considerable confusion exists in the minds of surgeons, physicians, hospital administrators, lay hospital boards, bacteriologists, epidemiologists, sanitary engineers, architectural engineers, attorneys, judges, and others about how these infections originate. Moreover, the increasing costs associated with the care of surgical patients with infections, the progressive threat of malpractice claims, and the growing demands of an informed and often "oversold" public have become important matters of concern.

In the meantime, the controversy over the relative importance of the aerial and contact spread of infection has continued from the last half of the 19th century to the present. Von Bruns and von Bergmann became convinced that contact was the principal method for spread of infection, and by their evidence persuaded Lord Lister to abandon his carbolic acid spray of the operating room environment. Ultraviolet light, lithium oxide, electrical precipitation of bacteria-laden dust particles, and various types of laminar flow were since developed; however, they have been relatively unsuccessful and are of limited value as currently used. It would seem that our profession still tends to avoid the application of pertinent knowledge and that we evade the discipline and inconvenience necessary for the effective control of infection.

More recently, another development of considerable concern has been a significant change in the pattern of infections, which has been recognized since 1956. This has included an increasing incidence of gram-negative bacillary infections, often by bacteria considered to have little or no virulence; a greater prevalence of infections by fungi and viruses; an increased awareness of the importance of gram-negative anaerobic infections, principally by the bacteroides; and a resurgence of virulent infections by *Staphylococcus aureus.*

In consideration of these problems and others, the Board of Regents of the American College of Surgeons appointed a Committee on Control of Surgical Infections of its Pre- and Postoperative Care Committee with the charge that matters relevant to the continuing occurrence and importance of infections in surgical patients be studied and that something be done about the Committee's findings. This Committee, therefore, planned four symposia on surgical infection in order to establish an authoritative data base upon which this *Manual on Control of Infection in Surgical Patients* was developed in 1976 for operating room and hospital use. Sharing in the concern over these problems have been the Center for Disease

Control, the American Hospital Association, the United States Public Health Service, other major surgical societies, nursing societies, societies concerned with infection and chemotherapy, and the new Surgical Infection Society. New data developed during the ensuing 8 years have made updating and publication of this revised edition necessary.

BIBLIOGRAPHY

ALTEMEIER WA: Control of wound infections. J R Coll Surg Edinb 11:271, 1966

ALTEMEIER WA: Bacteriology of surgical infections: Clinical and experimental considerations. Vingt-quatriene Congres de la Societe Internationale de Chirurgie, Moscow, 1971

ALTEMEIER WA: The significance of infection in trauma (Scudder Oration). Bulletin of the American College of Surgery 57(2):7, 1972

ALTEMEIER WA: Surgical infections: Incisional wounds. In Bennett JV, Brachman PS (eds): Hospital Infections, p 287. Boston, Little, Brown & Co, 1979

ALTEMEIER WA: Perspectives in surgical infections. Surg Clin North Am 60(1):1–4, 1980

ALTEMEIER WA: Sepsis in surgery. Arch Surg 117:107, 1982

ALTEMEIER WA: Hospital acquired infections: A personal perspective. In Polk H (ed): Clinical Surgery International, Chap 13. New York, Churchill Livingstone, 1982

ASHURST APC: The centenary of Lister (1827–1927): A tale of sepsis and antisepsis. Ann Med Hist 9(3):202, 1927

BENNETT JV, BRACHMAN PS (eds): Hospital Infections. Boston, Little, Brown & Co, 1979

BRACHMAN PS, DAN BB, HALEY RW, HOOTON TM, GARNER JS, ALLEN JS: Nosocomial infections: Incidence and cost. Surg Clin North Am 60(1):15, 1980

BURKE JF: Wound infection and early inflammation. Monographs in Surgical Sciences 1:301–345, 1964

CRUSE PJE, FOORD R: The epidemiology of wound infection. Surg Clin North Am 60(1):27, 1980

HAMPTON O, PARKER J: Observations on battle fractures of the extremities. Surgery 15:869, 1944

HOWARD JM et al: Postoperative wound infections: The influence of ultraviolet irradiation of the operating room and of various other factors. Ann Surg 160 (Suppl):1,1964

ILLINGWORTH CW: Lister centenary lecture: Lister and the Glasgow School of Surgery. Scott Med J 6:1, 1961

LISTER J: On a new method of treating compound fractures, abscesses, etc., with observations on the conditions of suppuration. Lancet 1:357, 1867

LISTER J: On the effects of the antiseptic system of treatment upon the salubrity of a surgical hospital. Lancet 1:4, 1870

LISTER J: On the antiseptic principle in the practice of surgery. Br Med J 2:242, 1867

MELENEY FL, WHIPPLE AO: A statistical analysis of a study of the prevention of infection in soft part wounds, compound fractures, and burns with special reference to the sulfonamides. Surg Gynecol Obstet 80:263, 1945

PASTEUR L: Memoire sur la fermentation alcoolique. Paris. Imprimerie de Mollet-Bachelier, 1860

POLK, HC: Overview of surgical infections. In Hospital Acquired Infections in Surgery. Baltimore, University Park Press, 1977

REYHER C: Die Antiseptische Wundbehandlung. Kriegschirugie (Sammlung Klinischer Vortrage, Leipzig) 45:1207, 1878

SCHIMMELBUSCH C: Die Durchführung der Aseptis in der Klinik des Herrn Geheimrath von Bergmann, in Berlin, Arch f klin Chir 42:123, 1891

VON BERGMANN E: Ueber antiseptische Wundbehandlung. Deutsch Med Wchnschr 8:559, 1882

VON BERGMANN E: Die antiseptische Wundbehandlung in der Königlichen Chirurgischen, Universitäts-Klinik zu Berlin. Jahrb klin. Chir 1:147, 1889

WALTER CW: Evolution of asepsis. In Aseptic Treatment of Wounds, pp 4–21. New York, Macmillan, 1948

WILLIAMS REO, SHOOTER RA (eds): Epidemiology and control. In Symposium on Infection in Hospitals, London, 1962. Philadelphia, FA Davis, 1963

2

One of the salient features of hospital life is infection, and many infections are of surgical significance. The development of an understanding of the cost and nature of hospital-acquired infections is, therefore, an essential part of clinical surgery.

The ubiquity of infectious agents in man's environment, their propensity for invading the body; their potential for producing significant pathophysiological effects on various body functions; their remarkable adaptability to newer forms of treatment; and the necessity for excluding their presence or controlling their growth to permit surgical treatment and wound healing—all affect surgical practice and the cost in personnel, equipment, and money necessary to prevent or control infection. Moreover, the expanding horizons of surgery have often depended upon the development and application of special methods to overcome the hazards of postoperative infections. In this regard, it is important to remember that every operation is an experiment in applied and practical microbiology.

The modern hospital environment is indeed very important during a person's illness or injury. Modern medical practice has resulted in the concentration within hospitals of large numbers and varieties of patients. Some of these patients are admitted for the treatment of established infections that developed in the home or in the community ("community based" infections). Others have an increased susceptibility to infection as a result of trauma, associated chronic debilitating diseases, various surgical procedures, and intimate exposure to the antibiotic-resistant hospital reservoir of bacteria. Many of these patients develop infections while they are in the hospital ("hospital based" infections).

For these reasons and others, as noted in Chapter 1, infection has continued to be a serious problem of worldwide scope, and a health hazard of great significance and expense. Infections developing in surgical patients have continued to produce important effects on the final result of the surgical treatment, on morbidity, and on mortality. Delayed healing, disability, deformity, and even death have resulted

Incidence and Cost of Hospital-Acquired Infection

from infection. In addition, the patient's quality of life, both physical and psychological, has often been affected.

Microbiology has made significant contributions to the advancement and safety of surgery through the development of the germ theory of surgical infections, antiseptic and aseptic technique, passive and active immunization, and antimicrobial therapy. Each of these has had revolutionary effects on the practice of surgery. A variety of stressful forces imposed upon microorganisms during the past 40 years, however, have produced reactions in the microbial world that, in turn, have influenced the pattern and nature of infections seen in the practice of surgery.

After the general use of modern antibiotic therapy for approximately one third of a century, it has become apparent that the overall incidence of infection in the surgical patient has not decreased and that many related problems are still present. As discussed in Chapter 1, this is somewhat misleading because we are now able to operate upon many patients on whom we would not have been able to 10 or 20 years ago because of the risk of infection. Also, as some types of infection have been prevented or brought under control, others have taken their places. Consequently, questions such as the following have been asked: "Why has the acceptance of the germ theory in surgical practice not decreased the overall incidence of infection in surgical patients during the past 40 years? Why has the daily practice of aseptic and antiseptic technique not yielded a greater decrease in infectious complications? Why has the general use of antibiotic therapy not eliminated wound- and hospital-acquired infections as a threat to the surgical patient? Are surgeons using antimicrobial agents correctly and to their greatest advantage? Should there be more control over the clinical introduction and general use of these agents?"

Such questions have emphasized the obvious need for a more comprehensive understanding of the significance of infection, a better understanding of the variables contributing to its development, and greater knowledge of the factors that influence the antimicrobial effect of the many agents now available for infection prevention or control. In addition, the increasing number of hospitalized patients who are at high risk of developing infection must also be kept in mind — the newborn and the elderly, diabetics, cancer patients, transplantation patients, those undergoing open heart and hip replacement operations, and severely injured, burned, or seriously ill persons. Others are put at high risk as a result of their therapy with immunosuppressive agents, anticancer drugs, and steroids. Consequently, a concentrated study is needed of the complexities of the hospital community, the action and interaction of personnel and patients, and the mechanisms of the transmission of significant bacterial contamination to patients.

Antimicrobial therapy has undoubtedly increased the complexity of surgical infection control. This increase in complexity has been caused not only by the effect of antibiotics on bacteria but also to a large extent by the over-reliance and overdependence of surgeons and nurses on the supposed effectiveness of antibiotics. Moreover, the rising costs of surgical care, the urgency of the treatment of many patients with life-threatening diseases or extensive injuries, and the demands of large numbers of patients requiring treatment in a short period of time have often tended to produce compromises in treatment and administrative controls.

Other considerations affecting the incidence and types of infections common to surgical patients have been the hospital reservoir of antibiotic-resistant bacteria, the duration of preoperative hospitalization, the complex pre- and post-operative diagnostic and supportive therapeutic procedures, the type of operation, the duration of the operation, and the many opportunities for contamination and infection of wounds by the operating room and ward personnel. The resistance of the patient and the biology of his response to infection must be taken into consideration (Chap. 5).

Economic and legal problems have also been increasing at an alarming rate. The cost of hospital infections to the patient and to society in general, the escalation of the cost of insurance liability, plaintiff settlements, and the growing list of legal issues must be considered as aspects related to the overall problem of infection in the clinical practice of surgery.

INCIDENCE

There is still considerable divergence of viewpoints on the incidence of infections in surgical practice (Table 2-1). One reason for the confusion is the tendency to include all types of wounds or operations under one category. It is generally recognized that usually from 40% to 60% of the patients in general hospitals are surgical. Approximately 30% of hospitalized surgical patients either have established infections at the time of admission or develop some type of infection during their hospital stays. In 1963 it was estimated that of the approximately 25,000,000 patients admitted to hospitals in the United States, over 1,000,000 developed postoperative or hospital-acquired infections.

The overall wound infection rate of 7.4% used in these estimations was the incidence for *all types* of operative wounds as determined during a 2½-year collabora-

Table 2-1. **Incidence of wound infection as reported from various countries.**

Author	Year	Country	No. of Operations	Rate (%)
Robertson	1958	Canada	1917	9.3
Williams	1959	England	722	4.7
Public Health Lab. Service	1960	England	3276	9.4
Roundtree	1960	Australia	198	14.0
Myburgh	1964	S. Africa	Not noted	17.0
National Research Council	1964	U. S.	15613	7.4
Clarke	1967	England	382	13.6
Cruse & Foord	1980	Canada	62939	4.7

(After Cruse PJE, Foord R: The epidemiology of wound infection. Surg Clin North Am 60(1):27, 1980)

Table 2-2.   Incidence of Infection in Relation to Wound Classification.

	Percentage of Total		Incidence of Wound Infection	
	NAS-NRC Study*	Foothills Hospital Study†	NAS-NRC Study*	Foothills Hospital Study†
Total	15,613	62,937	7.4%	4.7%
Clean	74.8%	75%	5.1%	1.5%
Clean-contaminated	16.6%	15%	10.8%	7.7%
Contaminated	4.3%	7%	16.3%	15.2%
Dirty	3.7%	3%	28.0%	40.0%
Unclassified	0.5%			

* Howard JM et al: Postoperative wound infections: The influence of ultraviolet irradiation of the operating room and of various other factors. Ann Surg (Suppl) 160(2):9–192, 1964

† Cruse PJE, Foord R: The epidemiology of wound infection: A 10-year prospective study of 62,939 wounds. Surg Clin North Am 60:27–40, 1980

tive study of 15,613 consecutive operative procedures done in five American university centers with the support of the United States Public Health Service and under the aegis of the National Academy of Sciences–National Research Council (NAS–NRC). The operative wounds thus studied were designated *clean, clean-contaminated, contaminated,* or *dirty.* Both elective and emergency operations were included (Table 2-2).

In the 11,690 clean elective operations in this series, the average wound infection rate was 5.1%, but the average rate for all types of operations was 7.4%. Comparable data reported by Cruse in a study of 62,939 wounds are noted in Table 2-2. It also became apparent that the incidence of infection varied with the type of operation.

Noteworthy, too, was the fact that the incidence of postoperative wound infection was increased three- to fivefold or more *whenever one of the major tracts was transected or resected* during a planned elective operation, when compared to elective operations without such procedures. For example, the incidence of infection following hernioplasty was 1.9%, whereas it was 6.1% for hysterectomy, 6.9% for cholecystectomy, 10% for partial colectomy, and 10.1% for subtotal gastrectomy (Table 2-3).

Farber and Wenzel have reported on prospective statewide surveillance of postoperative wound infection rates after 44,687 selected surgical procedures performed in Virginia from January 1, 1977 to May 31, 1979. The results of this survey are presented in detail in Table 2-4.

The incidence of hospital-acquired or nosocomial infections, other than postoperative wound infections, is also of considerable current significance. In addition to the data collected by Cruse and Foord (Table 2-1), other data have been derived from community hospital surveillance studies in the United States by Brachman and his associates at the Center for Disease Control (1980). The Epidemiology Program

Table 2-3. Incidence of Infection Following Selected, Commonly Performed Operative Procedures.

Operative Procedure	Number of Procedures	Incidence of Infection (%)
Herniorrhaphy*	1312	1.9
Thyroidectomy	406	2.2
Hysterectomy	628	6.1
Cholecystectomy	756	6.9
Partial colectomy	220	10.0
Subtotal gastrectomy	288	10.1
Appendectomy	551	11.4
Nephrectomy	127	17.3
Radical mastectomy	227	18.9

* Including inguinal, femoral, and epigastric; excluding incisional and ventral
(Adapted from NAS–NRC Study of Postoperative Wound Infections, 1964)

of the Center for Disease Control cooperated with 82 community hospitals in conducting their surveillance programs. The hospitals were located throughout the United States and varied in size from 187 to 375 beds. Each had nurse infection surveillance officers who maintained a day-to-day check of all patients within their institutions by making routine ward rounds and by reviewing the individual case report forms and bacteriological records.

Of the 82 hospitals, 5 were categorized as municipal, 12 as university, 4 as federal, and 60 as community. The nosocomial infection rate in surgical patients in municipal hospitals was found to be approximately 7%, in university hospitals 5.7%, in federal hospitals 5.6%, and in community hospitals 4.3%. Urinary tract infections were the most prevalent, accounting for 39% of the overall incidence; surgical wound and skin infections accounted for 32%, respiratory tract infections for 16%, primary bacteremia for 4%, nonsurgical cutaneous infections for 4%, and burn infections for 1%.

In a review of hospitalized patients with nosocomial infections caused by gram-negative organisms, Altemeier and associates (1976) found urinary tract infections to be the primary source in 53%, with continuous indwelling catheters and urinary tract instrumentation also being important etiologic factors. Brachman and his associates also reported in a previous study (1970) that the incidence of hospital-acquired infections in community hospitals did not show any significant monthly variation. This finding was at variance with some of the reports in the literature in which a higher incidence was seen in winter months. Their studies also confirmed those of Altemeier, Davis, Ehrenkranz, and others that gram-negative infections had become the most serious problem, accounting for between 50 and 70% of hospital-acquired infections throughout the United States — and probably throughout the world.

(Text continues on p. 14)

Table 2-4. Postoperative Wound Infection Rates After Selected Surgical Procedures

Procedure	University Hospital (N=1)		Community Hospitals <100 Beds (N=7)	
	No.	%	No.	%
Appendectomy	16/294*	5	24/506*	5
Ruptured	5/24	21	9/64	14
Nonruptured	10/251	4	8/388	2
Cholecystectomy	9/331	3	9/516	2
Herniorraphy	5/513*	1	13/633*	2
Complicated	1/10	10	1/28	4
Uncomplicated	4/498	1	1/521	0.2
Colon resection	10/132	8	7/71	10
Splenectomy			0/8	
Thyroidectomy			0/30	
Above-knee amputation			4/33	12
Below-knee amputation	8/62	13	3/28	11
Total abdominal hysterectomy (abdominal wound infection)	22/269	8	16/513	3
Total vaginal hysterectomy (cuff infection)	17/235	7	8/275	3
Cesarean section	106/514	21	17/465	4
Total hip replacement	3/100	3	1/33	3
Total knee replacement	4/87	5	0/39	
Meniscectomy	0/592		0/127	
Laminectomy	13/358	4	2/176	1
Femoropopliteal bypass	3/60	5	1/9	11
Aortofemoral bypass	1/36	3	0/9	
Nephrectomy	3/65	5	0/13	
Radical neck dissection	7/59	12		
Total	3,707		3,484	

* Incomplete classification within group.
(After Farber BF, Wenzel RP: Postoperative wound infection rates: Results of prospective statewide surveillance. Am J Surg 140:343–346, 1980)

| Community Hospitals | | | | Federal Hospitals (N=2) | | All Hospitals (N=38) | |
| 100–300 Beds (N=21) | | >300 Beds (N=7) | | | | | |
No.	%	No.	%	No.	%	No.	%
147/3,075*	5	78/1,626*	5	1/21	5	266/5,522	5
73/257	28	48/164	29	0/2		135/511	26
63/2,126	3	29/1,301	2	1/19	5	11/4,085	3
116/3,098	4	58/2,323	3	8/75	11	200/6343	3
43/2,381*	2	32/2,899*	1	3/352*	1	95/6,778	1
5/198	3	7/143	5	0/9		14/388	4
23/2,577	1	21/2,179	1	0/146		48/5,899	1
91/682	13	90/745	12	1/31	3	199/1,661	12
7/123	6	2/99	2	0/2		9/232	4
3/326	1	0/327		0/15		3/698	0.4
20/188	11	10/133	8	11/55	20	45/409	11
13/148	9	16/114	14	4/46	9	44/398	11
129/3,271	4	61/2,760	2			228/6,813	3
51/1,177	4	17/720	2			93/2,407	4
136/2,911	5	52/1,678	3			311/5,568	6
5/363	1	3/228	1	0/24		12/748	2
7/185	4	6/93	7	1/13	8	18/417	4
10/993	1	1/500	0.2	0/20		11/2,232	0.5
24/1,356	2	22/1,406	2	0/3		61/3,299	2
9/137	7	9/196	5	1/32	3	23/434	5
8/124	7	3/73	4	0/19		12/261	5
8/111	7	4/132	3	0/4		15/325	5
2/12	17	8/50	16	1/21	5	18/142	13
20,661		16,102		733		44,687	

Community hospitals represent the majority of hospitals in the United States, and the incidence of infections identified in them by these studies indicates that such hospitals are involved in the problem. While they do not have as large staffs or as well-equipped diagnostic facilities as larger academic institutions, they do have the same problem with an overall incidence of hospital-acquired infections of approximately 4% to 5%.

COST

It is frequently implied that the quality of medical care in the United States is lagging behind other advances in our society. One area claimed to be such a "quality gap" is that of hospital-acquired infections. Since the quality of medical care is related to its cost-effectiveness, it has been a matter of concern to physicians, hospital administrators, insurance carriers, and government agencies as well as surgeons.

As early as 1935, Meleney noted that postoperative infection doubled the length of hospitalization of surgical patients. More recently, the cost of postoperative wound infection has been addressed in a study by Green and Wenzel. They used the data base in the University of Virginia Hospital computer to identify matched controls by patient age, sex, operation performed, pathologic findings, and underlying disease processes that could have altered the patient's risk of infection. They defined postoperative wound infection as the presence of pus at the incision site. The increased hospital stay and the resulting increased direct cost of hospitalization from postoperative wound infection were determined after six commonly performed operations including appendectomy, cholecystectomy, colon resection, total abdominal hysterectomy, cesarean section, and coronary artery bypass graft. The duration of hospitalization and the actual hospital bill for each patient with a postoperative wound infection were compared with the same data for each control patient. Green and Wenzel's findings indicated that wound sepsis approximately doubled the postoperative stay and added significantly to the expense of hospitalization; the mean additional cost ranged from $443 for cholecystectomy to $2602 for coronary artery bypass graft.

Brachman and associates (1980) in their National Nosocomial Infection Study investigated costs along with the prolonged hospital stay associated with hospital-acquired infections. Their investigations indicated that the average surgical wound infection added 7.4 extra days and more than $800 to the bills of infected patients in 1975 and 1976.

Another recent prospective study by Haley and associates was reported by Brachman to show that the rate of nosocomial infections was 5.4% and the average resultant increase in hospital stay was 7.4 days. The average additional cost was $839, with the range being zero to $7900.

Dr. William Foege, Director of the Center for Disease Control, reported before a Senate – Labor – HHS Appropriations Committee budget hearing that two million Americans who enter hospitals each year (5% of all admissions) acquire infections unrelated to their original condition. These infections result in 80,000 deaths each year, add approximately $1.5 billion to the nation's health care costs, and add an average of 4 days to the hospital stay.

These and other observations emphasize the economic burden of postoperative and other nosocomial infections in hospital practice. Unfortunately, the inflationary spiral of the present time will almost certainly continue to escalate medical costs related to these complications. Consequently, methods and programs to correct the magnitude of these costs are important matters for surgeons to consider.

Legal Considerations

Consideration must also be given the malpractice and professional liability aspects of surgical infections. The seriousness, growing frequency, and complexity of litigation related to surgical infections were reported at the First Symposium on Control of Surgical Infections by Halter for the Medical Malpractice and Physicians' Liability Committee of the American College of Surgeons.

The issue of infectious complications in surgical practice as the basis of malpractice claims has been especially difficult. Currently most suits have charged negligence on the basis of failure to perform an examination, obtain a culture, or order a test or an x-ray in time to have made an early diagnosis so that effective treatment could have been instituted. Failure to remove a bandage and examine an operative wound when the patient had fever or complained of pain have been regularly rewarded by successful claims. Failure to order a culture of drainage of purulent material and to order chest x-rays in cases of suspected pneumonia have led to similar legal results. An understanding of the importance of these clinical practices is necessary for good patient care and the self-protection of surgeons.

More complex issues have arisen as the legal profession has become more knowledgeable in their understanding of cross-infection in patients sharing the same room, equipment, or other facilities. The necessity for an active infection control program and a plan for patient isolation in each hospital has become generally recognized. The physician remains liable for the action of supporting and paramedical personnel under his direction even when at times these may be remote from his observation.

The basis for the malpractice and professional liability problem is not totally understood, but the rising case loads of civil suits pending in our courts has suggested that we are in the process of *becoming a nation of litigants*. The public has grown to expect compensation for any injury and many postoperative complications, in some cases even in the absence of any evidence of negligence. Indeed, it has become increasingly apparent that the people of this nation expect no poor results or complication from their treatment. A number of other factors have led to this state of unjustified malpractice suits, including the medical profession's own efforts to "put its best foot forward," and the unrealistic interpretation and "oversell" of medical results by the press lay magazines or television. In this age of heart transplants, limb reimplantations, and many other almost unbelievable surgical feats, it has been difficult for patients to accept anything less than perfection in what they consider to be lesser procedures. It must be realized by all that medicine is, at best, an *inexact science,* if in many cases it is a science at all, and the public should be apprised of this fact. Still another reason has been a definite breakdown in the doctor–patient relationship and the "busy doctor" syndrome due to the ever-increasing demands on the physician's time. As health care has become more sophisticated and more institutionalized, with providers consisting of teams of primary care physicians, consultants, and technicians, the practice of medicine has become much less personal, and the close physician–patient relationship has continued to deteriorate. Under these conditions unhappy and dissatisfied patients or their families are more likely to start litigation than before. Sanderson has indicated that the real challenge for health care professionals in the 1980s will be in the area of public relations.

Another important factor has been the inadequate policing of our own profession, as pointed out by Halter and others. There is some evidence that the medical profession has been lax in policing the activities of a relatively small number of physicians whose performance has been less than adequate. The continuing practice of such representatives of the profession yields grist for the mills of those who seek compensation for all less-than-perfect results of treatment. Shively emphasized the importance of positive and aggressive action to reduce the number of suits, and indicated that the reduction of malpractice insurance premiums cannot be accomplished without the cooperation of the Fellowship, the legal profession, the insurance companies, and the public.

It can be concluded that if a surgeon is well acquainted with the principles of informed consent, the need for good medical records, proper acceptance of operating room responsibilities, the significance of hospital and staff legal accountabilities, and the need for excellent rapport with his patients, the chances of his being a defendant are greatly minimized. It is also important for surgeons to make renewed efforts to rebuild their image in the public eye by cultivating closer physician–patient relationships. In the final analysis, efforts along these lines will yield better results, both in terms of promoting good medical practice and resolving the problem of malpractice litigation related to the complications of infection, than all of the innumerable hours spent on risk management and loss control.

BIBLIOGRAPHY

Altemeier WA: The significance of infection in trauma (Scudder oration). Bull Am Coll Surg 57(2):7, 1972

Altemeier WA: Have we lost our way? Am J Surg 129:1, 1975

Altemeier WA: Surgical infections: Incisional wounds. In Bennett JV, Brachman PS (eds): Hospital Infections, p 287. Little, Brown & Co, Boston, 1979

Altemeier WA: Perspectives in surgical infections. Surg Clin North Am 60(1):5, 1980

Altemeier WA: Hospital acquired infections: A personal perspective. In Polk H (ed): Infection and the Surgical Patient, Chap 13. New York, Churchill Livingstone, 1982

Altemeier WA: Sepsis in surgery. Arch Surg 117:107, 1982

Altemeier WA, Culbertson WR, Fullen WD, McDonough JJ: *Serratia marcescens* septicemia. Arch Surg 99:232, 1969

ALTEMEIER WA, LEVENSON S: Trauma Workshop Report: Infections, immunology, and gnotobiosis. J Trauma 10:1084, 1970

BARRETT FF, CASEY, JI, FINLAND M: Infections and antibiotic use among patients at Boston City Hospital, Feb. 1967. N Engl J Med 278:5, 1968

BRACHMAN PS, DAN BB, HALEY RW, HOOTON TM, GARNER JS, ALLEN JS: Nosocomial infections: Incidence and cost. Surg Clin North Am 60(1):15, 1980

BROTE L, GILLQUIST J, TARNVIK A: Wound infections in general surgery: Wound contamination, rates of infection and some consequences. Acta Chir Scand 142(2):99–106, 1976

BURNS SJ, DIPPE SE: Postoperative wound infections detected during hospitalization and after discharge in a community hospital. Am J Infect Control 10(2):60, 1982

CHEYNE WW: Suppuration and septic diseases. Wood's Medical and Surgical Monographs 8:94, 1890

COLES B, VAN HEERDEN JA, KEYS TF, HALDORSON A: Incidence of wound infection for common general surgical procedures. Surg Gynecol Obstet 154(4):557, 1982

CRUSE PJE, FOORD R: The epidemiology of wound infection. Surg Clin North Am 60(1):27, 1980

CRUSE PJE, FOORD R: A five year prospective study of 23,649 surgical wounds. Arch Surg 107:206, 1973

DAVIS JH: Staphylococcal infection in surgical patients. Am Surg 33:642, 1967

EHRENKRANZ NJ: Surgical wound infection occurrence in clean operations. Am J Med 70:909, 1981

FABRY J, MEYNET R, JORON MT et al: Cost of nosocomial infections: Analysis of 512 digestive surgery patients. World J Surg 6:362–365, 1982

FARBER BF, WENZEL RP: Postoperative wound infection rates: Results of prospective statewide surveillance. Am J Surg 140:343–346, 1980

FARRAR SM, MACHEAD CM: Staphylococcal infections in a general hospital. Am J Hygiene 72:38, 1960

FOEGE W: Hospital costs cited. Council of Teaching Hospitals Report, pp 12–13. April–May 1982

GOODE AW, GLAZER G, ELLIS BW: The cost effectiveness of dextraromer and eusol in the treatment of infected surgical wounds. Br J Clin Pract 33(11–12):325, 1979

GREEN JW, WENZEL RP: Postoperative wound infection: A controlled study of the increased duration of hospital stay and direct cost of hospitalization. Ann Surg 185:264, 1977

HASSELGREN PO, HOLM J: Sources and routes in postoperative wound infections. Acta Chir Scand 147:99–103, 1981

HOWARD JM et al: Postoperative wound infections: The influence of ultraviolet irradiation of the operating room and of various other factors. Ann Surg 160(Suppl):1, 1964

KASS EH: Antimicrobial drug usage in general hospitals in Pennsylvania. Ann Intern Med (Suppl, Pt 2) 89:800–801, 1978

LEISSNER KH: Postoperative wound infection in 32,000 clean operations. Acta Chir Scand 142(6):433–439, 1976

MELENEY FL: Infection in clean operative wounds. Surg Gynecol Obstet 60:264, 1935

NATIONAL COMMUNICABLE DISEASE CENTER: Hepatitis surveillance. Report No. 30, April 21, 1969

NATIONAL ASSOCIATION OF INSURANCE COMMISSIONERS: Malpractice Claims: 1977, 1980 (Milwaukee, Wisconsin). Medical Insurance Feasibility Study. San Francisco, Sutter Publication, 1977

PINNER RW, HALEY RW, BLUMENSTEIN BA, SCHABERS DR, VON ALLMEN SD, MCGOWAN JE: High cost nosocomial infections. Infect Control 3(2):143, 1982

POLK, HC: Overview of surgical infections. In Hospital-Acquired Infections in Surgery. Baltimore, University Park Press, 1977

QUINN RW, HILLMAN JW: An epidemic of streptococcal wound infections. Arch Environ Health 11:28, 1965

SANDERSON RR: Medical malpractice: 1981. Legal Aspects of Medical Practice 9:1–4, 1981

SANDUSKY WR: The Burden of Sepsis. Presidential Address. Am Surg 48(1):1–4, 1982

SCHECKLER WE: Hospital costs of nosocomial infections: A prospective three-month study in a community hospital. Infect Control 1(3):150, 1980

SHIVELY FL JR: Professional liability—an overview. Bull Am Coll Surg 58(9):13, 1973

SHIVELY FL JR: A report from the Governors' Committee on professional liability. Bull Am Coll Surg 59(3):20, 1974

SNOW E: Report on the Governor's Committee on professional liability. Bull Am Coll Surg 1971

VITAL STATISTICS RATE IN THE UNITED STATES: 1900–1940. In Adjusted Death Rates and Other Indexes of Mortality, Chap 4. Washington, United States Government Printing Office, 1943

WALTER CW, KUNDSIN, RB, BRUBAKER MM: The incidence of airborne wound infection during surgery. JAMA 196:908, 1963

WILLIAMS REO, SHOOTER RA (eds): Infection in hospitals: Epidemiology and control In Symposium on Infection in Hospitals, London, 1962. Philadelphia, FA Davis, 1963

3

DEFINITIONS

Infection in clinical surgical practice is the product of the entrance, growth, metabolic activities, and resultant pathophysiological effects of microorganisms in the tissues of a patient. "Surgical" infections have at least four principal characteristics:

1. They often involve postoperative or postinjury wounds (Fig. 3-1).
2. The infection is unlikely to resolve spontaneously or with simple antibiotic treatment, and suppuration, necrosis, gangrene, prolonged morbidity, other serious effects, or death may occur if untreated surgically (Fig. 3-2).
3. Excision, incision, or drainage are often advantageous or necessary.
4. Surgical infections are usually polymicrobic but may be monomicrobic. They are often invasive with the rapid growth and regional or systemic spread of bacteria.
5. Their microbial etiology may be synergistic.

"Surgical" infection is also an inclusive term encompassing the diseases of all patients having surgical disorders with associated signs of infection. It includes the following:

1. Spontaneous infections for which patients are generally admitted to the hospital for surgical diagnosis and treatment
2. Wound infections, whether following trauma or surgical operations
3. Regional postinjury or postoperative infections
4. Systemic sepsis occurring after injury or operation
5. Coincidental infections in unrelated organs occurring during, or as a result of, postoperative or postinjury care
6. Various other infections whose management may require surgical treatment

METHODS OF CLASSIFICATION

Classification of infection is important because it aids in facilitating the search for the origin and causes of infection, permits earlier presumptive diagnosis before bacteriological results are available, indicates earlier and more effective methods of

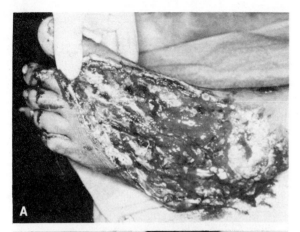

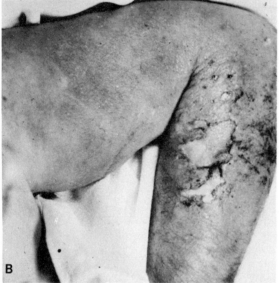

Fig. 3-1. (*A*) A post-traumatic severe infection of the foot and leg with extensive necrosis of the underlying tissues. (*B*) A patient with a life-threatening "community-based" infection caused by the beta hemolytic *Streptococcus* in a burn of the left arm. Note the extensive cellulitis of the forearm and arm. (*A*: U.S. Army Institute of Surgical Research, Brooke Army Medical Center, Fort Sam Houston, Texas; *B*: Cincinnati General Hospital)

treatment, and provides a plan for the collection of more meaningful data related to the nature and control of infections.

Surgical infections have also been classified on the basis of the source or base of the infection, the associated anatomical and pathophysiological changes, and the microbial etiology, as outlined below:

Classification of Surgical Infections by Location and Pathophysiological Changes
Wound Infection
    Cellulitis with erythema, swelling, or increased tenderness
    Suppuration or liquefaction of tissues
    Abscess
    Septic necrosis of tissues
    Septic thrombophlebitis in vicinity of local wound

Fig. 3-2. Three different wound infections are represented with varying types of suppuration. (*A*) Staphylococcal and mixed infection with abscess cavity and extensive cellulitis developing in a wound of the leg. (*B*) Postoperative crepitant cellulitis and fasciitis of the abdominal wall and flank complicating an operation for strangulated inguinal hernia. (*C*) Acid injury of hand with secondary infection and suppuration due to a mixed bacterial flora. Extensive debridement and antibiotic therapy were necessary to control the infection and preserve the hand. (U.S. Army Institute of Surgical Research, Brooke Army Medical Center, Fort Sam Houston, Texas)

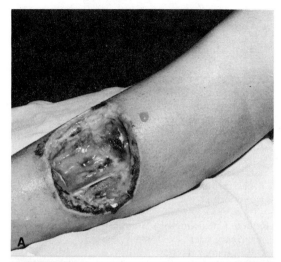

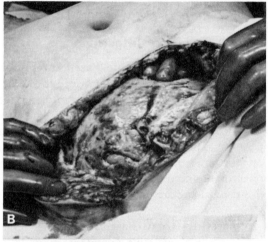

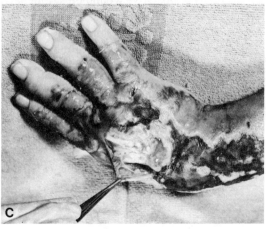

Regional Extension
  Direct extension through adjacent tissues
  Lymphangitis and lymphadenitis
  Thrombophlebitis
  Peritonitis
  Central nervous system infection, including meningitis and brain abscess
  Spreading fasciitis or necrotizing cellulitis
  Mediastinitis
  Retroperitoneal cellulitis

Organ or Visceral Infection

Systemic Infection
  Bacteremia
  Septicemia

Remote Coexisting or Complicating Infections
  Urinary tract
  Respiratory tract
  Skin, etc.

Source or Base of Infection

Community- or Home-Based Infection.   There are many infections that develop spontaneously or otherwise in the home or community. As many as 30% to 40% of patients admitted to a surgical service in a general hospital may have developed home-based infections (*e.g.,* acute appendicitis, acute cholecystitis, acute diverticulitis with perforation and peritonitis, acute perforated peptic ulcer with peritonitis, human or animal bite wounds, foreign bodies, *etc.*). Infections in this category are generally unrelated in their etiology to the hospital or to the hospital reservoir of microorganisms; they do not come within the assigned responsibility of this manual and are not discussed further.

Operating-Room-Based Infections.   Operating-room-based infections consist primarily of operative wound infections developing postoperatively as a result of surgical procedures performed in the operating room. For purposes of special discussion, because of their importance and the problems they currently present, they are considered separately from other hospital-acquired infections in this manual. The sources of these infections are both endogenous and exogenous.

Other Hospital-Based Infections.   Infections occurring in patients during hospitalization are considered to be hospital-acquired and are termed *nosocomial.* They are the result of microbial invasion of the body, most often by antibiotic-resistant and virulent microorganisms of the hospital environment (Chap. 10). Invasion may occur in the circumstances listed below:

· In patients in whom resistant bacteria have been selected by antibiotic usage
· Following diagnostic procedures such as angiography

- Following therapeutic procedures such as lower urinary tract catheterization or instrumentation
- In patients with tracheostomy or intravenous therapy, especially when continuous
- The emergence of virulent bacteria during antibiotic therapy and from other medications that enhance the growth of bacteria
- In patients with decreased resistance due to immunosuppression
- Antibiotic and other pharmacologic agent impairment of host defenses and selection of "resistant" bacteria
- Following prolonged hospitalization permitting replacement of the normal microbial flora with virulent or antibiotic-resistant bacteria of the hospital resevoir
- Following operations on high-risk, aged, or malnourished patients

Characteristics of Infection

Infection usually develops as a diffuse inflammatory process without suppuration (cellulitis), which is characterized by edema, erythema, pain, and interference with function. The tissues undergo cellular infiltration by red blood cells, leukocytes, histiocytes, and macrophages. *Suppuration* often follows, being the result of liquefaction of tissues and the formation of pus as an abscess. Abscesses are usually walled off by a pyogenic membrane that produces induration about the abscess. Cellulitis in varying degrees usually extends beyond the wall of the abscess. Regional infections may develop from the direct extension of microorganisms along areolar, fascial, muscular, or other anatomical planes.

Bacterial enzymes, including proteinases, aid in the process of tissue liquefaction. Collagenase, for example, produces liquefaction of collagen and may aid in the spread of infection along fascial barriers. Hyaluronidase may favor the spread of the septic process. Hemolytic streptococci may produce a fibrinolysin, another enzyme capable of retarding the walling off of streptococcal infections.

Thrombosis of local blood vessels and those adjacent to wounds frequently occurs and contributes to the local destruction and necrosis of tissues. If the thrombi are infected, small abscesses, areas of cutaneous gangrene, or septic gangrene of extremities may follow. Thrombophlebitis of regional veins communicating with local infections may occur and produce thrombi and septic emboli that gain their way into the circulating bloodstream. The hemolytic *Staphylococcus* is one organism that can develop a coagulase capable of causing septic thrombosis and embolization. Other microorganisms, notably the *Bacteroides* group, have the propensity for producing thrombophlebitis.

Bacteria and their metabolic products may be carried from the area of primary infection into the lymph fluid and distributed to larger areas through lymphatics and their related lymph nodes. In so doing, they may cause *lymphangitis* and *lymphadenitis,* either suppurative or nonsuppurative.

Other regional infections include *peritonitis, retroperitoneal phlegmon, empyema,* and central nervous system lesions such as *meningitis* and *brain abscesses.*

Necrotizing fasciitis is also usually of regional extent, as exemplified by acute crepitant cellulitis of the perineum, which spreads beneath Scarpa's fascia to involve the scrotum, abdominal wall, and flank.

Systemic infections occur through the dissemination of microorganisms from a distributing focus into the circulating bloodstream, resulting in either *bacteremia* or *septicemia.* In the case of a bacteremia, the primary focus distributes bacteria once or intermittently, resulting in their transient appearance in the blood. In a septicemia, the bacterial distribution is more or less constant, causing their continued presence in the bloodstream. The old concept suggested that the actual growth or reproduction of microorganisms within the circulating bloodstream was septicemia, in contrast with bacteremia, in which the microorganisms found it impossible to reproduce within the circulating bloodstream. The newer concept, however, indicates that the difference is in the rate of dissemination and density of broadcast from the distributing focus, with the rate being more or less constant in septicemia but intermittent or single in bacteremia.

Organ or visceral infections may be the result of penetrating injuries, postoperative complications, or metastatic involvement. Examples include those that develop in the liver, pancreas, biliary tract, lung, ovary, or kidney. Another type of infection that may be categorized anatomically occurs as a coexisting or complicating infection in remote areas of the body. Examples include acute tonsillitis or other upper respiratory infections, urinary tract infections, lower pulmonary infections, central nervous system infectious processes, postoperative parotitis, and infected decubiti.

Microbial Etiology

The precise and complete identification of microorganisms present in a surgical infection is important and advisable. Emphasis has frequently been placed on infections produced by the hemolytic *Staphylococcus aureus,* largely because of its epidemic potential and the ease of its cultivation. It must be remembered, however, that a considerable number of surgical infections are mixed bacterial infections produced by a variety of bacteria, both aerobic and anaerobic, gram-positive and gram-negative. The gram-negative bacilli and fungi have assumed increasing importance during the past 21 years (Chaps. 2 and 10). Apparently almost any microbe is capable of participating in a wound infection if the local factors are supportive to its colonization and growth, and if the immune mechanisms are suppressed. The various determinants of infection are discussed in Chapter 9.

The incidence of various fungal and viral infections has been steadily increasing with the expanding clinical use of steroids, immunosuppressive agents, and multiple antibiotic agents. Pruitt's reports have emphasized the importance of these nonbacterial infections in patients with extensive burns. Herpetic whitlow in ICU personnel is an example of a nonbacterial infection of this type.

Based upon clinical and laboratory research made on the Surgical Service of the University of Cincinnati during the past 36 years and a review of pertinent literature, an etiologic classification of surgical infections has been developed (see p 25). The numerous types of bacteria vary considerably in their comparative incidence and relative importance.

Microorganisms Causing Infections in the Surgical Patient

Aerobic and Facultative Bacteria
- Gram-positive cocci
  - Staphylococcus
    - *Staphylococcus aureus*
    - *Staphylococcus epidermis*
  - Streptococcus
    - *Streptococcus hemolyticus*
    - *Streptococcus faecalis*
    - *Enterococcus*
    - *Nonhemolytic streptococcus*
    - *Streptococcus viridans*
    - *Streptococcus pneumoniae*
      (*pneumococcus*)
- Gram-negative cocci
  - *Neisseria catarrhalis*
  - *Neisseria gonorrhoeae*
- Gram-positive bacilli
  - *Nocardia* species
  - *Bacillus* species
  - *Corynebacterium*
  - Diphtheroids
  - *Mycobacterium tuberculosis*
  - *Mycobacterium* atypical species
- Gram-negative bacilli
  - *Escherichia coli*
  - *Proteus* species
  - *Klebsiella* species
  - *Pseudomonas aeruginosa*
  - *Serratia marcescens*
  - *Enterobacter* species
  - *Hemophilus* species
  - *Citrobacter* species
  - *Salmonella* species
  - *Alcaligenes faecalis*

Microaerophilic Bacteria
- Gram-positive coccus
  - Streptococcus
    - Hemolytic
    - Nonhemolytic

Anaerobic Bacteria
- Gram-positive cocci
  - *Peptococcus* species
  - *Peptostreptococcus* species
- Gram-positive bacilli
  - *Clostridium perfringens*
  - *Clostridium novyi*
  - *Clostridium septicum*
  - *Clostridium bordelli*
  - *Clostridium tetani*
  - *Clostridium difficile*
  - *Actinomyces* species
- Gram-negative bacilli
  - *Bacteroides fragilis* group
  - *Bacteroides melaninogenicus*
  - *Fusobacterium* species

Nonbacterial Infections
- Fungi and yeasts
  - *Candida* species
  - *Asperigillus* species
  - *Fusarium* species
  - *Histoplasma capsulatum*
  - *Coccidioides* species
  - *Mucor* species
  - *Blastomyces* species
  - *Sporotrichum schenkii*
- Viruses
  - Herpes viruses
    - Herpes simplex, type 1
    - Herpes simples, type 2
    - Varicella-zoster
    - Cytomegalovirus
  - Hepatitis viruses
    - Hepatitis A
    - Hepatitis B
    - Hepatitis non-A, non-B
  - Paramyxovirus (mumps)
  - Poliovirus
  - Poxvirus (vaccinia)
  - Rabies virus
  - Measles virus

The relative frequency of the more prevalent pathogens found in postoperative wounds is illustrated in Tables 3-1 and 3-2.

Microbial Prevalence. The analysis of the incidence of microorganisms in 390 postoperatively infected wounds in a total of 1388 cultured in the USPH/NRC ultraviolet wound study (1960–1964) showed *Staphylococcus aureus* to be the most

Table 3-1. Frequencies of Recovery of Organisms from Cultures of Postoperative Drainage of All Wounds, by Postoperative Infection Status, Combined Five-University Hospitals

Organism	Recovered from Infected Wounds (Total: 390)	
	Number of Times Recovered	Frequency of Recovery (%)
Coagulase positive staphylococci	122	31.3
Coagulase negative staphylococci	123	31.5
Escherichia sp.	87	22.3
Proteus sp.	52	13.3
Pseudomonas sp.	51	13.1
Nonhemolytic streptococci	38	9.7
Aerobacter-Klebsiella	34	8.7
Paracolobactrum sp.	22	5.6
Alpha-hemolytic streptococci	14	3.6
Beta-hemolytic streptococci	8	2.1
Bacteroides sp.	7	1.8
Clostridium sp.	5	1.3
Anaerobic streptococci	1	0.3
Other	72	18.5
Unidentified	3	0.8
None	36	9.2

(Adapted and modified from Table 86 of Postoperative Wound Infections—The influence of ultraviolet irradiation of the operating room and of various other factors. Ann Surg (Suppl)160:1–192, 1964)

frequent, being isolated in 31.3% (Table 3-1). The enteric gram-negative bacteria *Escherichia* species, *Proteus* species, and *Pseudomonas* species had incidences of 22.3%, 13.3%, and 13.1% respectively. In addition, the incidence of *S. aureus* varied in the five participating hospitals between 23.2% and 47.2%. During the same period, Williams, McDonald, and Blower (1960) in another collaborative study in 21 hospitals showed *S. aureus* to occur in 60% of the postoperatively infected wounds. Barnes, Behringer, Wheelock, and Wilkins also reported a similar frequency of 65% (1961).

In the First National Nosocomial Study between January 1970 and August 1973, the results indicated probable changes in the microbial etiology of wound infections. Although there was a continuing relatively high incidence of *S. aureus*, that of *E. coli* was now essentially the same as that of the *S. aureus*, giving further evidence of the increasing incidence of the gram-negative bacilli as previously noted by Finland, Altemeier, and others.

For a number of reasons, including problems of transport and anaerobic culture, the incidence reported for an anaerobic pathogen such as *Bacteroides* probably does not represent its actual frequency.

Clinical Significance

Certain criteria should be established in order to provide objective definitions and understanding of surgical infections that will permit consistent evaluation and reports. Microbial wound studies alone are inadequate and frequently unreliable because of limitation of bacteriological laboratories, inadequate sampling and testing methods, or positive reports for secondary invaders or contaminants. It is not unusual for discharges to be reported sterile when cultured, even from wounds judged to be definitely infected. Neither is it unusual to recover organisms from wounds that are healing without infection. On the other hand, it is believed that classification based only on individual clinical judgment may be subjective and biased. It is therefore recommended that uniform clinical criteria be used to promote understanding and agreement among observers.

Surgical wounds are considered uninfected if they heal per primam without discharge. They are definitely infected if there is a purulent discharge even if organisms are not cultured from the purulent material (Chap. 11). Wounds that are inflamed without discharge and wounds that drain culture-positive serous fluid are considered possibly infected. Small stitch abscesses are excluded from definite or possible infections if (1) inflammation and discharge are minimal and confined to points of suture penetration, or (2) the incision heals per primam without drainage. However, in the belief that clinical judgment is most important in the diagnosis of wound infections, wounds may be judged infected or uninfected by the responsible surgeon, who should be free to diagnose infection that does not meet the above criteria but should not be allowed to judge a wound "uninfected" that does meet the above criteria for infection.

Contamination-Infection Risk

A wound classification based on a clinical estimation of bacterial density, contamination, and risk of subsequent infection was developed in the U.S. Public Health Service and National Research Council ultraviolet study. It was a modification of one used in a previous National Research Council–Office of Scientific Research and Development (NRC–OSRD) collaborative study of wounds in 1942–1946. This system as outlined on p 28 is now widely accepted as a standard classification of operative wounds. It is recommended for use in collating information about infections; relating infections to sources of contamination; assessing the degree of risk of infection; and determining if there is a need for antimicrobial therapy and, if so, the type of therapy.

Table 3-2.   Postoperative Wound Pathogens Reported by National Nosocomial Infections Study

Pathogen	Service		
	Surg.	Gyn.	Med.
Escherichia coli	4899	850	183
Staphylococcus aureus	5300	347	345
Pseudomonas aeruginosa	2612	105	166
Proteus mirabilis	1461	247	65
Bacteroides	986	203	35
*Proteus species**	794	171	55
B-Hemolytic streptococci†	400	95	20
Group-A streptococci	261	29	24
Clostridium perfringens	324	8	14
Other pathogens	9963	1342	579
Totals	27,000	3398	1486

* Species unknown
† Group unknown
(Reprinted from Table 16-5, Hospital Infections. From National Nosocomial Infections Study [NNIS], W ton, D.C., U.S. Public Health Service, January 1970 through August 1973)

Classification of Operative Wounds in Relation to Contamination and Increasing Risk of Infection

Clean
   Elective, primarily closed, and undrained
   Nontraumatic, uninfected
   No inflammation encountered
   No break in aseptic technique
   Respiratory, alimentary, genitourinary, or oropharyngeal tracts not entered
Clean-Contaminated
   Alimentary, respiratory, or genitourinary tracts entered under controlled conditions
      and without unusual contamination
   Appendectomy
   Oropharynx entered
   Vagina entered
   Genitourinary tract entered in absence of culture-positive urine
   Biliary tract entered in absence of infected bile
   Minor break in technique
   Mechanical drainage
Contaminated
   Open, fresh traumatic wounds
   Gross spillage from gastrointestinal tract
   Entrance of genitourinary or biliary tracts in presence of infected urine or bile
   Major break in technique
   Incisions in which acute nonpurulent inflammation is present
Dirty and Infected
   Traumatic wound with retained devitalized tissue, foreign bodies, fecal contamination,
      or delayed treatment, or from a dirty source
   Perforated viscus encountered
   Acute bacterial inflammation with pus encountered during operation

		Service		
Obst.	Ped.	Newborn	Total	Percent
226	53	24	6235	18.7%
104	90	43	6229	18.6%
18	46	4	2951	8.8%
72	9	2	1856	5.6%
55	7	0	1286	3.8%
43	6	2	1072	3.2%
26	4	3	548	1.6%
8	8	0	330	1.0%
7	2	0	355	1.0%
495	104	63	12546	37.6%
1054	329	141	33,408	99.9%

A *clean wound* is a nontraumatic, uninfected operative wound in which neither the respiratory, alimentary, or genitourinary tracts nor the oropharyngeal cavities are entered. Clean wounds are elective, primarily closed, and undrained wounds.

Clean-contaminated wounds are operative wounds in which the respiratory, alimentary, or genitourinary tract is entered without unusual contamination and under controlled conditions, or wounds that are mechanically drained.

Contaminated wounds include open, fresh traumatic wounds, operations in which there is gross spillage from the gastrointestinal tract, surgical procedures with a major break in sterile technique (*e.g.*, open cardiac massage), and incisions encountering acute, nonpurulent inflammation.

Dirty and infected wounds include old traumatic wounds and those involving clinical infection or perforated viscera. The very definition of this classification suggests that the organisms causing postoperative infection are present in the operative field before operation.

BIBLIOGRAPHY

ALTEMEIER WA: Control of wound infection. JR Coll Surg, Edinb 11:271, 1966

ALTEMEIER WA: Diagnosis, classification, and general management of gas-producing infections, particularly those produced by *Clostridium perfringens*. Proceedings of the 3rd International Conference on Hyperbaric Medicine, pp 481–490. Washington, DC, National Academy of Science, 1966

ALTEMEIER WA: Bacteriology of surgical infections, clinical and experimental considerations. Vingt-quatriene Congres de la Societe Internationale de Chirurgie, Moscow, 1971

ALTEMEIER WA: The significance of infection in trauma (Scudder Oration). Bulletin of the American College of Surgeons 57(2):7, 1972

ALTEMEIER WA: Infection control in the operating room and perioperative areas. In Roderick MA (ed): Infection Control in Critical Care, pp 63–71. Rockville, Aspen Systems Corp, 1983

ALTEMEIER WA: Surgical infections: Incisional wounds. In Bennett JV, Brachman PS (eds): Hospital Infections, Chapter 16, p 287. Boston, Little, Brown & Co, 1979

ALTEMEIER WA, BARNES BA, PULASKI EJ, SANDUSKY WR, BURKE JF, CLOWES GHA: Infections: Prophylaxis and management—A Symposium. Surgery 67:369, 1970

ALTEMEIER, WA, BERKICH E: Wound sepsis and dehiscence. In Hardy JD (ed): Critical Surgical Illness, pp 187–206. Philadelphia, WB Saunders, 1971

ALTEMEIER WA, TODD JC, INGE WW: Newer aspects of septicemia in surgical patients. Arch Surg 92:566, 1966

BARTLETT P, REINGOLD AL, GRAHAM DR et al: Toxic shock syndrome associated with surgical wound infections. JAMA 247:1148–1450, 1982

BRUCK HM, NASH G, FOLEY FD, PRUITT BA JR: Opportunistic fungal infection of the burn wound with Phycomycetes and *Aspergillus:* A clinical pathologic review. Arch Surg 102:476–482, 1971

CRUSE PJE, FOORD R: A five year prospective study of 23,649 surgical wounds. Arch Surg 107:206, 1973

CRUSE PJE, FOORD R: The epidemiology of wound infection. Symposium on Surgical Infections. Surg Clin North Am 60:27–40, 1980

CURRERI PW, BRUCK HM, LINDBERG RB, MASON AD JR, PRUITT BA JR: *Providencia stuartii* sepsis: A new challenge in the treatment of thermal injury. Ann Surg 177:133–138, 1973

DAVIDSON AIG, CLARK C, SMITH G: Postoperative wound infections: A computer analysis. Br J Surg, 58(5):333,1971

FINLAND M, JONES WF, BARNES MW: Occurrence of serious bacterial infections since introduction of antibacterial agents. JAMA, 170:2188, 1969

FOLEY, FD, GREENAWALD KA, NASH G, PRUITT BA JR: Herpesvirus infection in burned patients. N Engl J Med 281:652–656, 1970

HOWARD JM, BARKER WF, CULBERTSON WR, GROTZINGER PJ, IOVINE VM, KEEHN RJ, RAVDIN RG: Postoperative wound infections: The influence of ultraviolet irradiation of the operating room and of various other factors. Ann Surg 160(Suppl):1, 1964

KEIGHLEY MRB, BURDON DW: The etiology of surgical infection. Antimicrobial Prophylaxis in Surgery, pp 1–22. Pitman Medical Publishers, 1979

MELENEY FL: The study of the prevention of infection in contaminated accidental wounds, compound fractures, and burns. Ann Surg 118:171, 1943

MUSHER DM, McKINZIE SO: Infections due to *Staphylococcus aureus.* Medicine (Baltimore) 56:383–409, 1977

NASH G, ASCH MJ, FOLEY FD, PRUITT BA JR: Disseminated cytomegalic inclusion disease in a burned adult. JAMA 214:587–589, 1970

NASH G, FOLEY FD, GOODWIN NM JR, BRUCK HM, GREENAWALD KA, PRUITT BA JR: Fungal burn wound infection. JAMA 215:1664–1666, 1971

NASH G, FOLEY FD, PRUITT BA JR: Candida burn wound invasion: A cause of systemic candidiasis. Arch Pathol Lab Med 90:75–78, 1970

NAZARI S, DIONIGI R, COMODI, DIONIGI P, CAMPANI M: Preoperative prediction and quantification of septic risk caused by malnutrition. Arc Surg 117(3):266, 1982

POLK HC: Overview of surgical infections, Chap 1, pp 1–18. In Hospital Acquired Infections in Surgery. Baltimore, University Park Press, 1977

PRUITT BA JR: Infections of burns and other wounds caused by *Pseudomonas aeruginosa.* In Sabath LD (ed): Pseudomonas aeruginosa, pp 55–70. Hans Huber, 1980

WILLIAMS REO, SHOOTER RA (eds): Infection in hospitals: Epidemiology and control In Symposium on Infection in Hospitals, London, 1962. Philadelphia, FA Davis, 1963

4

EPIDEMIOLOGY

An understanding of the epidemiologic aspects of hospital-acquired (nosocomial) infections in surgical patients is necessary for effective surveillance. It is important to realize that the pattern of hospital-acquired infections during the past 15 years has shifted from *Staphylococcus* as the major offender to a group of aerobic gram-negative bacilli (see Chaps. 2 and 10). This phenomenon, however, has not decreased the need for staphylococcal control in the hospital environment. Furthermore, in recent years *Staphylococcus epidermidis* and methicillin-resistant *Staphylococcus aureus* have emerged as important pathogens causing postoperative wound infections. In addition, one must keep in mind that the full scale of microbial agents, including viruses, fungi, and protozoa, are potential sources of nosocomial infections (Chap. 3). Burn infections provide an excellent example of this phenomenon. Prior to 1940, the Group A *Streptococcus* organisms represented the major microbial problem in burns. With the development of antibiotics and environmental controls, the coagulase-positive *Staphylococcus aureus* emerged as the major microbial problem in burns, only to be followed by aerobic gram-negative bacilli including *Pseudomonas* and *Providencia* species, as well as true fungi, even the *Candida albicans* and herpes simplex virus.

Other types of microbial infections to be considered are those caused by anaerobic organisms, principally *Clostridia, Bacteroides,* and *Peptostreptococcus.* More recently, anaerobic infections in general have been reported with increasing frequency. Wound botulism has also been described. It is uncertain whether this development is related to altered host resistance in critically ill patients or to improved laboratory techniques for isolation and identification of these bacteria. Experience suggests that both causes have been factors.

Certain common factors are important determinants in the occurrence of opportunistic *nosocomial infection.* First, these infections tend to develop in people with anatomical, biochemical, or physiolog-

Epidemiology and Surveillance of Infection in Surgical Patients

ical defects in their defense mechanisms. Second, they occur within an environment in which antibiotic-resistant bacteria are prevalent. The organisms responsible for the frequently encountered nosocomial infections include *Staphylococcus aureus, Escherichia coli, Pseudomonas, Klebsiella, Enterobacter, Proteus, Serratia, Providencia, Herellea* species, and *Flavobacterium* species, all of which are ubiquitous, can survive at room temperature or under refrigeration, and have the propensity to acquire resistance to antibiotics (Chap. 10).

Man is the major reservoir for *Staphylococcus aureus.* Newborn infants are essentially free of staphylococci at the time of delivery. However, 7% acquire staphylococci in the nose within 24 hours of birth, and 88 % are carriers by the seventh day of life. The staphylococci are almost always those of the hospital environment and not those of the mothers. In examinations of a nonhospital adult population, it has been found that about 50% carry staphylococci in the nasopharynx. In a population of adults who work in hospitals, however, about 40% to 60% carry staphylococci in the nose. More recent studies suggested that the incidence of pencillin-resistant strains at times may reach 90% in such a population, and some may become carriers. It is important to emphasize that the reservoir of hospital-acquired methicillin-sensitive *S. aureus* postoperative wound infections is frequently the nares of operating room personnel. However, the reservoir of methicillin-resistant strains appears to be the infected or colonized wounds of other patients. Gram-negative bacilli of the hospital environment may also be picked up and harbored in the nares or gastrointestinal tract of hospital personnel. The importance of carriers in the pathogenesis of infection has been emphasized by Walter.

Notwithstanding these various studies, routine culture of hospital personnel has not been recommended by the Center for Disease Control (CDC). However, if a local problem develops and hospital personnel are epidemiologically involved in an outbreak of staphylococcal infection, immediate bacteriological detection, treatment, and follow-up are indicated. Persons who have dermatitis or a draining lesion, such as a furuncle or paronychia, are great hazards and they should be removed from patient contact. The goal of therapy is to eliminate an epidemiologically significant microbial strain from the carrier and in the surgical environment. A cream consisting of neomycin, polymyxin B, and bacitracin applied intranasally, three to four times daily, has been found to suppress *Staphylococcus aureus* in about 70% to 90% of carriers. However, reappearance of the same or a different strain of *Staphylococcus aureus* occurs in many treated persons within 1 to 2 months, and retreatment may become necessary if the previously treated strain reappears or if infection in exposed patients continues to occur. Infection of the lower enteric tract, prostatitis, and uterine cervicitis may also be sites of infection in *Staphylococcus aureus* carriers.

Staphylococcal infections can be spread by direct contact with contaminated patients, personnel, or fomites. Other sources of infection are pets, stored clothing, toys, beds, and bedding. The coagulase-positive *Staphylococcus aureus* may also be recovered from the environment, making it important to keep the environment as clean as possible by using effective housekeeping techniques (see Chap. 14). Since the spread of such organisms is primarily from and by people, handwashing is the single most important means of minimizing the spread of infection, providing it is carried out before and after patient contact, *even when gloves are used.* Disinfection of hands is also useful. Walter has indicated that the use of a squirt or sponge of isopropanol is effective, even for nails; it prevents chapping, can be done without special equipment, and is quick and pleasant. To prevent drying he has recommended that cetyl alcohol be added.

People are also the reservoir for many gram-negative microorganisms, and hand-washing and other hygienic practices can be helpful in minimizing their spread. Standing water and alcoholic or aqueous solutions can become reservoirs of many gram-negative organisms, including *Pseudomonas, Serratia, Enterobacteriaceae, Herellea,* and *Flavobacteria.* Such solutions are frequently found in multiple containers around the patient's bed. It should be noted that covered pans or jars containing aqueous or alcoholic solutions of germicides may lose their efficacy because of adsorption, dissipation, inactivation, or volitalization of the agent. Residual germicide must be provided for, articles must be clean, and the bore of the equipment, material, or instrument must be filled. Likewise, dip basins, containers of water for irrigating suction catheters, open glass vials of medication, saline or water bottles, and nondisposable shaving equipment serve as ready sources for spread of gram-negative organisms and should be discarded after a single use. Recently, there have been two outbreaks of infection in hospitals traced to iodophors contaminated by organisms of the genus *Pseudomonas.*

Indwelling urethral catheters and urinary tract instrumentation are associated with a high incidence of gram-negative urinary tract infection, as reported by Kunin and other investigators. Martin has estimated that there may be as many as 30,000 deaths a year in the United States from gram-negative bacteremia associated with prolonged catheter use. Altemeier and associates found that 53% of cases of gram-negative septicemia had their source of origin in the urinary tract. Data from the National Nosocomial Infection Study (1971–1974) indicated that approximately 40% of all nosocomial infections involved the urinary tract. The most important means of control of this type of infection is the use of a closed-drainage system and the prevention of reflux of bacteria from the collection reservoir along the catheter and back into the bladder (Chap. 10). The rigorous use of closed drainage systems can greatly reduce the retrograde entry of microorganisms into the bladder and urinary tract. The system may also be contaminated by opening it to collect urine samples, the highest risk occurring when it is opened for irrigations. The daily application of antibiotic ointment to the urethral meatus has not been shown to reduce the rate of catheter-related tract infections. Furthermore, the routine use of antiseptics in drainage bags of catheterized patients in acute care hospitals has not reduced the rate of associated urinary tract infections. Bladder irrigations are to be avoided, but if they become necessary a "three-way" system should be used (Chap. 10).

Intravenous lines for physiological monitoring, prolonged administration of fluids and medications, and hyperalimentation may also be sources of septicemia caused by gram-negative, gram-positive, or fungal microorganisms. Recommendations for their control are considered further in Chapter 10.

The nebulization equipment for respirators may also serve as a frequent source of contamination of the respiratory tract unless adequately cleansed and properly maintained. Anesthesia equipment may also present problems, because the design makes sterilization very difficult, and aseptic precautions may be inadequate.

Other troublesome infections are caused by the agents of viral hepatitis; these agents are transmitted either by fecal–oral contamination, or by inoculation from contaminated blood serum or (in the case of type B and types non-A, non-B) various other materials. There are special epidemiologic problems with the viral hepatitis agents because of the variable incubation periods. Moreover, patients may have subclinical cases of the disease and be inapparent hazards to hospital personnel, especially interns and residents, nurses, and laboratory workers. Hemodialysis units and renal transplant services are particularly high-risk areas for non-A, non-B viral hepatitis as well as for Type B viral hepatitis. If the disease is acquired in the hospital, the patient may be discharged long before it becomes evident, and its occurrence may never be known to the hospital where it was acquired. Any physician observing a recent postoperative patient with hepatitis should report this to the operating surgeon and the hospital or hospital epidemiologist concerned.

SURVEILLANCE

Searching for different sources of infection may be helpful as a preventive measure. Routine monitoring, such as culturing of personnel, skin in the operative area, the wounds themselves, the floors and walls of operating theaters, and the air in the operating room, is not considered to be cost-effective and is not recommended. However, extensive bacteriological sampling (epidemiologically directed) is recommended by the Center for Disease Control of Atlanta when a cluster of infections appears or there is other evidence of a problem.

Careful, routine, and periodic checks on the effectiveness of sterilizing equipment and the degree of contamination of inhalation therapy and anesthesia equipment should be carried out. The sterilizing effectiveness of autoclaves, hot air ovens, and ethylene oxide sterilizers should be checked regularly by processing standard spore strips or specially prepared dirt samples containing spores, and subsequently culturing them to see if they are sterile. The Bowie-Dick test is useful to check on the effective penetration of packs by steam in high vacuum autoclaves (Chapter 16).

Regular testing for hepatitis B surface antigen ($HB_s Ag$) in blood products for transfusion remains important.

The Joint Commission on the Accreditation of Hospitals has published guidelines and standards for infection prevention, control, surveillance, and reporting to ensure that the lives and well-being of patients and hospital personnel are protected. The Committee on Control of Surgical Infections of the Pre- and Postoperative Care Committee of the American College of Surgeons agrees with these guidelines, which include the following:

1. The appointment of an infection control committee
2. The development, evaluation, and revision on a continuing basis of the procedures and techniques used for meeting established sanitation and asepsis standards

3. The development of a practical system for reporting, evaluating, and keeping records of infections among patients and personnel
4. The provision of facilities for the isolation of certain infected patients
5. The development of written standards for hospital sanitation and medical asepsis
6. The maintenance of an adequate microbiology service
7. The prevention of contamination of foods
8. The periodic review of the use of antibiotics as they relate to patient care

Items 2 and 5 are considered in Chapters 8, 9, 10, and 17, and item 8 in Chapter 11. Item 3 involves surveillance, identification, and accurate reporting of infections that require the attention of the infection control committee and the full cooperation of the medical staff with the infection control officer or epidemiological practitioner.

The Hospital Infection Control Committee

The hospital infection control committee is vested with the responsibility for the control of infections within the hospital and for the evaluation of the infection potential of the related environment. Close collaboration with the chief of surgical services and the chief of medical services is desirable and important for effective effort.

The hospital infection control committee should consist of medical staff members from various disciplines as well as representatives from the administration, the microbiology laboratory, and the nursing service. The infection control practitioner and the hospital epidemiologist, if such exist, should attend the meetings. When possible, the hospital infection control committee should include a surgeon, an epidemiologist, a bacteriologist or pathologist, a pediatrician, an internist, a nurse, and a hospital administrator. The chairman should have a special interest and knowledge in the area of infection and its control. Representatives of the dietary service, the pharmacy, central supply service, housekeeping, and maintenance should be consulted as indicated and should be invited to attend meetings when appropriate. The committee should meet on a scheduled basis and hold additional meetings when necessary. The work of the committee is most meaningful if a specific agenda is planned for each meeting. The committee should report regularly to the executive committee of the hospital medical staff. Selected data may be disseminated to other members of the medical staff when indicated, care being taken to ensure confidentiality because of the privileged nature of such information and its possible misuse.

Development of Written Standards for Medical Asepsis and Hospital Sanitation

The hospital committee on control of infection should develop and continuously revise as necessary written standards for hospital sanitation and medical asepsis. A system for monitoring, surveillance, and reporting must be developed, and the data generated by such a system analyzed and applied to decrease the risk of infection and improve the quality of patient care.

For the development of a practical system of reporting, evaluating, and keeping records of infections among patients and personnel, *effective surveillance* is necessary. Effective surveillance requires the timely identification and prompt reporting of infections as they occur in any hospital patient. This involves monitoring of patients, hospital personnel, and the hospital environment according to the standards noted above. Surveillance may be used to define the endemic level and types of infection as they occur in a given hospital. Surveillance also identifies clusters of infection and epidemics as they occur. If a hospital experiences one or two cases of infection caused by an unusually rare organism or an organism having an unusual sensitivity pattern, consideration should be given to initiation of an epidemiologic investigation. Determination of the source or origin of any infection is a difficult problem, and epidemiologic studies may be necessary to determine such sources and to identify various environmental hazards.

The epidemiologic survey required to isolate the source of a cluster of infections may be laborious and time-consuming, and requires the cooperation of the hospital staff, the microbiology laboratory, the infection control committee, and an epidemiologist. The epidemiologic approach often involves comparing infected with noninfected patients in an attempt to uncover those factors that differ significantly between them. The Centers for Disease Control (CDC) may provide assistance in studying hospital epidemics. Local and state health departments may also be called upon to assist hospitals in epidemiologic investigations. Such an investigation was carried out in one outbreak of postoperative infections caused by Group A beta-hemolytic *Streptococcus*. Its time of onset strongly indicated the operating theater as the source. Hospital and operating room personnel were cultured to detect nasal or pharyngeal carriers of Group A *Streptococcus*. The organisms uncovered, however, were of a different type than those isolated from the infections. Assessment of individual operating room attack rates related to the attending personnel in the operating rooms suggested that an anesthesiologist was associated with these infections. When extensively cultured, this person was found to be a disseminating anal carrier of Group A beta-hemolytic *Streptococcus* with the epidemic M and T antigenic patterns.

Surveillance may improve patient care, diagnosis, and personal hygiene by emphasizing the frequency and importance of hospital-acquired infections. It also permits detection of alterations in endemic flora and may emphasize problem areas in which modifications of control measures may be necessary. Additionally, it may permit evaluation of the effectiveness of changes in procedures and policies. Recent studies by the Centers for Disease Control (the Senic study) have shown that reporting of operation-specific postoperative wound infection rates may be associated with subsequent reduction in rates.

Maximum usefulness of surveillance data requires that the flow of information be current, continuous, and promptly available to appropriate and authorized personnel. The simplest way to collect the required data is to construct a form on which the epidemiologic or microbiological data of significance can be entered. The extent of the information collected depends upon specific interests and the resources and personnel available. At a minimum, entries should include date of onset, causative organism, antibiotic sensitivity, type of wound, name, identifying number, age and sex of patient, hospital service, primary diagnosis, identity of attending personnel, selected host and therapeutic factors that predispose to the infection, dates and type of surgical procedures, time of onset with reference to admission and to surgery, and complications. Morbidity and mortality data related to the infection, should such occur, would also be useful.

An effective and successful system to collect this information uses an infection control practitioner who works under the supervision of a physician on the infection control committee. A large, active surgical service may justify a full-time surgical infection control nurse, whereas a smaller surgical service could be monitored by a nurse reviewing infections for the entire hospital. The infection control nurse may also be used to monitor the adherence to infection control policies and practices related to both patient and equipment care. This nurse should also conduct in-service training as deemed necessary and approved by the infection control committee.

The above information on nosocomial infections should be obtained not only from regularly scheduled visits to the wards and interviews with attending personnel but also from the microbiology laboratory. Temperature and vital sign charts, as well as medication charts, may also provide indications that an otherwise unappreciated infection exists. Spontaneous reporting by other hospital personnel may be unreliable because of the other demands upon their time. The nurse epidemiologist, however, can devote full time to providing factual data in a usable, readily retrievable, easily interpreted, and ethical form.

The responsibilities of the hospital epidemiologist and the infection control committee include the following:

1. Identification and recording of postoperative wound and nosocomial infections on a systematic and current basis
2. Monthly reporting and analysis of nosocomial infections
3. Conduct of epidemiologic investigation of all significant clusters of infection
4. Development and implementation of infection control measures
5. Conduct of in-service training programs on infection prevention and control
6. Notification, as required by law, of local health departments of "reportable" infectious diseases seen in the hospital
7. Review of environmental cleanliness, including monitoring programs for inhalation, anesthesia, and physical therapy equipment
8. Supervision of bacteriological monitoring to ensure the quality of the specimens obtained and the techniques involved

Another facet of surveillance is the analysis of the data that has been collected. To the best of its ability, the hospital infection control committee should distinguish between infection acquired in the hospital and that acquired outside, and should differentiate between colonization and infection. This includes the classification of the infection by source — community-based, operating-room-based, or hospital-based other than operating-room-based (Chap. 3) — and involves the identification of characteristics in a group of infected patients that predisposes them to infection.

Statistical assessment of differences in attack rates is one of the first steps in identifying an epidemiologic problem. Attack rate is defined as the number of cases of a given infection divided by the population-at-risk in a given interval of time. The population-at-risk must be ascertained from records of admission to a hospital on a given ward or from ward census data. The number of patients undergoing a given surgical procedure can be obtained from the operating room logbook, and can then be related to the total number of patients operated upon during a given time period and the specific personnel involved. After determination of the at-risk population, the number of patients with a given infection is divided by that larger population to obtain the attack rate.

Analysis of the data obtained should also include an interpretation of the degree or significance of the infection — whether it is minimal or insignificant, moderately severe, or serious (Chap. 3). Reporting of the surveillance data must be facilitated by the construction of a *site-pathogen table,* in which the services or wards with unusual infections can be easily identified. Such a table can be constructed for each surgical subspecialty that is large enough to justify such an analysis. Wound infection and attack rates also can be related to the type of operation performed and to the attending surgeon, and that information supplied to the individual concerned.

The surveillance studies should also include periodic reports of antibiotic sensitivities of any causative organisms isolated in order to assist in the selection of the appropriate antimicrobial therapy. (See Chap. 11 for examples of antibiotic profiles.)

Another useful function of the hospital infection control committee is the periodic review of the hospital's bacteriological services, either in-house or out-of-house, to determine whether such services are of good quality and are readily available, either in the hospital or in an outside laboratory. Bacteriophage typing, when needed, may be sought through official local and state health agencies if such is not available in the hospital.

The committee should conduct programs to educate medical staff and hospital employees on the importance of reporting to responsible authorities when they have skin infections and acute upper respiratory infections, and to provide in-service training programs as indicated, particularly for new employees. A high turnover of personnel requires active in-service training programs in asepsis, hand-washing, isolation, and so forth. Since a hospital may be considered responsible for the negligence of its employees, provision for supplying adequate periodic training and supervision of hospital employees becomes important in the acceptable practice of medical asepsis.

Computer Aids

The analysis of epidemiologic data is time consuming and complex enough to warrant the use of a computer. It is, of course, essential that the computer program be designed to provide the information needed by the infection control committee. It is necessary for criteria and specific definitions of infection to be developed prospectively in collaboration with the physician staff members (see Chap. 3). The programming and computer processing of the data should be planned and carefully supervised by the responsible physician.

Table 4-1. Monthly Infection Report of Hospital Infections

For the Month of _____ 19____

	Number	Percent of Discharges
Number of patients with one infection	_____	_____
(a) postoperative wound	_____	_____
(b) hospital-acquired (nosocomial)	_____	_____
Number of patients with two infections	_____	_____
(a) postoperative wound	_____	_____
(b) hospital-acquired (nosocomial)	_____	_____
Number of patients with three or more infections	_____	_____
(a) postoperative wound	_____	_____
(b) hospital-acquired (nosocomial)	_____	_____
Total	_____	_____

	Number	Percent
Total Number of Infections		
Present on Admission	_____	_____
Developed After Admission	_____	_____
(a) postoperative wound	_____	_____
(b) hospital-acquired (nosocomial)	_____	_____

Infections Developed After Admission (By Service)

Ward or Floor	Service	Number of Discharges	Number of Infections	Attack Rate
_____	_____	_____	_____	_____
_____	_____	_____	_____	_____
_____	_____	_____	_____	_____
_____	_____	_____	_____	_____
_____	_____	_____	_____	_____

Type of Infections Developed After Admission		Attack Rate
Wound	_____	_____
Urinary Tract	_____	_____
Respiratory	_____	_____
Skin and Subcutaneous Tissue	_____	_____
Intravenous Route and Blood	_____	_____
All Other	_____	_____

(Sample report from University of Cincinnati Medical Center)

Ideally, at least a monthly report should be generated and made available to the physicians in the hospital. This report should include the overall rates of postoperative wound and nosocomial infections by ward and specialty; the type of operation; a site–pathogen table when indicated; attack rates for wound infections related to the type of surgical procedure; and summaries of special investigations of infections carried out during that month (Table 4-1).

Administrative support for the infection control committee should be provided so that effective action can be taken based on the information received. This support is necessary so that clearly defined problem areas can be promptly addressed.

Surveillance of patients for late-occurring infections, including hepatitis, is more difficult to carry out with accuracy after discharge from the hospital, but the hospital committee on infection control should make provisions for a follow-up inspection of high-risk patients and their wounds.

BIBLIOGRAPHY

ALMEIDA JD, KULATILAKE AE, MACKAY DH et al: Possible airborne spread of serum-hepatitis within a haemodialysis unit. Lancet 2:849, 1971

ALTEMEIER WA: The surgical conscience. Arch Surg 79:167, 1959.

ALTEMEIER WA, CULBERTSON WR, HUMMEL RP: Surgical considerations of endogenous infections — sources, types and methods of control. Surg Clin North Am 48:227, 1968

ALTEMEIER WA, CULBERTSON WR, FULLEN WD, McDONOUGH JJ: *Serratia marcescens* septicemia. Arch Surg 99:232, 1969

ALTEMEIER WA, HUMMEL RP, HILL EO, LEWIS S: Changing patterns in surgical infections. Ann Surg 178:436, 1973

ALTEMEIER WA, TODD JC, INGE WW: Gram-negative septicemia: A growing threat. Ann Surg 166:530, 1967

BAILEY NTJ: The Mathematical Theory of Epidemics. New York, Hafner, 1957

BRACHMAN P: In Institutionally Acquired Infections. Atlanta, GA, National Communicable Disease Center, 1963

BRACHMAN PS: Nosocomial infection control: An overview. Rev Infect Dis 3(4):640–648, 1981

BRUUN JN, BOE J, SOLBERG CO: Disinfection of the hands of ward personnel. Acta Med Scand 184:417, 1968

BURKE JF: Identification of the sources of staphylococci contaminating the surgical wound during operation. Ann Surg 158:898, 1963

BURKE JF, CARRIGAN EA: Staphylococcal epidemiology on a surgical ward. N Engl J Med 264:321–325, 1964

BYRNE EB: Viral hepatitis: An occupational hazard of medical personnel, experience of the Yale–New Haven Hospital, 1952 to 1965. JAMA 195:362, 1966

CDC GUIDELINES ON INFECTION CONTROL: Infect Control 3(1):52–82, 1982.

CLAESSON B, BRANDBERG A, NILSSON LO, KOCK NG: Quantitative recovery of contaminating bacteria at operation and the relation to postoperative infection in intestinal surgery. Acta Chir Scand 147(4):285–288, 1981

CROSSLEY K, LANDESMAN B, ZASKE D: An outbreak of infections caused by strains of *Staphylococcus aureus* resistant to methicillin and aminoglycosides. II. Epidemiologic studies. J Infect Dis 139(3):280–287, 1979

CRUSE PJE, FOORD R: A five year prospective study of 23,649 surgical wounds. Arch Surg 107:206, 1973

DAVIDSON AIG, CLARK C, SMITH G: Postoperative wound infection: A computer analysis. Br J Surg 58:333, 1971

DAVIS, JM, WOLFF B, CUNNINGHAM TF, DRUSIN L, DINEEN P: Delayed wound infection: An 11-year survey. Arc Surg 117(2):113–117, 1982

EDWARDS LD: The epidemiology of 2056 remote site infections and 1966 surgical wound infections occurring in 1865 patients: A four year study of 40,923 operations at Rush– Presbyterian–St. Luke's Hospital, Chicago. Ann Surg 184(6):758–766, 1976

FARBER B, KAISER DL, WENZEL RP: Relation between surgical volume and incidence of postoperative infection. N Engl J Med 305:200–204, 1981

FARBER BF, WENZEL RP: Postoperative wound infection rates: Results of prospective state-wide surveillance. Am J Surg 140(3):343–346, 1980

FLOURNOY DJ, MUCHMORE HG, FRANCIS EB: Nosocomial infection linked to handwashing. Hospitals 53(15):105, 1979

GREEN MS, RUBINSTEIN E, AMIT P: Estimating the effects of nosocomial infections on the length of hospitalization. J Infect Dis 145(5):667–672, 1982

GREEN JW, WENZEL RP: Postoperative wound infections: A controlled study of the duration of hospital stay and direct cost of hospitalization. Ann Surg 185:264–268, 1977

HARLEY RW: The usefulness of a conceptual model in the study of the efficacy of infection surveillance and control programs. Rev Infect Dis 3(4):775–780, 1981

HASSELGREN PO, SALJO A, FORNANDER J, LUNDSTAM S, SARETOK T, SEEMAN T: Postoperative wound infections—a prospective study in a newly opened hospital. Ann Chir Gynaecol 69(6):269–272, 1980

HOSPITAL ACCREDITATION PROGRAM: Environmental services In Accreditation Manual for Hospitals, p 90. Chicago, Joint Commission on Accreditation of Hospitals, 1973

HOWARD JM ET AL: Postoperative wound infections: The influence of ultraviolet irradiation of the operating room and of various other factors. Ann Surg 160(Suppl):1, 1964

KALLINGS LO: Program for surveillance and intervention in specific problem areas of nosocomial infections. Rev Infect Dis 3(4):721–727, 1981

KENDALL DG: Deterministic and stochastic epidemics in closed populations. In Berkeley Symposium on Mathematical Statistics and Probability. Berkeley, University of California Press, 1956

KRUGMAN S, GILES JP, HAMMOND J ET AL: Infectious hepatitis. Evidence for two distinctive clinical, epidemiological, and immunological types of infection. JAMA 200:365, 1967

LEDGER WJ: Prevention, diagnosis, and treatment of postoperative infections. Obstet Gynecol 55(5):2039–2069, 1980

LEISH DA: An eight year study of postoperative wound infection in two district general hospitals. J Hosp Infect 2(3):207–117, 1981

LeRICHE WH, BALCOM CE, BELLE GV: The Control of Infection in Hospitals. Springfield, IL, Charles C Thomas, 1966

MOSLEY JW: The surveillance of transfusion-associated viral hepatitis. JAMA 193:1007, 1965

M'TERO SS, SAYED M, TYRELL DA: Quantitative studies on preventing the spread of micro-organisms in a hospital isolation unit. J Hosp Infect 2(4):317–328, 1981

POLK HC JR, LOPEZ-MAYOR JF: Postoperative wound infection: A prospective study of determinant factors and prevention. Surgery 66:1,97, 1969

PRINCE, AM et al: Immunologic distinction between infectious and serum hepatitis. N Engl J Med 282:987, 1970

RAHMAN M: Outbreak of Streptococcus pyogenes infection in a geriatric hospital and control by mass treatment. J Hosp Infect 2(1):63–69, 1981

REPORT TO MEDICAL RESEARCH COUNCIL BY THE SUBCOMMITTEE ON ASEPTIC METHODS IN OPERATING THEATRES OF THEIR COMMITTEE ON HOSPITAL INFECTION. Lancet 1:705, 763, 831, 1968

SHOOTER RA, TAYLOR GW, ELLIS G, ROSS JP: Postoperative wound infection. Surg Gynecol Obstet 103:257, 1956

STEWART GT: Epidemiology of drug-resistant infections. In Antimicrobial Agents and Chemotherapy, p 245. American Society of Microbiology, 1967

VALENTI WM, MENGUS MA: Nosocomial viral infections. IV. Guidelines for cohort isolation. The Communicable Disease Survey. Collection and transport of specimens for virus isolation and considerations for the future. Infect Control 2(3):236–245, 1981

VILLAREJOS VM, VISOND KA, GOTIERREZ A, RODRIGUEZ A: Role of saliva, urine, and feces in the transmission of Type B hepatitis. N Engl J Med 291:1375, 1974

WALTER, CW, KUNDSIN RB: The bacteriologic study of surgical gloves from 250 operations. Surg Gynecol Obstet 129:949, 1969

WALTER CW, KUNDSIN RB, PAGE L, HARDING AL: The infector on the surgical team. Clin Neurosurg 14:361, 1967

WALTER CW, RUBENSTEIN AD, KUNDSIN RB, SHILKRET MA: Bacteriology of the bedside carafe. N Engl J Med 259:1198, 1958

WENZEL RP: The emergence of methicillin resistant *Staphylococcus aureus.* Ann Intern Med 97:440–442, 1982

WENZEL RP, HUNTING RJ, OSTERMAN CA: Postoperative wound infection rates. Surg Gynecol Obstet 144:749–752, 1977

WENZEL RP, OSTERMAN CA, HUNTING RJ et al: Hospital acquired infections. I. Surveillance in a university hospital. Am J Epidemiol 103:253–260, 1976

WILLIAMS REO, BLOWERS R, GARROD LP, SHOOTER RA: Causes and prevention. In Hospital Infection, 2nd ed, Chap 18. London, Lloyd Luke, 1966

WILLIAMS REO, SHOOTER RA (eds): Infection in hospitals: Epidemiology and control. In Symposium on Infection in Hospitals, London, 1962. Philadelphia, FA Davis, 1963

WOLINSKY E, LIPSITZ PJ, MORTIMER EA, RAMMELKAMP CH: Acquisition of staphylococci by newborns, direct versus indirect transmission. Lancet 2:620, 1960

5

The prolonged morbidity and high mortality of sepsis more than justify preventive and therapeutic measures for the control of infection among the surgical patients of any hospital. Not only are individual septic patients relieved of life-threatening complications, but also a reservoir of infection may be eradicated. From a clinical standpoint, such measures, to be effective, depend largely upon knowledge of the biological effects of infection in the body as well as familiarity with the bacteriology of invading organisms. Understanding of these matters permits the competent surgeon to recognize the deleterious effects of bacterial invasion and to deal with them by appropriate supportive or therapeutic means.

Four major aspects of the pathophysiology of infection are of clinical importance:

1. The nature, source, and invasive qualities of microorganisms dictate the steps to be taken to reduce the number and virulence of bacteria to which the patient may be exposed.
2. The inflammatory and immunological responses of the invaded body, as well as the dose of microorganisms, play a major role in determining whether an infection will become established. In addition to breaks in the epithelial barriers of the body, devitalized tissue and foreign bodies predispose to infection in many instances.
3. Survival or death of the infected patient is directly related to the balance between the injury inflicted by the infection and the physiological responses that preserve life until the septic process can be brought under control and eliminated.
4. Finally, continued energy metabolism and synthesis of proteins are essential to the maintenance of immunocompetence, healing of wounds, and preservation of the structure of vital organs. These functions are dependent upon an adequate supply of energy fuel substrates and amino acids for protein building blocks. In contrast with normal starvation, amino acids derived from muscle protein degradation are employed for accelerated synthesis of special proteins in the liver and other visceral tissues. When this pattern of physiological and metabolic responses to sepsis is inadequate, the usual outcome is overwhelming infection, progressive multisystem failure, and death.

The Pathophysiology of Infection

Surgical infection involves the lodgment and propagation of the infecting microorganism, not only in the wound but also in other tissues of the body. In addition to local necrosis and cell death caused by invasive infection, septicemia as well as blood-borne toxic products released by microorganisms or injured tissue may cause serious cellular damage and abnormal metabolism in distant organs. A series of characteristic physiological, metabolic, and immunological responses occur which are directed toward defense and continuation of vital organ function. These alterations are induced by endocrine and neurological activity and by a series of circulating peptides derived from sites of inflammation and tissue injury. Whereas the modest elevation of metabolic rate in uneventful recovery from clean surgery imposes no more than an 8% increase in circulatory and respiratory work, the septic state imposes serious stresses upon the circulatory, respiratory, and other systems. In septic patients who recover, the metabolic rate is elevated between 30% and 40%, while cardiac output averages 72% above the normal resting value. In patients whose cardiovascular systems are unable to satisfy the demands of the high peripheral circulation, vasoconstriction, shock, and further injury to vital organs, such as the liver and kidney, may occur. Hypoxemia secondary to interstitial pneumonitis and subsequently bronchopneumonia may further tax all systems. Additionally, the use of fuel substrates and the enzymatic pathways of cellular energy production are altered from the economic pattern of simple starvation in which protein is conserved.

For convenience, the course of sepsis can be divided into three phases:

1.   Invasion
2.   Localization of the septic process
3.   Resolution and recovery

It is important to realize that these phases are not clearly separable but that they merge, and the progression toward recovery may be reversed at any time. In the early stage of "invasive sepsis," immunological and inflammatory reactions tend to isolate and contain the infectious process. Many stresses remain, however, even when the infection is localized, and these may impair the function of other organs (*e.g.,* the lung, heart, kidney, liver, and gastrointestinal tract). Toxic products may continue to enter the circulation by diffusion into the lymphatics and capillaries, and act directly or indirectly upon organs (Chap. 3). "Resolution" of the septic process by drainage or resorption of pus and sloughing of necrotic tissue will lead to healing. Recovery is completed by the restoration of tissue depleted by metabolic demands. Throughout this sequence of events, death may occur if the factors of injury overpower the protective reactions.

MECHANISMS OF INVASION

The pathogenic potential of bacteria depends upon their ability to invade, survive, and multiply within host tissues; inhibit host defense mechanisms; and cause overt damage to the host by destroying tissues. Quantitatively, the number of certain specific organisms required to produce cell necrosis and label the process as "invasive infection" is often quoted as $10^5/g$ of infected tissue or milliliter of biological fluid. In addition to a direct effect on cells, certain bacteria possess or manufacture substances such as exotoxins, aggressins, "impedins," enterotoxins, and endotoxins that may also injure tissue. Pneumococcal capsular polysaccharide, which acts as an antiphagocytic agent, and streptococcal M protein, a cell wall antigen, have been demonstrated to exert potent cytotoxic effects upon both platelets and polymorphonuclear leukocytes and to exhibit a paracoagulation reaction with plasma fibrinogen resulting in fibrin precipitation. Staphylococci produce coagulase as well as substances harmful to leukocytes, including leukocidin, an exotoxin, and a thermostable, nonantigenic component distinct from leukocidin. Antibiotic resistance, bacterial synergism, and the occurrence of L forms of bacteria may complicate the infectious process.

Exotoxins may be of significance in a number of surgical infections caused by such bacteria as *Streptococcus pyogenes, Staphylococcus aureus,* the clostridia of gas gangrene and tetanus, and the pneumococci. Exotoxins, some of which are simple antigenic proteins, are produced by organisms during their growth and are both locally and systemically toxic. Examples are erythrogenic toxin, streptolysins O and S, streptokinase, and hyaluronidase of the streptococci. Hemolytic staphylococcal alpha exotoxin interacts with and lyses lipoprotein membranes. Clostridia release alpha toxin with lecithinase activity, and the recently described Toxin A of certain *Pseudomonas* organisms may also exert deleterious effects. The actions of exotoxins are multiple, and include direct dilatation of vessel walls by the toxin of *Clostridium welchii.* Lysis of red cell membranes by the hemolysins of gram-positive organisms and certain gram-negative rods also occurs.

Endotoxins (lipopolysaccharides in the membrane structure of gram-negative bacilli) may be important in some surgical infections. The lipid component or toxic portion, known as "Lipid A," consists of even-numbered fatty acids, saturated and unsaturated, attached by glucosamine and other amide linkages to the carbohydrate backbone. The endotoxin molecules, which are of varying sizes, are unique.Carbohydrate fatty acid bonds are not found in other biological compounds. The polysaccharide portion corresponds to the O antigen of the gram-negative bacilli. The molecule also contains phosphoric acid. Lipid A, embedded by hydrophobic bonds in the center of the bacterial membrane bilayer structure, is exposed or released only upon death of the organism when membranes are broken down. Although endotoxins do play a role in invasion by local injury to cells at the site of infection, the most important concern is the serious and often lethal effects of these substances with their widespread dissemination throughout the body, resulting in injury to many tissues, either by direct action or by the agents they activate.

Another important category of surgical infections is that produced by two or more bacterial species with symbiotic and synergistic survival, and proliferation of two or more organisms in tissues. Finally, antimicrobial agents may cause the appearance of spheroplasts, or L forms, cell wall variants that are resistant to antibiotics, rendering them extremely difficult to eradicate.

Regardless of their origin, when bacteria gain a foothold at a point within the body where their numbers and virulent potential exceed the capacity of the local tissues to destroy them, they may multiply and destroy tissue unless contained by the immunological and inflammatory responses.

HOST RESISTANCE

Local Defense and the Inflammatory Response

The lysosomes of injured cells, particularly those of the granulocytes and macrophages, contain peptidases and other enzymes that activate the inflammatory response. Prekallikrein from the tissues and blood is converted to kallikrein, a specific peptidase, which is capable of activating the kinins. Of particular importance is bradykinin, which causes venular contraction, increase of endothelial membrane permeability, and opening up of intercellular junctions of the capillary and venular endothelium. The elevated filtration pressure and the augmented capillary permeability may lead to edema with the escape of water, proteins, and cells into the interstitial spaces. Prostagladins also play an important role in this process.

Platelet aggregation may release vasoactive factors having effects similar to those of bradykinin. Additionally, platelet prothrombin promotes clotting. Clotting, further induced by tissue thromboplastin and by the activation of Hagemen factor (Factor XII), in the interstitial spaces and in the immediately adjacent capillaries as well as in the lymphatics, serves to wall off the region of invasion. Furthermore, plasma proteins containing antibodies and complement alter the invading organisms. Macrophages and granulocytes attracted by leukotactic substances act by phagocytosis to limit infection.

The ultimate resolution of an inflamed septic focus depends on the removal of foreign matter, including the debris of bacteria and cells. Usually this is effected by drainage or by lysis of microorganisms and resorption, after which tissue continuity can be restored by the deposit of collagen. Then, healing of specialized structures occurs.

Immunohumoral and Cellular Factors of Host Resistance

Human beings are continually exposed to a variety of potentially pathogenic organisms. Surgical and traumatic wounds are especially important among the routes by which bacteria enter the internal milieu of the body, since few if any are sterile. Fortunately, these bacteria usually are effectively killed and removed from sites of contamination by means of the process of inflammation (Fig. 5–1).

The plasma proteins contain many substances important to host defense, including several types of specific antibody and serum complement components. Immunoglobulin G (IgG) antibodies are by far the most important in antimicrobial defense, but immunoglobulin M (IgM) may play a role in fungal and certain gram-negative infections. When the bacteria have antigenic determinants that will combine with certain of these antibodies, the physical character of the antibody is altered in such a

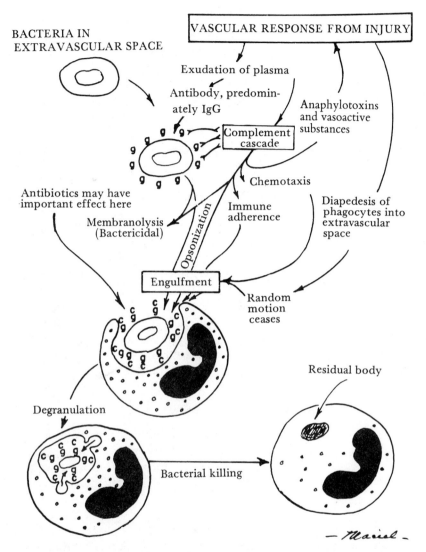

BACTERIA IN
EXTRAVASCULAR SPACE

VASCULAR RESPONSE FROM INJURY

Exudation of plasma

Antibody, predomin-
ately IgG

Anaphylotoxins
and vasoactive
substances

Complement
cascade

Chemotaxis

Antibiotics may have
important effect here

Immune
adherence

Diapedesis of
phagocytes into
extravascular
space

Membranolysis
(Bactericidal)

Opsonization

Engulfment

Random
motion
ceases

Residual body

Degranulation

Bacterial killing

— Mansel —

Fig. 5-1. Early physiological events in response to bacterial contamination. Note the important interrelationships between specific antibody, complement, and the phagocytic cells in destruction of bacteria. (Altemeier WA, and Alexander JW: Surgical infections and choice of antibiotics. In Sabiston Jr DC [ed]: Christopher's Textbook of Surgery, 10th ed, p 320. Philadelphia, WB Saunders, 1972)

way as to activate the cascading sequence of the complement reaction. In the classical pathway of complement, there are 12 distinct proteins (9 components). Recently, it was discovered that the alternative pathways exist for entry into the complement cascade at the level of the third component (C3). Once considered relatively unimportant, the alternative pathway now appears to be a major component of natural nonspecific resistance to infection. Activation of complement has many important biological functions, including immune adherence, membranolysis, chemotaxis, agglutination of bacteria, opsonization of bacteria, and release of vasoactive substances. In this sense, antibody provides specificity for activation of the complement sequence that, in turn, is the effector mechanism for promoting phagocytosis of all bacteria and even direct killing of a few species of lysis.

Phagocytic cells (neutrophils, mononuclear phagocytes, and the reticuloendothelial cells) readily phagocytize opsonized bacteria by an active process of engulfment. Once bacteria are inside the phagocytic cells, they are protected from the lethal action of both bacteriostatic and bactericidal antibiotics. Killing of ingested bacteria then depends upon host defense mechanisms, including intracellular destruction by a process analogous to the digestion of food within the stomach. Digestive and hydrolytic enzymes, superoxides, halides, and perhaps other yet-to-be-defined antibacterial substances kill and digest bacteria of susceptible species. Although various bacteria differ considerably in their ability to resist intracellular killing (*e.g.,* the tubercule bacillus is highly resistant), the process for each is essentially the same. When bacteria are phagocytized by mononuclear phagocytes, the antigens may be incompletely degraded; these antigens later stimulate lymphocytes to synthesize specific antibodies directed against antigenic structures of the bacteria. Neurtrophils are short lived and their usefulness is quickly expended. Dead neutrophils are removed by mononuclear phagocytes, but if the number of dead neutrophils exceeds the capability for removal, the lesion may take the form of a localized purulent collection with characteristic abcess formation.

Abnormalities of Immune Mechanisms

Abnormalities of the antibacterial immune mechanisms may be conveniently divided into three categories: those affecting inflammatory response, those affecting phagocytic function, and those affecting humoral factors. Each of these may be of critical importance in predisposing a patient to the development of invasive bacterial invasion.

Abnormalities of the Inflammatory Response. Before phagocytic cells can remove bacteria from a site of contamination, they must be deposited in sufficient numbers to cope with the size of the inoculum. Anything that interferes with their deposition or with the physical contact of phagocyte and bacterium will enhance the development of an infection. Deficient blood supply, the presence of ischemic or dead tissue, suture material, foreign bodies, hematomas, and seromas all effectively prevent the deposition of phagocytic cells at these sites, and markedly reduce the number of bacteria necessary to cause the development of an infection. As an example, less than 100 bacteria can cause an infection when introduced with a silk suture into a small wound, but 10,000 times as many bacteria are required to cause an infection in a similar wound in the absence of a foreign body (Elek and Conen). In addition to the presence of foreign bodies and collections of blood or fluid within the wound, which physically prevents delivery of phagocytic cells to critical areas, other factors are of importance in effecting the inflammatory response. Among these are the administration of vasopressor agents, which causes reduction of blood flow to an area; radiation injury; uremia; severe nutritional deficiencies, which inhibit the synthesis of antibodies and other essential proteins; and a number of drugs such as adrenocortical steroids, opium, salicylates in high doses, and ethanol.

Abnormalities in Phagocytic Function.   Phagocytic cells are an essential component of the host resistance mechanisms. Without normally active phagocytic cells, a person would soon die of overwhelming sepsis, as examplified by the diseases associated with severe neutropenia. Neutrophils and tissue macrophages are the most important of the phagocytic cells, since they are the first and predominant cells to collect at a site of bacterial contamination. Not only are the number of neutrophils delivered to a site of an inflammatory response of great importance, but their functional status also plays a crucial role. Patients with severe thermal injury and with certain nutritional deficiencies associated with severe trauma or sepsis have significant abnormalities, including defects of bactericidal and chemotactic capacity. The degree of abnormality of neutrophil function in these conditions appears to relate directly to the incidence and severity of life-threatening infections. In some surgical patients, sepsis appears to be related to physiological abnormalities of neutrophil function that may be accentuated by certain conditions, such as the administration of adrenocortical steroids and continued stress. Corticosteroids are believed to enter the bilayer of macrophages, thereby stiffening the membrane. Not only does this reduce their phagocytic capability but also prevents the macrophages from being activated by C3A and C5A. Thus, lysozomal enzymes and peroxides, which play a role in injury of various tissues, are not released in the usual way. A first-rate example of the latter is the amelioration of adult respiratory distress syndrome (ARDS) by steroids. However, it must be borne in mind that the beneficial effects of such steroids may be far outweighed by the accompanying reduction in bacterial killing and the danger of widespread infection. Nutritional depletion, particularly that of protein, appears to play a decisive role in some of these acquired defects. The role of the reticuloendothelial system is less clear in the early protective response to infection, but it is of major importance in the clearance of bacteria from the bloodstream and the removal of blood-borne toxins.

Abnormalities of Opsonins.   Patients with genetic inability to synthesize complement components or specific antibody are uncommonly encountered in surgical practice, but surgeons should be aware of these conditions. Several acquired defects in the complement system have recently been described that have been associated with injury. One of these, which occurs following burn injury, appears to result from activation of C3 by damaged tissue or necrotizing infection. This may produce complement degradation products that inhibit cellular function. Recently, it has been clearly demonstrated by Heideman, and associates that bacteria, necrotic tissue, and even endotoxin can activate the complement cascade through the alternative pathway. In severe sepsis, complement components from C3 onward are consumed, resulting in low blood concentrations. When C3, C5, and C4 were reduced below 50% of normal for more than 1 week, 95% of the patients became bacteremic with a high mortality. Drainage of abscesses or removal of gangrenous tissue usually resulted in a restoration of complement concentrations toward normal with clinical improvement. Antibody is an essential component in preparing bacteria for phagocytosis and initiating the complement sequence. Resistance to specific types of infections may be increased by specific immunization, and the absence of antibody for a specific organism may increase the organism's potential for invasiveness. Conversely, the administration of hyperimmune gamma globulin may be beneficial in the treatment of certain systemic infections. However, in surgical patients, the deficiency of opsonic proteins in itself is rarely a predisposing cause of septic complications.

SYSTEMIC INJURY IN SEPSIS: ALTERED FUNCTION AND RESPONSES OF ORGAN SYSTEMS

At least four mechanisms exist by which invading bacteria may adversely affect distant organs throughout the body:

1. Bacteremia or septic emboli may lead to invasion by "seeding" and abscess formation in remote tissues. This may occur particularly in liver, lung, kidney, bone, brain, and injured areas.
2. Endotoxins or exotoxins produced by certain bacteria may affect cellular function directly. For example, endotoxin injures hepatocytes sufficiently so that they are unable to continue the process of converting lactate and amino acids to glucose. The result of an endotoxin infusion in experimental animals is that within 12 to 18 hours progressive hypoglycemia occurs.
3. Local necrosis at the site of infection results in the release of proteolytic enzymes from the lysosomes of destroyed cells; these enzymes are capable of breaking down proteins to form toxic peptides and other products. Additionally, both endotoxin and the peptidases from injured tissues can activate a variety of circulating vasoactive peptides; induce intravascular clotting and plasmin activity, or cause platelet aggregation and release; affect both systemic and pulmonary vascular resistance; alter membrane function; and change energy metabolism.
4. Disseminated intravascular coagulation (DIC) may also occur, resulting in an accumulation of fibrin-split products and a consumption of platelets. In the blood, another series of powerful vasoactive substances, the kinins, may also be activated. It has been found in studies by Attar and associates that kinins are present in the blood of septic patients. Studies by Colman and O'Donnell suggest that peptidases, whether activated by endotoxin or tissue injury secondary to infection, may act as mediators of many reactions.

Autonomic Nervous System, Hormones, and Other Circulating Mediators

The dynamic balance between forces of injury and responses leading to survival with recovery of the septic patient occurs through a complex series of physiological and biochemical events. The reactions of various systems are controlled in part by the autonomic nervous system, by hormones, and by circulating peptides derived principally from elements of the immunological – inflammatory system. In almost all respects the neuroendocrine function during sepsis is similar to that observed in other stressful situations, such as severe exercise, hypoxia, hypovolemia, hypotension, trauma, or pain. In general, secretion and blood concentrations of the following hormones are elevated above normal: insulin, glucagon, growth hormone, the corticosteroids, aldosterone, antidiuretic hormone, and the catecholamines. However, in the presence of hypoxia or low cardiac output, which stimulate catecholamine release, blood insulin falls to low levels because of adrenalin suppression of pancreatic beta cell degranulation.

A variety of physiological and metabolic responses are mediated by peptides and prostaglandins released into the bloodstream from macrophages, platelets, and other elements of the immunological system associated with sites of inflammation or injury. In addition to the classical antigen – antibody activation of complement, bacteria, necrotic tissue, and endotoxin are all capable of activating the complement cascade through the alternate pathway. C3A and C5A, short-lived fragments of C3 and C5, stimulate both platelets and macrophages. The aggregated platelets accumulate in the lung and other tissues. There, they release a series of vasoactive and vasodepressive substances, notably prostaglandins E2 and F2a, as well as thromboxane and prostacyclin. Normally, thromboxane produced by platelets, which is vasoconstrictive in action, is opposed in its action by prostacyclin produced by vascular endothelium. On the other hand, this mechanism may be overwhelmed in the presence of a very large production of thromboxane, which may then be released into the circulation. The prostacyclin has a greater half-life, and when released into the circulation, may produce a series of vasodepressive effects that include reduction of peripheral resistance and venous return, and probably myocardial depression. Other vasoactive factors released by platelets include serotonin, adenosine diphosphate (ADP), adenosine triphosphate (ATP), and histamine in humans. At first glance, it would appear that treatment with aspirin or other drugs that reduce prostaglandin synthesis by inhibition of cyclooxygenase activity might be useful. Except in limited circumstances, such as management of pulmonary embolism and the prevention of thrombosis, this practice is not favored at present because of bleeding and other untoward reactions.

The macrophages and circulating granulocytes are also stimulated by activated complement. When antigen – antibody complexes are present, this activity leads to phagocytosis. But in the absence of phagocytosis this group of macrophages may be stimulated to release superoxides and lysozomal proteolytic enzymes. These potent agents may well injure otherwise normal tissue such as the lung, the liver, the kidney, or possibly even the myocardium. Endogenous pyrogen (EP; otherwise known as "interleuken" or "leucocyte endogenous mediator") secreted by activated macrophages induces fever and also promotes synthesis of the acute reactive proteins in the liver. The macrophages also probably produce the circulating small glycopeptide (molecular weight 4200) described by Clowes that induces degradation of muscle protein and the release of amino acids for protein synthesis in the wound and visceral tissues.

Circulatory Function

Patients who do well and recover from sepsis are apt to have low peripheral vascular resistances and high cardiac outputs. Cardiac indices of 3.5 to 6 are not unusual (Table 5 – 1). In addition to increased circulatory demand occasioned by extra work of breathing and an elevated metabolic rate (usually 30% to 40% above normal), the vascular resistance is low and blood flow is accelerated in otherwise nonaffected tissues, particularly muscle.

Several explanations for the apparent general vasodilation and low resistance have been advanced. Microanatomic shunts probably open up in the mesentery. Certainly, arteriovenous connections exist in the skin and are usually open when required for body cooling to maintain a given body temperature. This is true except

Table 5-1.   Comparison of Uneventful Surgical Convalescence with Survival or Death from Sepsis (Average + Standard Deviation or Range)

	Uneventful Convalescence (30 Patients)		Septic Survivors (37 Patients)
	Maximal Response	Conva- lescence	Onset Day 1
Hemodynamic			
Cardiac index (liters/min/M²)	3.6 ± 0.3	3.2 ± 0.2	3.0 ± 1.9
CVP	5.0 ± 2.0	3.0 ± 3.0	2.0 ± 5.0
Arterial BP mean	86 ± 12	88 ± 10	73 ± 16
Central venous pressure	5 ± 3	5 ± 3	8 ± 4
Pulmonary arterial mean pressure	19 ± 3	17 ± 4	23 ± 4
Left atrial (wedge) pressure	8 ± 3	8 ± 3	10 ± 4
Respiration			
Arterial PO₂ breathing 40% O₂	76 ± 8	105 ± 6	72 ± 15
Arterial PCO₂	36 ± 6	38 ± 4	30 ± 8
Metabolism			
Metabolic rate (Cal/M²/24 hrs)	980 ± 210	928 ± 146	
Body temperature (°F PR)	100.6 ± 1.2	100.6 ± 0.8	101.4 ± 1.5
Arterial blood pH	7.36 ± .03	7.42 ± .05	7.39 ± .06
Buffer base (mEq/liter)	−2 ± 5	−1 ± 4	−4 ± 3
Excess lactate (mM/liter)	1.4 ± 1.2	0.5 ± 0.2	1.9 ± 0.6

when fever is rising. Circulating vasodilator substances have been demonstrated. Prostaglandins and possibly certain peptides from the site of tissue injury, or even the toxins of certain bacteria such as the clostridia are known to reduce vascular resistance. There is also ample evidence of the increased production of metabolites, which are vasodilators. A change in muscle metabolism occurs during sepsis. Abnormally large quantities of lactate are produced from the glucose taken up, even in the presence of adequate oxygen delivery. It has been suggested that oxygen delivery is impaired due to reduced 2, 3 diphosphoglycerate in erythrocytes or to tissue edema. Oxygen consumption, measured as the product of cardiac index times arterial-mixed venous difference, is proportional to the metabolic rate in those patients who are in the usual "hyperdynamic state." Under these conditions, lack of

Septic Survivors (37 Patients)		Septic Deaths (21 Deaths)		
Maximal Response	Conva- lescence	Onset Day 1	Maximal Response	Premortem (1 Day)
4.7 ± 1.6	4.1 ± 1.0	3.1 ± 2.2	4.9 ± 1.0	2.3 ± 1.3
7.0 ± 4.0	5.0 ± 3.0	4.0 ± 5.0	12 ± 6.0	17 ± 6.0
88 ± 15	91 ± 12	59 ± 21	87 ± 17	58 ± 24
10 ± 5	10 ± 3	6 ± 5	14 ± 3	16 ± 6
28 ± 5	20 ± 1	24 ± 5	32 ± 5	26 ± 6
14 ± 4	9 ± 4	11 ± 6	17 ± 2	16 ± 3
71 ± 13	94 ± 9	68 ± 16	61 ± 14	58 ± 16
27 ± 7	33 ± 4	28 ± 5	26 ± 10	43 ± 9
1206 ± 221	1141 ± 151		1271 ± 245	1186 ± 178
101.8 ± 1.8	100.3 ± 1.1	101.3 ± 1.7	102 ± 1.6	99 ± 2.3
7.48 ± .06	7.45 ± .04	7.39 ± .08	7.44 ± .11	7.21 ± .10
−2 ± 3	−1 ± 4	−5 ± 5	−7 ± 5	−11 ± 4
1.5 ± 0.7	0.7 ± 0.3	2.0 ± 0.8	2.2 ± 1.6	3.1 ± 1.6

oxygen availability does not appear to be a cause for vasodilation or lactate production except when cardiac output is low (see Metabolic Alterations).

On the other hand, a state of septic shock exists when the cardiovascular system is unable to satisfy the elevated circulatory demand. Thus, a patient with a low or even a normal resting cardiac index may be in shock. As in any other low cardiac output state, there is an intense response of the sympathoadrenal system. Epinephrine and norepinephrine are secreted. The cardiac function increases in response to beta adrenergic stimulation, and vasoconstriction is caused by alpha adrenergic stimulation. The patient appears gray or even mottled. In addition to the increased demand for circulation, there appear to be at least three principal causes of septic shock: (1) hypovolemia due to translocation of fluid into edema spaces; (2) an increase in pulmonary vascular resistance in the presence of hypoxia due to pulmonary shunting, which may cause right heart failure; (3) myocardial depression. These phenomena are all illustrated by the data in Table 5 – 1.

Hypovolemia is usually manifested by reduced central venous and left atrial (wedge) pressures. Intravenous fluid infusion is the readily apparent form of treatment, but there is very real danger of overtreating with too much fluid, which can increase pulmonary edema and raise the left atrial pressure to too great an extent. The problem of elevated pulmonary vascular resistance is dealt with below; the treatment is respirator support. Myocardial depression is evident when the usual response to an elevation of left atrial pressure fails to cause a greater cardiac output. Hechtman and his colleagues constructed clinical starling curves in septic patients. Left atrial pressure was raised progressively by infusions of 25% salt-poor albumin. The cardiac index rose in certain septic patients to a lesser extent than might be expected as the wedge pressure increased. Often a peak was reached at 14 to 15 cm H_2O. Beyond that point, cardiac index and stroke work decreased, giving evidence of left heart failure. The treatment of this condition is to keep the left atrial pressure at the level of maximum output and to infuse beta adrenergic agents such as low-dose dopamine. Shoemaker and Siegel as well as other investigators have demonstrated a close correlation between death and a reduction of oxygen consumption due either to low flow or to failure of tissues to take up oxygen.

Respiratory Responses

Gas exchange in septic patients (uptake of oxygen and excretion of carbon dioxide) is seldom greater than 50% above the normal resting value. This modest elevation of ventilatory requirement would pose no problem if it were not for the untoward pulmonary complications that are prone to occur under these conditions. In recent years, a syndrome characterized by hypoxemia, interstitial edema, and reduced compliance of the lung has been recognized, because its association with wounds and the attendant shock in casualties of the Vietnam War, the term "shock lung" was applied. However, various authors have demonstrated a much greater association with sepsis (approximately 90%) or tissue trauma (approximately 62%) located anywhere in the body. More appropriately, this clinical pattern is now referred to as "adult respiratory distress syndrome" (ARDS).

ARDS passes through three distinct clinical and pathologic phases unless progress is arrested by healing and appropriate therapy:

Phase I (interstitial edema). Twelve to 24 hours after the onset of sepsis, hypoxemia, often with a mild degree of respiratory alkalosis, is accompanied by a relatively clear chest roentgenogram which at most may show evidence of pulmonary edema. These changes are illustrated by the data in Table 5–1 under the "onset Day 1" of septic patients. They represent a combination of pulmonary shunting with adequate ventilation. Subsequently, compliance is reduced as edema increases, recognizable by the necessity of greater peak inspiratory pressure to maintain ventilation. Pulmonary vascular resistance tends to rise as shunting increases. Lung biopsies from such patients and from experimental animals disclose interstitial edema of alveolar septa, margination of leucocytes with macrophage infiltration, and numerous but non-confluent collapsed alveoli. The lesion is associated with circulating agents capable of inducing increased capillary permeability and edema in a perfused normal animal lung. Evidence is accumulating that the agents are associated with stimulation of macrophages and platelets by activated complement to release agents that damage vascular endothelium. Surfactant production by type II alveolar macrophages is also reduced, in part accounting for the diffuse alveolar collapse. As pointed out by Teplitz, these abnormalities all represent the pulmonary inflammatory response to any noxious stimulus.

Phase II (bronchopneumonia and atelectasis). As the pulmonary dysfunction increases, pulmonary infection supervenes. The roentgenogram reveals the picture of bronchopneumonia or collapse of one or more segments or lobes of the lung. The shunt becomes worse, manifested by increased hypoxemia, often accompanied by some degree of CO_2 retention, which is evidence of impaired ventilation. Powers and his associates demonstrated that the degree of pulmonary shunting was inversely proportional to the functional residual capacity (FRC). Pulmonary vascular resistance increases further, and compliance decreases to an even greater extent. The work of breathing becomes so great that a respirator often is a necessity to maintain ventilation and gas exchange. Histological examination at this stage shows large areas of consolidation with fluid and polymorphonuclear leucocytes in both the alveoli and the interstitial spaces. Bacteria are visible and culturable, which they are not in Phase I. In advanced stages of bronchopneumonia, shunts of 30% or more are not uncommon (normal: 3% to 6%), as illustrated in Figure 5–2, when the PaO_2 was only 60 mm Hg while the patient received 40% oxygen. PaO_2 rose to only 120 mm Hg when breathing 100% oxygen. At low cardiac outputs, when the lung lesion limits oxygenating capacity, increased oxygen extraction and low mixed venous PO_2 values increase the A–a PO_2 gradient. Thus, both the degree of shunt and the cardiac output are of importance in determining the PaO_2.

Phase III (pulmonary fibrosis). If Phase II persists for a prolonged period of several weeks, requiring continuous respiratory support, the interstitial fibrin becomes organized to fibrous tissue as collagen is deposited. The lung remains poorly compliant, the work of breathing is great, and it may become impossible to wean the patient from the respirator. This is end-stage pulmonary failure accompanied by high pulmonary vascular resistance. Cor pulmonale may develop.

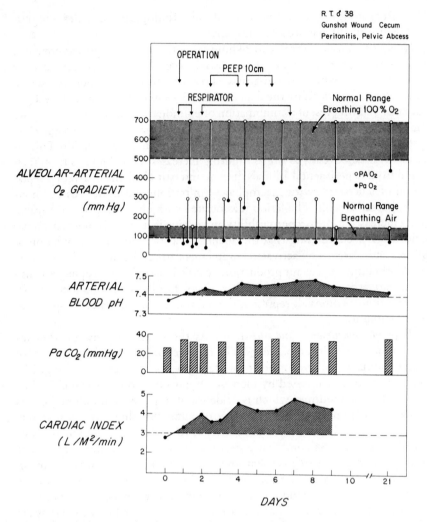

Fig. 5-2. Progressive development of pulmonary shunting in a patient with generalized peritonitis secondary to a neglected bullet wound of the cecum, sustained one day before admission. Note the progressive alveolar–arterial oxygen tension gradient on various respiratory gas mixtures (FIO$_2$: 0.4, and 0.2). Also illustrated are the beneficial effects of PEEP to supplement respiratory support with a volume ventilator in reestablishing a normal ventilatory perfusion ratio. (Clowes GHA Jr: Unpublished record)

Treatment is in great measure dependent upon respiratory support with a well-adjusted volume-rate controlled respirator operating through a cuffed endotracheal tube. Every effort must be made to maintain the respirator as sterile as possible. In general, the carbon dioxide tension of the arterial blood is regulated by ventilation (tidal volume × rate) and the arterial oxygen tension is dependent on the concentration of oxygen in the respiratory gas mixture. Considerable pressures must be employed, at times up to values as high as 60 cm H_2O, in order to effect adequate gas exchange. In the presence of severe shunting (hypoxemia with large alveolar–arterial gradients), positive end expiratory pressure (PEEP) will be required. Two beneficial effects of the respirator may then be obtained: (1) collapsed alveoli may be expanded to reduce shunting as FRC is increased, as shown in Figure 5–2, and (2) the work of ventilation may be reduced. However, it is important to remember that PEEP in excess of 15 cm H_2O may result in reduced cardiac output because of impairment of venous return and an increase of pulmonary capillary resistance in overdistended alveoli. It is also probable that circulating agents (possibly prostaglandins) released from overstretched alveoli may be vasodepressant, and reduce both venous return and myocardial function. Circulatory function must be monitored carefully when PEEP is employed. The important point is oxygen delivery to tissues. If there is a modest increase of arterial oxygen content, but cardiac output is severely depressed, a net loss of oxygen availability occurs.

An important aspect of dealing with this life-threatening pulmonary complication is its prevention, when possible. This is accomplished in two ways. The first is to remove the source of sepsis at the earliest opportunity by incision and drainage or excision. The second is to employ a respirator prophylactically for one or more days after an operation in which a septic situation, such as perforated gut, figures prominently. By so doing, alveoli are less likely to collapse and the metabolism of all parts of the lung are better maintained. Secretions can be easily removed. However, a respirator has serious disadvantages as well, including possible introduction of contamination and infection and progressive weakening of the respiratory muscles. Therefore, it should be discontinued as soon as possible when the patient can maintain adequate spontaneous ventilation.

Water, Electrolytes, and Renal Function

Invasive sepsis is commonly accompanied by hypovolemia due to edema or third space formation at the site of inflammation. In addition, an increase of capillary permeability is apt to occur in noninvolved tissues, particularly lung, subcutaneous, and skeletal muscle. Such translocation of fluid from plasma to the extravascular space tends to accentuate fluid and electrolyte shifts between body compartments. Moore, Randall, and their colleagues have estimated the alterations of fluid compartments found in the presence of invasive sepsis. By comparison with predicted normal values, the extracellular water (ECW) may rise to 130% or more. This change is, in part, at the expense of intracellular water (ICW), which may decrease to 90% of normal and much more as the lean body mass is depleted by septic starvation. Serum sodium concentration may decline to values ranging from 120 to 130 mEq/liter. Potassium derived from the declining cellular mass will be excreted to prevent hyperkalemia, unless renal failure supervenes. Conversely, respiratory alkalosis may be accompanied by low serum K, which should be prevented or treated vigorously in patients receiving digitalis therapy.

In a young, normally responsive patient, a reduction of blood volume to 20%

below normal will result in a reduction of venous return and cardiac output to the extent that the sympathoadrenal system can no longer preserve blood pressure. Catecholamine secretion is grossly accelarated. Hypotension with vasoconstriction of both veins and arteries occurs. In general, renal function appears to be closely related to the state of the circulation. Oliguria occurs with hypotension, due either to reduced blood volume or to a primary low cardiac output. Vasoconstriction is reflected in the reduced glomerular perfusion and urine production, a situation observed in other forms of hypovolemic low output shock. Usually, prompt restoration of circulating fluid volume by the administration of saline solution results in an elevation of cardiac output sufficient to satisfy the high circulatory demand. An increased urinary output usually follows.

Renal function is important not only for the maintenance of body water volume and electrolyte concentrations but also for excretion of waste products. Although earlier studies suggested that renal plasma flow depression was a sensitive and reliable index of kidney damage in sepsis, recent experiments by Hermreck and Thal and by Rector and associates have indicated that despite an apparent reduction of glomerular flow and filtration, true renal plasma flow is elevated in the septic state. The latter investigators found that despite the reduction of glomerular filtration rate (GFR) to 80% and clearance of para-aminohippuric acid (PAH) to 73%, the average total renal blood flow amounted to 171% of the expected normal and accounted for 21% of the total cardiac output in these patients. Thus, it appears that the kidney may share the hyperdynamic circulatory state and may not have a reduced blood flow in the critically ill septic patient, as has long been assumed from studies in other forms of shock in which vascular resistance is high.

Thus, the changes in renal function during sepsis are, in general, manifestations of renal adaption to the altered systemic circulation. In the high output or "hyperdynamic state," perfusion of the glomeruli and tubules may be normal. However, in septic shock, as in ordinary hypovolemic shock, a reduction of blood volume leads first to constriction of the efferent glomerular arterioles. GFR continues, but tubular reabsorption is grossly increased due to the low pressure and high osmotic values in the peritubular tissue. Subsequently, with increasing hypotension the afferent glomerular arterioles are constricted, with a profound reduction in GFR. Perfusion of the renal cortex is low whereas perfusion of the renal medulla increases. In fact, total renal blood flow may be increased under these conditions.

Energy and Protein Metabolism

Recovery from sepsis is ultimately dependent upon continued function and structure of vital organ systems as well as synthesis of proteins essential to immunocompetence and healing. Under these conditions, the regulation of energy fuel substrates and amino acid use differ in important ways from the patterns observed in normal fed and fasted people. In the septic state energy expenditure is elevated 25% to 50% above normal. Although fat still remains a major source of energy, protein contributes a somewhat greater proportion. Other metabolic alterations occur, including a higher rate of hepatic gluconeogenesis and lactate production by muscles. Muscle protein degradation proceeds at rates three to five times that of normal fasting. The increased supply of amino acids released from the periphery are delivered to the liver and other visceral tissues where they are employed in the synthesis of "the acute reactive proteins," the production of antibodies, wound healing, and the assembly of a host of other proteins that are scarcely present under normal conditions.

This entire pattern of metabolic events is under the control of the hormones, the same that regulate the metabolism in normal daily life. However, there are certain notable additions that cause modifications: largely, the peptides released at the site of injury or inflammation and the toxic agents derived from bacteria or from injured and necrotic tissue. The altered direction of fuel use and protein metabolism is greatly influenced by the state of sepsis, by the acute phase of shock (the so-called ebb phase), or in the more chronic state of adaption to the infection process (the so-called flow phase). Finally, the nutritional condition and the presence or absence of feeding also play major roles in establishing the metabolic state of affairs.

Energy Requirements.   The basal metabolic rate of a 70-kg man is about 1800 Cal/day (25.7 Cal/kg/day). Kinney and associates found that the resting metabolic expenditure (RME) of patients with intra-abdominal sepsis was 25% to 45% above normal. Long suggested that an additional increase of 20% should be added for activity. It was estimated that RME averaged 30.17 Cal/kg/day with a total daily need of 42 Cal/kg/day. This value is close to that found by a number of investigators as the caloric intake needed to produce a positive nitrogen balance when an adequate supply of amino acids is provided. Certain special situations exist in which caloric expenditure is greatly increased, as in extensive burns in which energy expenditure may be doubled. Extra calories will then be required, but there is no merit in providing a caloric excess that only results in excess fat deposit.

The general pathways by which body fuels are converted within the mitochondria to usable energy are presented in Figure 5–3. High-energy phosphate bonds are both the means for storing energy for immediate cellular use and the biological medium of energy exchange within the cell. All cellular functions requiring energy derive it from adenosine triphosphate (ATP). An an indicator of the tremendous energy exchange, the conversion of adenosine diphosphate (ADP) to ATP involves the transfer of 7700 Cal/mole during the process of oxidative phosphorylation. Oxygen is the hydrogen acceptor required for the ultimate oxidation of body fuels (carbohydrate, fat, and protein) to carbon dioxide and water. In the relative absence of oxygen, when PO_2 of tissue is below 10 mm Hg, only two ATP molar equivalents are produced by the anaerobic degradation of glucose to lactate, in contrast to the 36 equivalents produced in the full carboxylic acid cycle oxidation of pyruvate. Utilization of the energy released by oxidation depends upon integrity of the cytochrome system to complete the production of ATP. An example of how this process may be disturbed is reduction of ATP production resulting from damage to liver oxidative phosphorylation, as observed by Mela experimentally both *in vivo* and *in vitro* when hepatocytes were exposed to endotoxin.

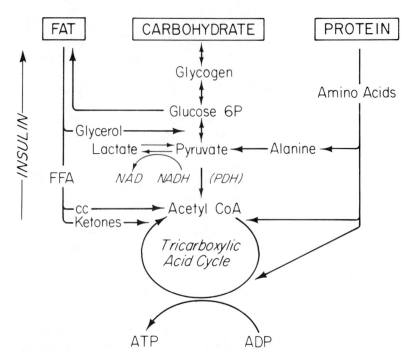

Fig. 5-3. Endogenous body fuel sources and their pathways of metabolism. It should be observed that insulin suppresses lipolysis and promotes the synthesis of protein and glycogen. On the other hand, glucagon stimulates glucogenesis by the liver and release of glucose into the circulation. Lipolysis and proteolysis are stimulated by catecholamines, which also suppress insulin secretion.

The available energy fuels stored in the body of a normal adult are approximately as follows:

Carbohydrate in the form of hepatic glycogen: 200 g (800 Cal)
Protein: 6 kg (24,000 Cal)
Fat: 15 kg (130,000 Cal)

Expressed as percentages of body weight, these values are carbohydrate 0.2%, protein 18%, and fat 20%. Of the protein, less than half is being actively turned over by proteolysis and resynthesis. By the time 50% of that portion of available protein is degraded to release amino acids, death has usually occurred. Thus, it is evident that the protein reserve that can be used for fuel purposes is very limited. Furthermore, the above values may be grossly reduced by inadequacy of preceding diet, by vitamin or mineral deficiency, or by other forms of depletion during illness.

Control of Energy Metabolism. Significant differences exist in the regulation of body fuel utilization in normal and septic states. In fasting, hepatic glycogen is quickly exhausted. As much as 75 g of protein are degraded daily at the outset of normal starvation to furnish amino acids for hepatic glucogenesis. This is the equivalent of 10 g to 15 g of nitrogen, excreted per day as urea. However, as blood glucose declines from normal values of 7mM/ml (125 mg%), so too does insulin secretion. At blood insulin concentration below 22 μU/ml, lipolysis is accelerated. Free fatty acid (FFA) oxidation increases proportionally as their concentration in the blood rises to more then 2 mM/liter. FFAs are oxidized directly by muscle. Hepatic beta oxidation of FFAs not only furnishes energy for the liver but also produces ketones, the concentrations of which also rise in the plasma. After a brief period of adaption, ketones become the preferred fuel of many tissues, including the central nervous system; the exceptions are the cells of the circulation. As the adaption occurs, fewer and fewer amino acids are mobilized, to the extent that nitrogen excretion declines to less than 5 g/day (the equivalent of about 30 g of protein).

In septic states fat still remains the major fuel. However, Duke and associates found that the proportion of energy supplied by protein in patients with peritonitis, as reflected by urea excretion, was greater than normal, Although it seldom exceeded 15% to 20% of the total. By contrast, with the normal state adaptation does not occur and nitrogen loss continues. The usual daily urinary 15-g to 25-g nitrogen excretion (80%–85% urea) is the equivalent of 75 g to 150 g of protein. At that rate it is possible quickly to exhaust the protein reserve.

Various explanations have been offered for this paradoxical wastage of the valuable and limited protein store. It is clear from the work of Kinney, Gump, Long, and their colleagues that an infusion of glucose does not inhibit hepatic ureagenesis and gluconeogenesis. It is more probable that deamination and oxidation of amino acids continues to be essential for clearance of excess amino acids, mobilized in response to other stimuli. The result of gluconeogenesis from lactate and amino acids is shown in Table 5–2. Even in fasted states blood glucose concentrations tend to be high, accompanied by insulin concentrations in excess of 30 μU/ml. Despite this moderate hyperglycemia and hyperinsulinemia, oxidation of glucose in muscles does not increase above normal. In part this lack of response to insulin and glucose intolerance has been referred to as the "pseudodiabetes" of sepsis. In contrast with muscle, adipose tissue responds to insulin in septic patients by an increased glucose oxidation and reduced lipolysis. A significant proportion of excess glucose is converted to fat in the liver.

Hormones.   Insulin, referred to by Cahill as the "overall fuel control in mammals," regulates energy metabolism by increasing the rate of glucose utilization and controlling the rate of free fatty acid release. Insulin promotes energy storage by conversion of glucose to glycogen and fat. The plasma free fatty acids are either oxidized (minimum 20% to 30% of FFA production) or are re-esterified to triacylglycerides in adipose tissue. The rate of turnover is proportional to the concentrations of plasma FFA and insulin. Insulin also induces synthesis of proteins in muscle, liver, and other tissues. In sepsis, insulin is prone to exceed 25 to 30 μU/ml.

In the high output hyperdynamic state of sepsis, the blood concentration of glucose is also moderately elevated, and in response, so too is insulin, as shown in

Table 5-2.   Concentrations of Oxygen, Substrates, and Metabolites (Value ± Se)

	Normal Resting (Overnight Fast)	Septic (6-Hr Fast)
Oxygen (ml % blood)	15.1 ± 1.3	13.8 ± 1.8
Glucose (μM/liter arterial plasma)	4510 ± 390	7883 ± 968
Lactate (μM/liter arterial plasma)	690 ± 120	1180 ± 246
Free fatty acid (μEq/liter arterial plasma)	1021 ± 91	513 ± 96
Ketones (μM/liter arterial plasma)	634 ± 128	163 ± 141
Amino acids (μM/liter arterial plasma)	2656 ± 225	1772 ± 239
Insulin (U/ml)	22 ± 4	36 ± 6

(Clowes et al: Amino acid and energy metabolism in septic and traumatized patients. JPEN 4(2):195, 1980)

Table 5–2. Free fatty acid and ketone concentrations tend to be reduced. Amino acids are released from peripheral tissues, particularly from muscles at rates three to five times those of normal fasting. Glucagon secretion by the pancreatic alpha cells is stimulated, and plasma concentrations ranging from 200 to 600 μU/ml are found in septic patients, in contrast with normal values ranging from 50 to 125 μU/ml. The principal effects of glucagon are glycogenolysis and the induction of hepatic gluconeogenesis. There is little evidence that glucagon stimulates muscle protein degradation. Growth hormone and glucocorticoids, both of which are antagonistic to the action of insulin, are also secreted in greater quantities. Glucocorticoids, when injected into animals to produce blood concentrations similar to those found under stress conditions, result in an increased proteolysis of muscle tissue as reflected by 3-methyl-histidine excretion. However, a far stronger stimulus to an elevation of net degradation of muscle protein appears to be the proteolysis-inducing factor described by Clowes. The muscle metabolism is altered so that there is both an increase of muscle glucose uptake and a proportionally greater production of lactate with virtually no elevation of glucose oxidation. This finding indicates a depression of pyruvate dehydrogenase activity, which occurs as the oxidation of leucine increases, a situation similar to the inhibition of glucose oxidation by free fatty acids.

The metabolic events in the septic surgical patient are modified as well by other hormones, which are secreted in different proportions, based in part upon the state of the circulation and respiration. In the presence of shock or severe hypoxemia the catecholamines are high. Insulin secretion is reduced by catecholamine suppression of beta cell degranulation. Catecholamines also promote calorigenesis, lipolysis, and glycogenolysis. Thus, under conditions of hypotension, FFA, glucose, and amino acids are all mobilized and blood levels are high. It was in order to restore blood insulin to more effective levels that the administration of glucose, potassium, and

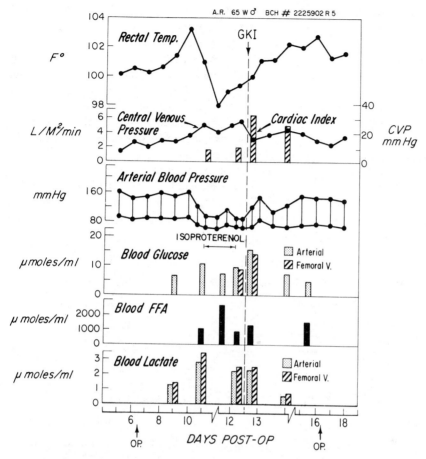

Fig. 5-4. The course of a patient with pelvic cellulitis after iliac endarterectomy secondary to reexploration and an infected hematoma. On the 10th day, the patient went into a state of "septic shock" with a cardiac index of 1.8 L/M² per minute and hypotension. Although isoproterenol failed to correct the circulatory insufficiency, a dramatic response occurred after the infusion of glucose, potassium, and insulin. Bearing in mind that serum insulin is apt to be high with high cardiac output and low with low output shock, this case also illustrates the behavior of blood glucose, FFA, and lactate in high and low output states. A pelvic abscess was drained on the sixteenth day, followed by ultimate recovery. (Clowes GHA Jr, O'Donnell TF Jr, Ryan NT, Blackburn, GL: Energy metabolism in sepsis: Treatment based on different patterns in shock and high output state. Ann Surg 179:684, 1974)

insulin was proposed as a means of treating septic shock. An example of its successful application is presented in Figure 5–4.

Changes in Amino Acid Metabolism. Protein and amino acid metabolism in septic patients also differs in important respects from the normal pattern. Some years ago Lust demonstrated experimentally that, in normal starvation, amino acids are mobilized as needed for gluconeogenesis from visceral tissues. The muscle mass is protected. By contrast, in sepsis or stress the muscle protein is degraded to a far greater extent for delivery of amino acids to visceral tissues for protein synthesis. Recently, this finding has been confirmed experimentally by Ryan and Lindberg, and clinically by Beisel, Clowes, and Rosenblatt. All of these investigators have found acceleration of visceral amino acid uptake. This is illustrated by data in Table 5–2; you will note that amino acid concentrations are lower than normal whereas visceral clearance or uptake is accelerated despite an accelerated rate of muscle amino acid release. The liver becomes greater in size as its protein structure increases; the same is true of other actively metabolizing organs.

The net degradation of muscle protein and release of amino acids from the peripheral tissues in fasted septic patients is elevated three to five times above that observed in normal fasted people. The principal stimulus to an acceleration of muscle protein degradation appears to be a circulating glycopeptide derived from stimulated macrophages. Although a portion of these amino acids is being oxidized,

Fig. 5-5. Control of protein metabolism in sepsis.

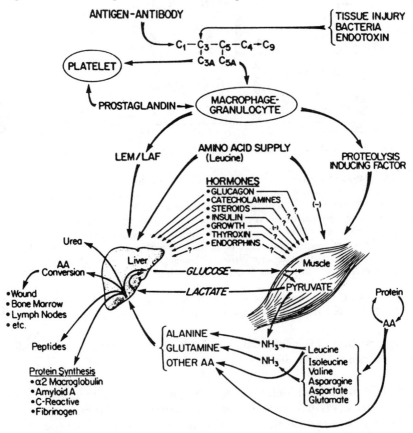

a far greater quantity of available amino acids is being transferred to the liver and other visceral tissues for synthesis of proteins essential to survival and recovery. This process is illustrated in Figure 5–5. Insulin, with the permissive action of corticosteroids, stimulates protein synthesis in the liver. However, the greatest stimulus to the acute hepatic response is Interleuken I (endogenous pyrogen, LEM). This agent, apparently from macrophages, has been described by Dinarello and Powanda. The hepatic production of the so-called acute reactive proteins (fibrinogen, alpha-2 macroglobulin, amyloid A, complement, and others) rises dramatically. Some of these proteins are protective against tissue injury by the patient's own immune system; others are defensive in nature. Certain amino acids are converted to other amino acids in the liver to be used elsewhere for synthesis of antibodies, proliferation of leukocytes and their enzymes, healing the wound, and so forth. Amino acids which remain in excess are deaminated, oxidized, or converted to glucose; otherwise, toxic concentrations of various amino acids would occur. In all probability this is the best explanation for the continued protein wastage of sepsis and the nonsuppressibility of gluconeogenesis.

It is evident, then, that in sepsis the liver plays a central role in amino acid metabolism in four ways:

1. Protein synthesis
2. Peptide synthesis
3. Conversion of amino acids
4. Deamination of amino acids and urea synthesis for oxidation or gluconeogenesis

Apparent liver failure is not uncommon in septic states, especially with intra-abdominal infection. The large bowel is a source of endotoxin, as are intraperitoneal abscesses. As previously mentioned, endotoxin may injure hepatocytes directly, or the combination of bacteria, dead tissue, and endotoxin may activate complement to stimulate the production of cytotoxic agents by macrophages, of which there are a great number in the liver. Cholestatic jaundice may occur 3 to 6 days after the onset of sepsis. Thus, it becomes important to measure the hepatocyte function to determine how effectively amino acids may be employed by the hepatocytes for the production of acute reactive proteins, complement, and other proteins essential to survival of hepatocytes and their organelles. Attempts to assess the ability of the visceral tissues to employ amino acids under these conditions by measuring plasma amino acid concentrations have met with some success. Cerra and his colleagues related death to the accumulation of amino acids that failed to enter the tricarboxylic acid cycle at the usual point. However, this took no account of protein synthesis. Clowes and Rosenblatt have demonstrated that the "central fractional clearance rate" of amino acids by visceral tissues is a very sensitive index of liver function. Failure to clear amino acids, especially the aromatic and sulfur-containing amino acids, accurately predicts loss of hepatocyte activity and is an indicator of impending death. Essentially, this value is the rate of clearance divided by the extracellular pool size of any given amino acids. Frequently, it has been found that liver function is much better than anticipated by physical signs or standard measurements, making it possible to resume parenteral alimentation.

The importance to survival from sepsis of energy metabolism and the supply of amino acids utilized by the liver and other visceral tissues is illustrated by the following examples:

1. Meakins, Christou, and their associates have demonstrated a relationship between protein malnutrition and loss of tissue immunity and granulocyte function.
2. Anergy is associated with reduced neutrophil adherence and chemotaxis.
3. Fibronectin synthesized by vascular endothelium may be depleted by DIC or other causes, with reduced phagocytosis and bacterial clearance.
4. When complement falls below 50% of normal due to consumption, bacteremia often follows.

These examples demonstrate that proteins important to defense against bacteria may be consumed in excess of production with possible lethal effects. Energy supply is closely related, since the majority of activities of living tissue, including protein synthesis, are energy dependent. Chaudry has demonstrated in rats a relationship of hepatic ATP reduction to inadequate macrophage function and bacterial clearance rates in the late stage of sepsis. Failure of either energy or protein metabolism is folowed by multisystem failure, overwhelming infection, and death.

NUTRITIONAL SUPPORT BY ENTERIC AND PARENTERAL ALIMENTATION

Sepsis combined with starvation poses a series of life-threatening metabolic dilemmas, the most important of which are as follows:

- Caloric expenditure increases 30% to 50% above normal.
- Continued protein degradation and nitrogen loss occur at a rate 3 to 4 times that of the normal adapted starved state.
- There is depletion and deficiency of essential fatty acids, minerals, and vitamins.
- Reduction of oxygen consumption by certain tissues occurs, along with loss of ability to oxidize energy fuel substrates for energy production.

Each of these can be prevented by adequate nutritional support, and some of them can be corrected in part, provided that tissue injury and death have not progressed to a point at which substrates and amino acids cannot be utilized. The first important point is that an early aggressive program of alimentation should be undertaken for any septic patient.

The basic requirements in the seriously ill patient to produce a balanced or slightly positive nitrogen balance are to supply a daily caloric intake that meets the total energy expenditure (approximately 42 Cal/kg/day) and to supply a mixture of amino acids equivalent to the daily loss of nitrogen (approximately 1.8 g of protein/kg/day). In addition, to preserve life and effect healing and recovery, essential fatty acids, trace minerals, and vitamins must be given. Aside from the volumes of intravenous fluids necessary, each of these requirements presents problems. Blackburn and Wolfe state, "Careful consideration is required to avoid abuse of this therapy through biochemical 'maneuveurs' that provide energy fuel substrates in a way that prevents their optimal use, and proper consideration of physiological and biochemical mechanisms is required."

The administration of amino acids is essential to supply the requirements for visceral and structural protein synthesis. With adequate caloric and amino acid supply, the breakdown of muscle protein and the peripheral release of amino acids can be markedly reduced. The problem lies in supplying the correct proportion of all amino acids needed for oxidation and protein synthesis. For example, leucine (one of the three branch-chain amino acids) becomes the preferred fuel in many tissues during sepsis. It is also needed for synthesis. However, in high concentrations it also has the ability to suppress muscle proteolysis. But, if it is given without adequate quantities of other essential amino acids, the liver and visceral tissues will be deprived of amino acids needed for synthesis.

BIBLIOGRAPHY

ALBRECHT M, CLOWES GHA JR: The increase of circulatory requirements in the presence of inflammation. Surgery 56:158, 1964

ALEXANDER JW, GOOD RA: Fundamentals of Clinical Immunology. Philadelphia, WB Saunders, 1977

ALEXANDER JW, MEAKINS JL: A physiological basis for the development of opportunistic infections. Ann Surg 176:273, 1972

ALEXANDER JW, STINNETT JD, OGLE CK, OGLE JD, MORRIS MJ: A comparison of immunologic profiles and their influence on bacteremia in surgical patients with a high risk of infection. Surgery 86:94–104, 1979

ALTEMEIER WA: Bodily response to infectious agents. JAMA 202:1085, 1967

ALTEMEIER WA, ALEXANDER JW: Surgical infections and choice of antibiotics. In Sabiston DC Jr (ed): Christopher's Textbook of Surgery, 11th ed, pp 340-362. Philadelphia, WB Saunders, 1977

ATTAR SMA, TINGEY HB, McLAUGHLIN JS, COWLEY RA: Bradykinin in human shock. Surg Forum 18:46, 1967

BEISEL WR: Magnitude of the host nutritional responses to infection. Am J Clin Nutr 30:1236-1247, 1977

BLACKBURN GL, BISTRIAN BR: Nutritional care of the injured and/or septic patient. Surg Clin North Am 56(5):1195, 1976

BLACKBURN GL, FLATT JP, CLOWES GHA JR, O'DONNEL TF, HENSLE TE: Protein sparing therapy during periods of starvation with sepsis or trauma. Ann Surg 177:588, 1973

BLACKBURN GL, WOLFE RR: Clinical biochemistry and intravenous hyperalimentation. In Recent Advances in Clinical Biochemistry, pp 197-228.

BLAISDELL FW, LIM RC, STALLONE RJ: The mechanism of pulmonary damage following traumatic shock. Surg Gynecol Obstet 130:15, 1970

BURKE JF, WOLFE RR, MULLANY CJ, MATHEWS DE, BIER DM: Glucose requirements following burn injury: Parameters of optimal glucose infusion and possible hepatic and respiratory abnormalities following excessive glucose intake. Ann Surg 190(3):274, 1979

CAHILL GF JR: Body fuels and their metabolism. Bull Am Coll Surg 55:12, 1970

CAHILL GF JR: Physiology of insulin in man. Diabetes 20:785-799, 1971

CERRA FB, SIEGAL JH, BORDER JR, et al: The hepatic failure of sepsis: Cellular versus substrate. Surgery 86:409-422, 1979

CERRA FB, SIEGAL JH, COLEMAN B, BORDER JR, McMENAMY RR: Septic autoconnibalism: A failure of exogenous nutritional support. Ann Surg 192(4):570-580, 1980

CHAUDRY IH, SCHLECK S, KOVACS KF, BAUE AE: Effect of prolonged starvation on reticuloendothelial function and survival following trauma. J Trauma 21(8):604, 1981

CHRISTOU NV, AND MEAKINS JL: Neutrophil function in anergic surgical patients: Neutrophil adherence and chemotaxis. Ann Surg 190(5):557-564, 1979

CLOWES GHA JR, GEORGE B, RYAN NT: Induction of accelerated proteolysis and amino acid release from skeletal muscle by a potent nonprotein factor in the plasma of septic patients. In McConn R (ed): Role of Chemical Mediators in the Pathophysiology of Acute Illness and Injury, pp 327-339. New York, Raven Press, 1982

CLOWES GHA JR, HEIDEMAN M, LINDBERG B, RANDALL HT, HIRSCH EF, CHUNG-JA C: Effects of parenteral alimentation on amino acid metabolism in septic patients. Surgery 88(4):531-43, 1980

CLOWES GHA JR, HIRSCH E, WILLIAMS L et al: Septic lung and shock lung in man. Ann Surg 181:681-692, 1975

CLOWES GHA JR, MARTIN H, WALJI S, HIRSCH E, GAZITUA R, GOODFELLOW R: Blood insulin responses to blood glucose levels in high output sepsis and septic shock. Am J Surg 135:577, 1978

CLOWES GHA JR, O'DONNELL TF, BLACKBURN GL, MAKI TN: Energy metabolism and proteolysis in traumatized and septic man. Symposium on Response to Infection and Injury. Surg Clin North Am 56:1169, 1976

CLOWES GHA JR, O'DONNELL TF JR, RYAN NT, BLACKBURN GL: Energy metabolism in sepsis: Treatment based on different patterns in shock and high output state. Ann Surg 179:684, 1974

CLOWES GHA JR, RANDALL HT, CHA CJ: Amino acid and energy metabolism in septic and traumatized patients. JPEN 4(2):195-205, 1980

CLOWES GHA JR, VUCINIC M, WEIDNER MG: Circulatory and metabolic alterations associated with survival or death in peritonitis: Clinical analysis of twenty-five cases. Ann Surg 163:6, 1966

COLEMAN RW, O'DONNELL TF, TALAMO RC, CLOWES GHA JR: Bradykinin formation in sepsis: Relation to hepatic dysfunction and hypotension. Clin Res 21:596, 1973

DINARELLO CA: Production of endogenous pyrogen. Fed Proc 38(1):52-56, 1979

DUKE JHR, JORGENSEN SB, BROELL JR, LONG CL, KINNEY JM: Contribution of protein to caloric expenditure following injury. Surgery 68:168, 1970

DUDRICK SJ, STEIGER E, LONG JM, RHOADS JE: Role of parenteral hyperalimentation in management of multiple catastrophic complications. Surg Clin North Am 50:1031, 1970

ELEK SK, CONEN PE: The virulence of *Staphylococcus pyogenes* for man: A study in the problems of wound infection. Br J Exp Pathol 38:573, 1957

FEARON DT, RUDDY S, SCHUR PH, MCCABE W: Activation of the properdin pathway of complement in patients with gram-negative bacteremia. N Engl J Med 292:937, 1975

FLECK A, MUNRO HK: Protein metabolism after injury. Metabolism 12:783, 1963

GOLDBERG AL, CHANG TW: Regulation and significance of amino acid metabolism in skeletal muscle. Fed Proc 37:2301, 1978

HAUSER WE JR, REMINGTON JS: Effect of antibiotics on the immune response. Am J Med 72(5):711-716, 1982

HECHTMAN HB: Adequate circulatory responses or cardiovascular failure. Surg Clin North Am 56(4):929, 1976

HEIDEMAN M: Complement activation *in vitro* By endotoxin and injured tissue. J Surg Res 26:670, 1979

HEIDEMAN M, SARAVIS CA, CLOWES GHA JR: Effects of nonviable tissue and abscesses on complement depletion and the development of bacteremia. J Trauma 22:527, 1982

HERMRECK AS, THAL AP: Mechanisms for the high circulatory requirements in sepsis and septic shock. Ann Surg 170:677, 1969

JONES CE, ALEXANDER JW, FISHER MW: Clinical evaluation of pseudomonas hyperimmune globulin. J Surg Res 14:87, 1973

KINNEY JM: Energy demands in the septic patient. In Hershey SG, DelGuercio LRM, McConn R (eds): Septic Shock in Man, Boston, Little, Brown & Co, 1971

KINNEY JM, ROE CF: The caloric equivalent of fever. I. Patterns of postoperative response. Ann Surg 156:610, 1962

LANSER ME, SABA TM: Opsonic fibronectin deficiency and sepsis: Cause or effect? Ann Surg 195(3):340, 1982

LEFER AM: Blood-borne humoral factors in the pathophysiology of circulatory shock. Circ Res 32:129, 1973

LINDBERG BO, CLOWES GHA JR: The effects of hyperalimentation and infused leucine on the amino acid metabolism in sepsis: An experimental study in vivo. Surgery 90(2):278-290, 1981

LONG CL, JEEVANANDAM M, KIM BM, KINNEY JM: Whole body protein synthesis and catabolism in septic man. Am J Clin Nutr 30:1340-1344, 1977

LONG CL, SPENCER JL, KINNEY JM, GEIGER JW: Carbohydrate metabolism in man: Effect of elective operations and major injury. J Appl Physiol 31:110, 1971

LUCAS CE: The renal response to acute injury and sepsis. Surg Clin North Am 56(4):953, 1976

LUST G: Effect of infection on protein and nucleic acid synthesis in mammalian organs and tissues. Fed Proc 25:1688-1694, 1966

McMENAMY RH, BIRKHAHN R, OSWALD G, REED R, RUMPH C, VAIDYANATH N, YU L, CERRA FB, SORKNESS R, BORDER JR: Multiple systems organ failure I. The basal state. J Trauma 21(2):99-114, 1981

MEAKINS JL: Pathophysiologic determinants and prediction of sepsis. Surg Clin North Am 56(4):847-857, 1976

MEAKINS JL, CHRISTOU NV, SHIZGAL HM, MACLEAN LD: Therapeutic approaches to anergy in surgical patients. Ann Surg 190(3):286, 1979

MELA L, BACALZO LV JR, MILLER LD: Defective oxidative metabolism of rat liver mitochondria in hemorrhagic and endotoxin shock. Am J Physiol 220:571, 1971

MOELLERING RC JR: Mechanism of action of antimicrobial agents. Clin Obstet Gynecol 22(2):277-283, 1979

MOORE FD, OLESEN KH, McMURREY JD, PARKER HV, BALL MR, BOYDEN CM: The Body Cell Mass and Its Supporting Environment. Philadelphia, WB Saunders, 1963

POWANDA MD, BEISEL WR: Leukocyte endogenous mediator/endogenous pyrogen/lymphocyte-activating factor modulates the development of nonspecific and specific immunity and affects nutritional status. Am J Clin Nutr 35(4):762-768, 1982

RANDALL HT: Fluid, electrolyte, and acid-base balance. Surg Clin North Am 56(5):1019, 1976

RECTOR F, GOYAL S, ROSENBERG JK, LUCAS CE: Sepsis: A mechanism for vasodilation in the kidney. Ann Surg 178:222, 1973

ROCHA DM, SANTEUSANIE F, FALOONA GR, UNGER RH: Abnormal pancreatic alpha-cell function in bacterial infections. N Engl J Med 288:700, 1973

ROSENBLATT S, CLOWES GHA JR, GEORGE B, HIRSCH E, LINDBERG B.: Exchange of amino acids by muscle and liver in sepsis: Comparative studies in vivo and in vitro. Arch Surg 118:167, 1983

RYAN NT: Metabolid adaptations for energy production during trauma and sepsis. Surg Clin North Am 56(5):1073, 1976

SABA TM, JAFFE E: Plasma fibronectin (opsonic glycoprotein): Its synthesis by vascular endothelial cells and role in cardiopulmonary integrity after trauma as related to reticuloendothelial function. Am J Med 68:577, 1980

SCHILLING JA: Wound healing. Surg Clin North Am 56(4):859, 1976

SHIZGAL HM: Total body potassium and nutritinal status. Surg Clin North Am 56(5):1185, 1976

SIEGEL JH, GOLDWYN RM, FRIEDMAN HP: Pattern and process in the evolution of human septic shock. Surgery 70:232, 1971

STRAUCH M, McLAUGHLIN JS, MANSBERGER A, YOUNG J, MENDONCA P et al: Effects of septic shock on renal function in humans. Ann Surg 165:536, 1967

TEPLITZ C: The core pathobiology and integrated medical science of adult acute respiratory insufficiency. Surg Clin North Am 56(5):1091, 1976

VITRO L, WEISEL RD, IRARRAZAVAL MJ, BERGER RL, HECHTMAN HB: Ventricular performance in sepsis and heart disease. Circulation 4,7,8(Suppl):228, 1973

WANNEMACHER RW JR: Key role of various individual amino acids in host response to infection. Am J Clin Nutr 30:1269-1280, 1977

WEISSMANN G, SMOLEN JE, HOFFSTEIN S: Polymorphonuclear leukocytes as secretory organs of inflammation. J Invest Dermatol 71:95, 1978

WILMORE D: Hormanal responses and their effect on metabolism. Surg Clin North Am 56(5), 1976

WILMORE DW, GOODWIN CW, AULICK LH, POWANDA MC, MASON AD JR PRUITT BA JR: Effect of injury and infection on visceral metabolism and circulation. Ann Surg 192(4):491, 1980

WRIGHT CJ, DUFF JH, McLEAN APH, MacLEAN LD: Regional capillary blood flow and oxygen uptake in severe sepsis. Surg Gynecol Obstet 132:637, 1971

6

The objectives of preoperative preparation of the patient are to improve his resistance to infection, reduce the total number of bacteria in sites of potential contamination and infection, and decrease the opportunities for bacterial entry into the physiological interior of the body. At the same time it is to be kept in mind that the gentle handling of tissues and accurate hemostasis are as important as asepsis in the prevention of most wound infections (Chap. 9).

These preoperative goals may not be reached in all surgical patients since many of the techniques require substantial periods of time and, therefore, their application to patients requiring an emergency operation may not be possible. In patients who are candidates for elective surgical procedures, careful implementation of the following principles should be considered.

PREADMISSION PREOPERATIVE PREPARATION AND HYGIENE

There are a number of measures that should be considered in the preoperative period for the prevention of postoperative infections in patients scheduled for elective surgical procedures. Among the possible methods of achieving this goal are shortening the preoperative period of hospitalization, controlling the patient's weight, correcting malnutrition, identifying and treating established remote infections, treating associated diseases, and maintaining general cleanliness.

Weight Control

The increase in the rate of wound infection and the increased hazard of pulmonary complications in the obese patient is proven. In obese patients preparing for elective surgery, it may be advisable to invest the time necessary to return the patient to acceptable weight prior to operation. It is noteworthy that severe obesity was found to be associated with an increased postoperative infection rate of 18.1% in

71

the National Academy of Science/National Research Council (NAS/NRC) five-university ultraviolet collaborative study, confirming the belief of many experienced surgeons in this regard (Howard).

Conversely, for the *malnourished* patient, improvement in the patient's state of nutrition is mandatory prior to elective surgery, since host resistance to infection may be impaired by starvation and by vitamin and protein deficiencies. In 67 severely malnourished patients who underwent surgery in the collaborative ultraviolet wound study, 22.4% developed wound infection, indicating the higher risk to infection of this type of patient. For those malnourished or undernourished persons whose usual route of food intake is blocked, calories, protein, vitamins, and other essentials should be provided parenterally until any metabolic deficits have been corrected. Fischer has pointed out that the relationship between nutritional support and the prevention or therapy of infections is a newly opened therapeutic field. There is evidence that in severely injured or burned patients, nonspecific host resistance is enhanced by the administration of an increased amount of protein. Similar data have been obtained in renal failure in the study carried out by Abel and co-workers and in a recently completed study by Cerra and co-workers in patients with hepatic disease, a finding supported by a multi-center Italian trial reported by Fiaccodori, and associates. The exact mechanism of such enhancement of resistance to infection is not clear; it may involve specific amino acids and their effects on specific host defense functions, or it may be a more nonspecific effect.

Remote Infections

The presence of any active infection should be searched for and identified prior to operation by detailed preoperative evaluation of the patient who is to undergo an elective operation. These infections may be entirely unrelated to the disease of concern, but they may contribute substantially to the risk of operative wound infection or to systemic infectious complications if unrecognized and untreated. The mechanism of spread may be either by dispersal over skin routes or by systemic routes. In both instances attempts at production of a barrier to its spread are less successful than eradication of the infection prior to operation. The presence of an acute upper respiratory infection, chronic ear infections, active skin infections such as furuncles, chronically draining sinuses, chronic dermatologic disease, acute or smouldering urinary tract infection, active peridontal disease, or chronic respiratory infections are strong reasons to consider deferring elective operations until control of such remote infections is accomplished.

In the unimmunized patient who has sustained trauma or burns, immunization against tetanus should be carried out according to guidelines of the American College of Surgeons (Walt).

Associated Noninfectious Conditions

A significant measure of benefit may also be gained by the correction or treatment of certain associated noninfectious conditions. Diabetes mellitus, uremia, and cirrhosis require special attention. As indicated earlier, chronic malnutrition states require dietary correction, judicious use of medication, and possibly hyperalimentation.

Specific training and advice can be offered on an outpatient basis. This includes deep breathing and coughing exercises to assist in postoperative pulmonary toilet, instruction on relaxation during micturition to help prevent the need for urinary bladder catheterization postoperatively, and instruction to avoid air swallowing to help reduce gastric distention postoperatively.

More specific disorders, such as benign prostatic hypertrophy, may require surgical correction to avoid urinary tract instrumentation and possible infection during the postoperative period. In patients with chronic pulmonary disease, thorough respiratory toilet and training in the use of intermittent positive pressure breathing devices, chest percussion, and postural draining techniques may do much to reduce respiratory tract infection. Specific advice and training can be offered the preoperative patient to enhance ventilation, initiate micturition, and correct aerophagia. When a patient is known to be a carrier of pathogenic microorganisms, control of this carrier state is of considerable importance (Chaps. 3, 4, and 10).

General Cleanliness

It is important to remove any dirt or soilage from the body surface through bathing or a shower, with special attention being given to the fingernails and toenails. The use of antiseptic soaps may be of additional value, as shown by Cruse; for example, his evaluation of the benefit of a preoperative shower with hexachlorophene soap in patients undergoing clean operations has shown a statistically significant improvement in infection rate. Such a study comparing three groups—those who had no preoperative shower, those who showered with ordinary bar soap, and those who showered with hexachlorophene soap—revealed infection rates of 2.3, 2.1, and 1.3% respectively.

POSTADMISSION PREOPERATIVE PREPARATION

After admission, it is important to continue the various measures described for the preadmission preparation for each patient. In addition, the possible effects of hospital environmental exposure of patients preoperatively should be kept in mind.

Exposure to the Hospital Environment and Length of Preoperative Stay

Consistent with the proper general care of the patient, his preoperative hospital stay should be as brief as possible. A direct correlation between the duration of preoperative hospital stay and the rate of postoperative wound infections has been demonstrated. For example, patients with electrolyte disorders, water imbalance, significant anemia, urinary or intestinal tract obstruction, or cardiac decompensation may require several days or more of treatment in the hospital before operation. Since bacteria migrate passively about hospitals on the hands and hair of hospital personnel, linens, air currents, and equipment, they may become part of the patient's flora and be implicated later in wound or other nosocomial infections. In the NAS/NRC ultraviolet study, the data showed that the rate of infection was approximately two times greater after 2 weeks' hospitalization and three times greater after 3 weeks' hospitalization, as compared with the rate in patients admitted 1 to 3 days preoperatively. Opportunities for contact spread from patients with existing infections to the preoperative patient must be kept to a minimum (Chaps. 7, 8, 10, 13, 14, and 17).

The patient approaching elective operation following long-term hospitalization and preparation may have had the bacterial flora of his various tracts significantly modified. Baseline cultures taken from the respiratory, genitourinary, or gastrointestinal tracts may be helpful in revealing the identity of microorganisms with unusual potential or capability for producing postoperative infections.

Immediate Preoperative Preparation

Management of Hair at the Operation Site.   Difference of opinion exists as to the most appropriate method of dealing with hair in the area of the proposed operative incision. The influence of hair management on the incidence of postoperative wound infection has been scrutinized by several observers.

In 1971 Seropian and Reynolds, studying 406 patients, reported that the postoperative wound infection rate was 5.6% in those shaved with a razor; 0.6% in those not shaved; and 0.6% in those in whom hair was removed by a depilatory cream. Two years later Cruse and Foord reported that the clean wound infection rate in patients who were shaved was 2.3%; in those not shaved but who had only pubic hair removed, 1.7%; and in patients who were neither shaved nor clipped, 0.9%.

By means of observations on 1013 patients reported in 1983, Alexander and his colleagues compared the influence of razor shaving and of clipping on the incidence of postoperative wound infection. Hair was removed from the operative area by one of four methods: shaving the night before operation; shaving the morning of operation; clipping the evening of operation; or clipping the morning of operation. The incidence of postoperative wound infection at time of discharge from hospital and at 30 days following operation is indicated in Table 6-1. Within the framework of this study, clipping the morning of operation is the preferred method.

If hair is to be removed, it should be done with care, avoiding skin injury or irritation. Shaving or even clipping may destroy some of the natural integumentary defenses, and may produce multiple superficial lesions containing exuded tissue fluids that favor or contain bacterial growth. This probability is the basis for the practice of shaving or clipping immediately prior to the time of the operation.

The area prepared must be adequate for the incision planned and for any possible extensions of it, as well as any possible additional incisions or points of exit of drains or tubes, the use of which may be necessitated by the procedure. An additional factor

(Text continues on p 81)

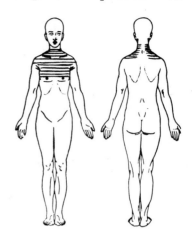

Thyroid prep. Extends from chin line to nipples, including axillary region. Extend to back of neck and upper shoulder as sketched.

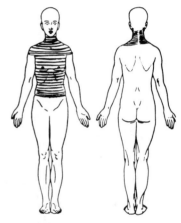

Parathyroid prep (as for sternal splitting). Extends from chin line to umbilicus, shoulder to shoulder in the front. Extend to back of neck and upper shoulder in back as shown. Prep laterally for chest tubes if so ordered.

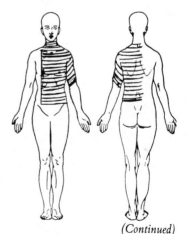

Thoracotomy prep. Extends from chin line to iliac crest, from nipple on unaffected side to at least 2 inches beyond the midline in back. Include axilla and entire arm to elbow.

(Continued)

Fig. 6-1. Skin preparation recommended for surgical procedures. (Modified from Walter CW: In Current Practice Bulletin No. 7-2-5. Boston, Massachusetts, Peter Bent Brigham Hospital, March, 1975)

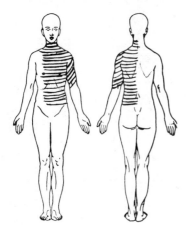

Mastectomy prep. Extends from upper neck to iliac crest, from nipple line on unaffected side to midline of back (affected side). Prep axilla and entire arm to elbow on affected side.

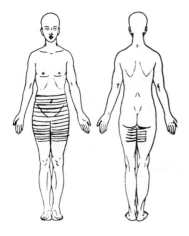

Lower abdominal prep (as for hernia, femoral vein ligation, femoral embolectomy). Extends from 2 inches above the umbilicus to mid-thigh, including the pubic area. Femoral ligation—prepare area to midline of thigh posteriorly. Hernia and embolectomy—prepare to costal margin and down to knee as ordered.

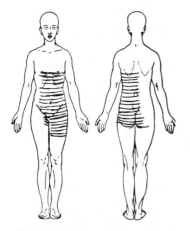

Flank prep (as for renal procedures, adrenalectomy, sympathectomy). Extends from nipple line to pubis and 3 inches beyond the midline in back. Prepare pubic area. Prepare upper thigh on the affected side.

Fig. 6-1,   Cont.

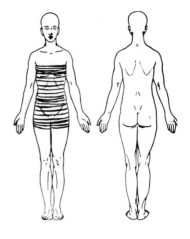

Abdominal prep. Extends from 3 inches above the nipple line to upper thighs, including pubis.

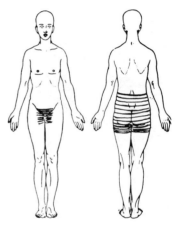

Perineal prep (as for hemorrhoidectomy, fistula-in-ano, pilonidal sinus). Extends from pubis, perineum and perianal area, from the waist in back to at least 3 inches below the groin.

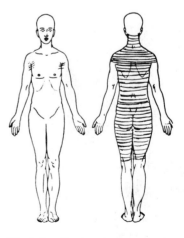

Spine prep. Extends from entire back including shoulders and neck to hairline and down to knees and to both sides, including axillae.

Fig. 6-1, Cont.

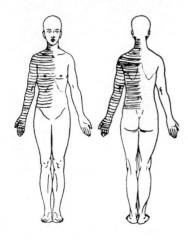

Shoulder prep. Extends from fingertips to hairline, midline chest to midline spine on operative side and to iliac crest, including axillae.

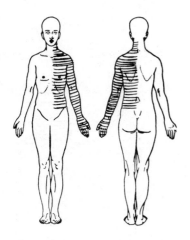

Upper arm prep. Extends from fingertips to neckline (hairline), on operative side from midline chest to midline spine, on operative side from axilla to iliac crest. Trim and clean fingernails. Use brush on hand and nails.

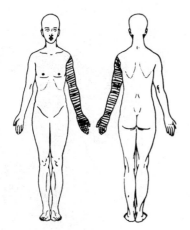

Hand prep. Extends from fingertips to shoulder. Trim and clean fingernails. Use brush on hand and nails.

Fig. 6-1, Cont.

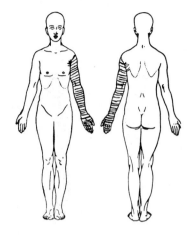

Forearm and elbow prep. Extends from fingernails to shoulder including axilla. Trim and clean fingernails. Use brush on hand and nails.

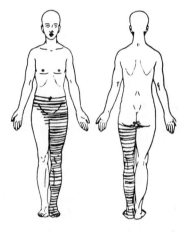

Saphenous vein ligation prep. Extends from umbilicus to toes of affected leg, or both legs. Include pubis and perineal area. Prep entire leg posteriorly.

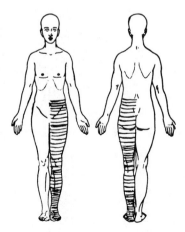

Thigh prep. Extends from toes to 3 inches above the umbilicus, midline front and back, including complete pubic area. Clean and trim toenails. Use brush on foot and nails.

Fig. 6-1, Cont.

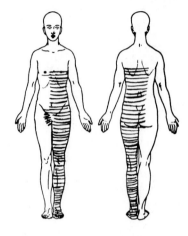

Hip prep. Extends from toes to nipple line to at least 3 inches beyond midline back and front, including complete pubic area. Clean and trim toenails. Use brush on foot and nails. Hip fractures—all preps done in the operating room.

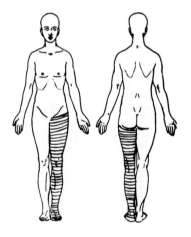

Knee and lower leg prep. Extends from entire leg, toes to groin. Clean and trim toenails. Use brush on foot and nails.

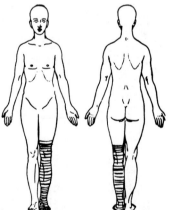

Ankle and foot prep. Extends from entire leg, toes to 3 inches above the knee. Clean and trim toenails. Use brush on foot and nails.

Fig. 6-1,   Cont.

Table 6-1.   Infection Rates and Preoperative Hair Management: Data from Alexander, Fisher, and Co-workers

	Infected At Discharge	Infected At 30 Days
P.M. Razor	14/271 (5.2%)	23/260 (8.8%)
A.M. Razor	17/266 (6.4%)	26/260 (10.0%)
P.M. Clipper	10/250 (4.0%)	18/241 (7.5%)
A.M. Clipper	4/266 (1.8%)	7/216 (3.2%)
Overall	45/1013(4.4%)	74/977 (7.6%)

(Data from Alexander JW, Fisher JE et al: The influence of hair removal methods on wound infections. Arch Surg 118:347–352, 1983)

to consider is the area to be covered by adhesive tape, which will adhere poorly to hair-bearing skin and may cause pain when removed.

Skin Degerming.   There is also considerable confusion and difference of opinion about the most effective methods of preparing the skin of the operative area and the most efficient types of degerming agents to be used. It must be kept in mind that while it is possible to sterilize all, or virtually all, of the instruments and other equipment used at operation, one cannot sterilize the skin either of the surgeon or of the patient's operative site without damaging or destroying it (Lowbury). The most that can be done to prevent contamination of wounds from these sources is to disinfect the skin by methods that usually leave some bacteria in the disinfected area. These bacteria, as Price showed many years ago, can be divided into "transient" and "resident" flora. The important practical distinction, though, is between superficial organisms, which can be almost completely removed either by washing with soap and water or by disinfection, and the more adherent organisms, which are much more effectively removed by disinfection than by washing. Most of the latter are undoubtedly residents, but some, for example *Clostridium perfringens,* are unlikely to multiply on the skin; these organisms are not residents, although they are undoubtedly adherent.

Heavy fecal contamination of the skin of the thighs and buttocks presents a hazard of gas gangrene in patients with poor blood supply having operations involving muscle and bone (*e.g.,* amputation for diabetic gangrene). In this situation a large proportion of *C. perfringens* spores can be destroyed on the skin by preoperative application of a compress soaked in povidone-iodine (Betadine) solution.

In 1965, 195 university and nonuniversity hospitals of wide geographic distribution were surveyed about their skin degerming practices. A significant change in the practices for degerming the *patient's* skin from the time that Price completed his study in 1948 had occurred. The use of the organic mercurials had decreased markedly, particularly in the university hospitals. The use of ethyl alcohol had also decreased considerably, and the use of Zephiran and quaternary ammonium compounds had to some extent diminished. Also, although the bis-phenols (hexachlorophene), of which pHisoHex and Septisol are probably the best known, are not bactericidal on contact and require a fairly protracted period to alter the bacterial floras, they were used without other degermers in a surprising percentage of instances. Another point of interest was related to *benzalkonium chloride* (Zephiran). The quaternary ammonium compound is a cationic degermer, and many have felt that the anionic environment left by washing with soap would vitiate the activity of Zephiran. Yet, in a surprisingly high percentage of institutions where Zephiran was used, there was no effort to rinse the skin of soap that had previously been applied.

On the basis of the presentations and discussions at the second and third symposia which it conducted, the Committee on Control of Surgical Infections prepared the following recommendations for the preparation of the operative area.

1. The preparation of the operative area should be done by a physician, a member of the operating team, a nurse, or an operating room technician who is knowledgeable and specially trained for this purpose. Sterile gloves should be worn during this procedure and sterile supplies used (Fig. 6-2 and 6-3).
2. The areas should initially be cleansed with soap, with a nonirritating detergent solution, or with a fat solvent.
3. A degerming agent should then be applied. Degerming agents commonly used for this purpose include iodine solutions, chlorhexidine, alcohol, quaternary ammonium compounds, and hexachlorophene.

Commonly Used Degerming Agents

Iodine and iodine compounds. Tincture of iodine is a time-honored degerming agent for skin preparation, but, because of sensitivity reactions and dermatitis, it has been largely replaced by iodine compounds known as iodophors. These compounds contain 1% to 3% elemental iodine. Release of the iodine accounts for germicidal action and also may cause hyperplasia of the thyroid. Iodine compounds are bactericidal and are effective against gram-positive and gram-negative organisms. Combined with a detergent, they are now popular and considered to be effective.

Chlorhexidine gluconate. Chlorhexidine gluconate (Hibiclens) is now approved by the U.S. Food and Drug Administration and is used widely. Chlorhexidine is for topical use only, and it offers a wide range of bactericidal activity, being effective against a wide spectrum of microorganisms. Its activity is reported not to be affected adversely by organic material (Lowbury).

Hexachlorophene preparations. Unlike the iodines, hexachlorophene (bis-phenol) preparations exert most of their effect on gram-positive organisms. They are often not bactericidal and require more prolonged contact to alter the bacterial flora. Their germicidal action depends on pH and solvent. They are being used less frequently.

Ethyl alcohol. Ethyl, or isopropyl, alcohol may be used as a 70% solution and is bactericidal for many gram-negative and gram-positive organisms.

Quaternary ammonium compounds. Benzalkonium chloride, cetylpyridinium chloride, and other quaternary ammonium compounds (cationic degerming agents) may be inactivated by anionic soaps, and they are more bacteriostatic than bactericidal. These solutions are not used frequently at this time.

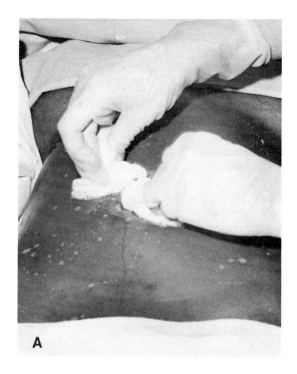

Fig. 6-2. *(A)* Preparation of the operating area is being done by a physician, using sterile gloves and sponges soaked in a detergent solution or liquid soap. In this case the "scrub" of the abdominal operative area lasted 10 minutes and was in preparation for a cholecystectomy. *(B)* The umbilicus frequently harbors dirt or other foreign material. This should be removed during the "scrubbing" preparation with sterile applicators soaked in the cleansing solution.

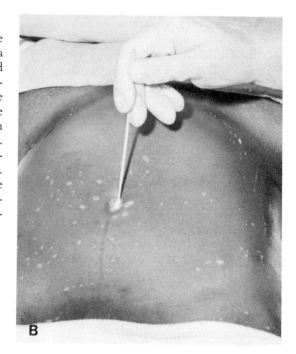

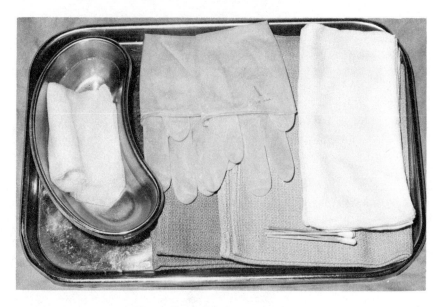

Fig. 6-3. A "prep" table with sterile cleansing solution, gauze sponges, and applicators ready for use by the physician, nurse, or operating room technician.

Most of the currently popular agents are acceptably benign if used in the prescribed manner, but certain persons develop allergic or atopic reactions to them. *Degerming agents may produce irritative effects on normal skin.* It should also be emphasized again that it is impossible to sterilize the skin of the patient's operative site without damaging or destroying it.

Improved removal and killing of bacteria on the skin of the operative site can be directly translated into a decrease in operative wound sepsis. For example, Cruse has reported data from a large number of patients. In the period 1967 to 1971, using a green soap and alcohol "skin prep" in the operating room, an infection rate of 2% was reported in 12,849 clean operations. In the 1971 to 1972 period, with the use of a povidone-iodine scrub on the ward, followed immediately by a preoperative paint with tincture of Hibitane, the infection rate fell to 1.2% in 1810 patients.

Techniques of Preparing the Operative Area.   The Committee on Control of Surgical Infections has concluded that preparation of the operative area should include washing, but the method of "washing" or "scrubbing" may vary considerably. The methods used effectively by different authorities and different surgical centers vary considerably. For this reason several examples are described below. At the same time it is also recognized that other methods may be used effectively and safely.

1. The following method is one used at the Massachusetts General Hospital for the preparation of the operative field. It depends upon two steps that must be carried out exactly as outlined to be effective.

    In the *first step,* surface dirt, loose skin, and other debris are removed by the scrubbing of the skin of the operative field for 2 minutes with soap and water by a member of the scrubbed surgical team before gowning, using sterile gloves and gauze sponges held by sponge forceps. The gauze sponges are changed frequently. Although this step does not kill bacteria, it is effective in defatting and removing skin debris.

    The *second step* is the degerming step and is carried out by the application of 70% isopropyl alcohol containing a red dye for marking. This step is accomplished by scrubbing for 2 full minutes with frequently changed sterile gauze sponges soaked with the alcohol solution. Excess alcohol may be removed from the operative site by blotting with a dry, sterile towel.

    In preparing the skin over breast tumors or areas of cellulitis, gentle washing is necessary, but 2 minutes for each step is maintained. Skin surfaces adjacent to the prepared areas are protected from becoming wet by sterile "soak" towels discarded at the end of the skin prep procedure.

    An alternate method used at Massachusetts General Hospital consists of a scrub of the operative with iodophor solution for 2 minutes.

2. On the Surgical Service of the University of Cincinnati Medical Center, one method used in elective cases is a 5- or 10-minute scrub of the skin of the operative area with an iodophor (Betadine) solution followed by the painting of the skin with an iodophor solution. This time may be decreased, however, particularly when the operation involves the face, an area of cellulitis or other active infection where the possibility of the spread of bacteria exists, or a breast tumor where there is the possibility of dissemination of tumor cells. The site of operation may also dictate modification in the overall technique. The face requires particular gentleness and care, especially around the eyes.

    The type of preparation depends upon whether the procedure is an elective or an emergency one, since the nature of the emergency may necessitate modifications. As an example, an open traumatic wound, heavily infiltrated with dirt and foreign matter, may require not only considerably longer than 10 minutes for preparation but also irrigation with copious amounts of saline solution. Care must be taken to avoid the application of antiseptics and detergents to open wounds because of their local irritating effects and the possibility of systemic toxicity due to absorption(see Chap. 9).

    The routine skin preparation that has been used on the surgical service of the University of Cincinnati has included the following steps, as described by Altemeier:

    a. After careful placement of the patient on the operating table to provide maximal exposure and a safe position, towels are placed about the operative area to collect any excess of the "prepping" solution.

    b. The area is then gently "scrubbed" for a specified period of time using iodophor solution, usually for 5 to 10 minutes, to remove surface debris, dirt, and desquamating skin and their microbial content.

c. The scrubbing is usually done by an ungowned member of the scrubbed surgical team wearing sterile gloves and using sterile gauze sponges provided from a "prep table" (Fig. 6-3). A nurse or a technician may also be used in some instances as an alternate for this purpose if so trained and supervised. The gauze sponges are changed frequently. Care is taken to wash all areas evenly.

Prepackaged sterile disposable prep sets are commercially available and are in general use in most hospitals. They contain all the required dry material for preoperative scrubs and they contribute to the uniformity of the scrub technique. Application is started at the site of the incision and spread peripherally to minimize contamination from outside the field (Fig. 6-4).

With the above method, incorporated with appropriate draping described below and surgical technique discussed in Chapter 9, a consistently low rate of infection at 0.7 to 0.9% in clean elective operative wounds had been obtained on the surgical services at the University of Cincinnati hospitals.

Other methods used effectively at Cincinnati by some members of the surgical staff include a similar 5- to 10-minute scrub with hexachlorophene solution or a chlorhexidine solution with occasional modification.

Fig. 6-4. Application of antiseptic degerming solution to operative area in the circular manner, progressing peripherally. In this instance, tincture of Ceepryn is being applied over the residual solution of 1 : 100 aqueous Ceepryn used for the 10-min preoperative cleansing.

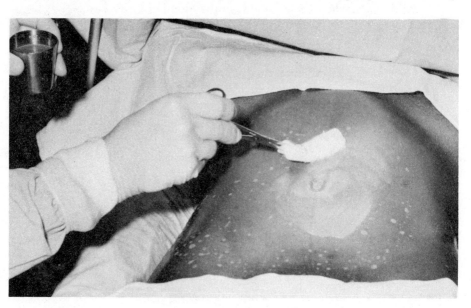

In the interest of *personnel training* and *cost effectiveness,* and for the purpose of developing a data base for clinical trials, it is considered desirable to establish one uniform technique within each institution if possible.

Draping. Appropriate draping is important as a means of demarcating, maintaining, and protecting a limited area prepared for the operation by cleansing and degerming techniques. It must be kept in mind that there are advantages to uniform drape design and application, including the saving of time, neatness, reduced contamination, decreased cost, and more accurate planning of required linen or other material. To accomplish a degree of standardization, each hospital should develop draping techniques and make them available to the operating team. The types of drapes in use include single-use prefabricated drapes (Fig. 6-5, *C*), and the conventional double-thickness linen towels and sheets (288-thread count) modified for use in various types of operations (Fig. 6-5, *A* and *B*). Plastic adhesive skin drapes may be particularly useful in excluding contamination from sinuses, fistulae, colostomies, and other contaminated or infected drainage tracts (Fig. 6-5, *E*).

Disposable or single use drapes. There exist considerable differences in opinion about the value and adequacy of disposable drapes for routine operating room use. Their use has increased considerably because of their ready availability, the escalation of costs of laundering and sterilizing linen drapes, and labor problems in providing a continuing supply of available linen drape material, especially for peak or unanticipated loads. Single-use drapes are gaining in popularity for the following reasons:

- Improved barrier properties
- Decreased linting
- Ready availability
- Competitiveness in cost
- Standardized application
- Ease in disposal of contaminated drapes
- Ease of stockpiling for use in unusual circumstances or in event of catastrophe
- Consistent packaging, and uniform supply and use procedures

The disadvantages of single-use drapes include the following:

- Proprietary variation
- Poor conformity to body contours
- Insufficient strength to permit manipulations of hip and extremities without tearing
- A possible fire hazard and an ecology problem presented by disposal
- Larger storage space needed because of increased bulk
- Hazard of electrification unless stored at the ambient temperature and humidity of the operating room

Linen drapes. Many surgeons continue to use "linen" drapes because of their conformity to body surfaces, their strength, and their adaptability to motion when required. When using linen drapes, consideration should be given to suturing to the

(Text continues on p 91)

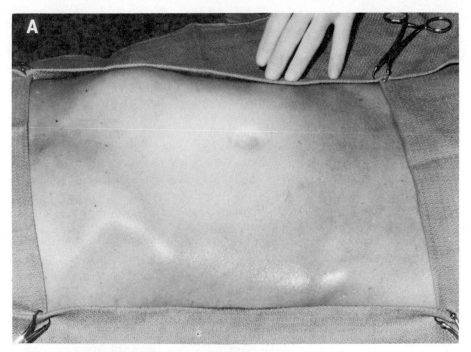

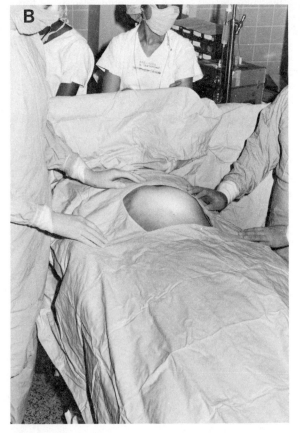

Fig. 6-5. *(A* and *B)* A patient is draped with sterile conventional double-thickness linen drapes and towels. *(C)* Single-use prefabricated drapes are used for an abdominal operation. They are particularly adaptable. *(D)* Plastic adhesive skin drapes (Steridrapes) may be applied over an area previously prepared by conventional linen draping. *(Continues on p 90.)*

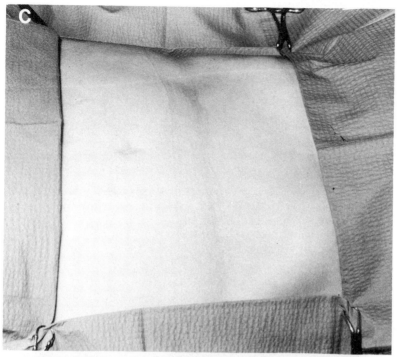

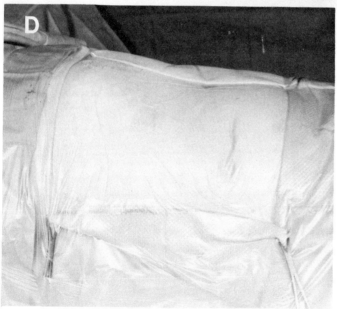

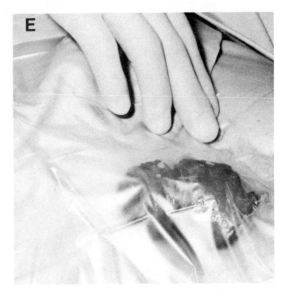

Fig. 6-5, Cont. (E) A plastic adhesive skin drape is used for the exclusion of fistulae, colostomies, and other contaminated or infected drainage tracts from the area of the operative incision. *(F)* The central edges of linen drapes bordering the operative area are sutured with interrupted silk sutures to prevent displacement of the drapes during the operation and consequent contamination of the operative wound.

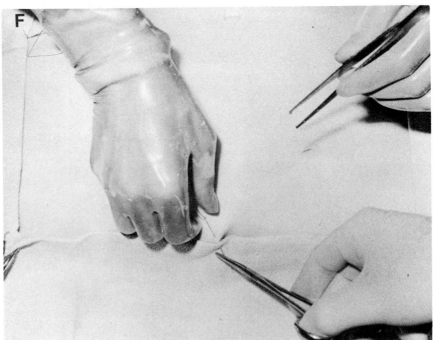

Table 6-2. Drapes and Clean Wound Infections

	Number	Number Infected	Percent
Cloth	11,893	186	1.5
Plastic	5,714	140	2.4

(Cruse PJE, Foord R: A five year prospective study of 23, 649 surgical wounds. Arch Surg 107:206, 1973)

skin the central edges bordering the operative area with interrupted silk sutures. This technique helps prevent displacement of the drape edges and resulting contamination of the operative wound (Fig. 6-5, *F*).

Another consideration is the avoidance of wetting linen drapes, since this may result in migration of bacteria from unprepared areas with contamination of the operative field. If the drapes should become wet during the surgical procedure, they should be covered promptly and effectively by another layer of sterile draping material. This is particularly true in long surgical procedures associated with ascites, hemorrhage, or other fluid transudates, or which require irrigation with saline solutions. Linen drapes must be laundered, kept in good repair, sterilized, and packed for use as needed in such a manner that their sterility is guaranteed (Chap. 16).

Adhesive drapes. Adhesive drapes are adhesive sheets of transparent plastic. Their use provides the opportunity of making the incision through the drape, the cut edges of which should remain adherent to the skin and keep the operative field sealed off from bacterial contamination arising from the adjacent skin edges.

It is hoped that the decrease in the number and types of skin bacteria, resident or transient, in the operative area after preoperative washing and degerming can be maintained and further decreased by the additional use of the adhesive drapes. Many surgeons have used, and are using, plastic skin drapes for this and other purposes (Fig. 6-5, *D*). One problem with their function as a protective barrier is that the edges loosen with time, allowing exposure to blood, tissue fluid, and sweat. Thus their effectiveness at the immediate wound edge is negated, since leakage of fluid may occur. Adhesive drapes have been found useful in some types of orthopaedic, neurosurgical, and plastic surgical procedures. They have also been found useful in isolating bacterial reservoirs, such as the stoma of a colostomy, a fistula, or infected areas from the surgical wound.

A number of reports, however, have noted no decrease in the number of wound infections occurring after the use of adhesive drapes when compared with conventional linen drapes (Cruse and Foord; Table 6-2; and Wheeler).

BIBLIOGRAPHY

Alexander JW, Fischer JE, Boyajian M, Palmquist J, Morris MJ: The influence of hair removal methods on wound infections. Arch Surg 118:347–352, 1983

ALTEMEIER WA: Symposium on hospital-acquired staphylococcal infection. Part III. Recommendations for control of epidemic spread of staphylococcal infections in surgery. Ann Surg 150:774, 1959

ALTEMEIER WA: Surgical antiseptics. In Block SS (ed): Disinfection, Sterilization, and Preservation, 2nd ed, Chap 32, pp 641–653. Philadelphia, Lea & Febiger, 1977

ALTEMEIER WA: Control of wound infections. JR Coll Surg Edinb 11:271, 1966

BALTHAZAR ER, COLT JD, NICHOLS RL: Preoperative hair removal: A random prospective study of shaving versus clipping. South Med J 75(7):799–801, 1982

BLANK IH, COOLIDGE MH: Degerming the cutaneous surface. I. Quaternary ammonium compounds. II. Hexachlorophene (G-(()). J Invest Dermatol 15(3), 1950

BLANK IH, COOLIDGE MH, SOUTTER L, RODKEY GV: A study of the surgical scrub. Surg Gynecol Obstet 91:577, 1950

CHISHOLM TC, DUNCAN TL, HUFNAGEL CA, AND WALTER CW: Disinfecting action of pHisoderm containing three percent hexachlorophene on the skin of the hands. Surgery 28:812, 1950

COURT-BROWN CM: Preoperative skin depilation and its effect on postoperative wound infections. J Coll Surg 26:238–241, 1981

CRUSE PJE, FOORD R: A five year prospective study of 23,649 surgical wounds. Arch Surg 107:206, 1973

CRUSE PJE, FOORD R: The epidemiology of wound infection: A 10-year prospective study of 62,979 wounds. Surg Clin North Am 60(1):27–40, 1980

HAMILTON HW, HAMILTON KR, LONE FJ: Preoperative hair removal. Can J Surg 20:269–275, 1977

HOWARD JM et al; POSTOPERATIVE WOUNDS INFECTIONS: The influence of ultraviolet irradiation of the operating room and of various other factors. Ann Surg 160(Suppl):1, 1964

KING TC, PRICE PB: An evaluation of iodophors as skin antiseptics. Surg Gynecol Obstet 116:361–365, 1963

LOWBURY EJL, LILLY HA, BULL JP: Disinfection of the skin of operative sites. Br Med J 5205:1039–1044, 1960

LOWBURY EJL, LILLY HA, BULL JP: Methods for disinfection of hands and operative sites. Br Med J 5408:531–536, 1964

POLOCK AV: Adhesive wound drapes. Lancet 2:883, 1970

POWIS SJA, WATERWORTH TA, ARKELL DG: Preoperative skin preparation: Clinical evaluation of depilatory cream. Br Med J 2:1166–1168, 1976

PRICE PB: The bacteriology of normal skin: A new quantitative test applied to a study of the bacterial flora and the disinfectant action of mechanical cleansing. J Infect Dis 62–63:301–318, 1938

PRICE PB: Fallacy of a current surgical fad—the three minute preoperative scrub with hexachlorophene soap. Ann Surg 134:476–485, 1951

PRUITT BA JR: Surgical dressings and drapes. In Lecture Outlines, Postgraduate Course on Pre- and Postoperative Care. Engineering in Surgery, pp 7–10. Presented at the 56th Clinical Congress, American College of Surgeons, October, 1970

SEROPIAN R, REYNOLDS BM: Wound infections after preoperative depilatory versus razor preparation. Am Surg 121:251, 1971

SIMMONS BP: Guidelines for the prevention and control of nosocomial infections. Washington, DC, U.S. Department of Health & Human Services, USPHS Center for Disease Control, 1981

SIESEL JH, CERRA FB, COLEMAN B, GIOVANNINI I, SHETYE M, BORDER JR, McMENAMY RH: Physiological and metabolic correlations in human sepsis. Invited Commentary. Surgery 86(2):163–193, 1979

TODD J, ALTEMEIER WA: Studies on the incidence of infection following open chest cardiac massage for cardiac arrest. Ann Surg 158:596–607, 1963

W<small>ALT</small> AJ (ed): Early care of the injured patient, 3rd ed, pp 68–72. Philadelphia, WB Saunders, 1982

W<small>HEELER</small>, MH: Abdominal wound protection by means of plastic drapes. In Strachan CJL, Wise R (eds): Surgical Sepsis. London, Academic Press, 1979

W<small>ILLIAMS</small> REO, S<small>HOOTER</small> RA (eds): Infection in hospitals; Epidemiology and control. In Symposium on Infection in Hospitals, London, 1962. Philadelphia, FA Davis, 1963

7

The strict enforcement of intelligent rules governing aseptic and antiseptic techniques within the operating room suite is of obvious importance in the prevention and control of infections in surgical patients. Although experienced operating room personnel are well aware of these rules and regulations, they must be ever mindful of them and alert to violations of any kind that might endanger the patient. Not only must they be aware of the necessity of setting an example by their own compliance with these rules, but they must also guard against violations by others, particularly inexperienced personnel such as students, consultants, observers, and various technicians whose exposure to the operating room and its rules may be limited or whose motivation toward adherence to those rules may be underdeveloped. All personnel who enter or work in the operating room should be given appropriate supervision and be governed by the same rules and regulations as the members of the surgical team.

Preparation of the Operating Team and Supporting Personnel

HEALTH AND HYGIENE

Patients, professional members of the surgical team, anesthetists, consultants, or supporting personnel, such as attendants and technicians, with active infections may present complex problems of control. It is a generally accepted practice that the members of the operating team and others working in the operating room must be free of transmissible bacterial infections. These include furuncles, carbuncles, dermatitis, psoriasis, draining sinuses, osteomyelitis, hydradenitis, ulcers of the skin, and unhealed wounds. Symptomless carriers of pathogenic organisms and personnel with obscure or hidden staphylococcal and streptococcal lesions may be difficult to identify and restrict (Walter).

As indicated in Chapter 4, many hospital personnel carry coagulase-positive staphylococci in the nose and throat. Although approximately 10% to 70% of hospital personnel in the operating room area have been shown to carry coagulase-positive *Staphylococcus aureus* in their nasal passages at various times, they are not necessarily dangerous as disseminators of this microorganism. With the careful and routine use of the precautions elaborated in this chapter, it is believed that most carriers are usually not hazardous to patients. However, a few persons will shed the organism in infectious numbers, and these individuals may become a hazard. Such carriers must be searched for when an obvious source of a cluster of infections is not found. The evidence indicates that the greatest danger lurks in the permanent heavy carrier or shedder who has evidence of active disease, such as furunculosis. Routine nasopharyngeal cultures of all personnel are not considered to be necessary unless an unusual number or "cluster" of infections occur in patients under their care (Chap. 4). If a staff member or other employee is found to be carrying staphylococci of the same phage type and antibiogram as that causing clinical infection in the cluster of patients with infections, he should be temporarily restricted from contact with patients until effectively treated. Care must be taken, however, not to label him as the source of the infections, since he may have contracted the carrier state or his infection from the patient.

A surgeon who has dermatitis on his hands and forearms cannot effectively reduce the bacterial count on his skin by scrubbing. If the second line of defense against infection is broken (*e.g.,* perforation of rubber gloves), increased and significant inoculation of the wound with many pathogenic microorganisms may occur. In addition to the upper respiratory tract and skin, the enteric tract and the genitourinary tract may be the sites of obscure infection and may harbor pathogenic bacteria such as *Staphlococcus aureus, Streptococcus,* or *Salmonella.*

In cases of demonstrated active and significant carrier states, the person should be treated not only for acute or chronic infections, but also for predisposing or contributing factors, such as diabetes, dermatitis, diarrhea, nasal abnormalities, or allergies. Antibiotic therapy and surgical treatment may be required in some instances. The advice of consultants with special expertise in the field of infections and infectious diseases may be useful.

In instances in which significant carrier or shedder states cannot be cleared up even with the most expert treatment, special individualized preventive measures or reassignment to duties without patient contact must be instituted.

OPERATING ROOM ATTIRE

Personnel in the operating room are considered to be the most common source of bacterial contamination. People exhale bacteria-laden droplets from their noses during forced respiration and expectorate them from their mouths when they talk. Desquamated epithelium is exfoliated from exposed areas of skin, and dandruff and bacteria are shed from exposed hair-bearing areas. Their clothing gives off lint, dust, and threads that carry viable microorganisms. The longer the hair, the more talking, or the more frequent coughing and sneezing, the greater the dissemination of bacteria.

For these reasons and others, it is generally recognized that barrier attire and draping against bacterial contamination of the surgical wound are necessary to minimize postoperative surgical infections from exogenous sources. Surgical drapes and gowns designed to reduce contamination of the operative site are essentially barriers to prevent nosocomial and exogenous infections.

With the advent of new materials, and particularly disposable attire and drape material, there has been further recognition that uniform methods for evaluating and testing the characteristics of the barrier are desirable. Materials should be tested for imperviousness to microorganisms under pressure, as well as for their folding, stretching, and comfort characteristics affecting their practical use. Additionally, the design and use of barrier materials must permit the exercising of good technique to prevent wound infection. The problems of inflammability and electrostatic charge deserve special consideration.

At the present time, the Committee on Control of Surgical Infections recommends that operating room clothing (including caps and masks) should be made of nonlinting material, must constitute an effective bacterial barrier, must be comfortable and allow free movement, must transmit heat and water vapor, must not be flammable, and must not have dangerous electrostatic properties.

All persons working in the operating suite must be appropriately attired and wear clean surgical scrub suits (in place of their street clothing); caps, masks, and shoe covers; and regularly cleaned boots or shoes whose use is restricted to the operating room (Fig. 7-1, B). Surgical scrub suits should be designed for maximum skin coverage as well as comfort. Sleeves of the operating room scrub suits must be short enough or turned up to allow adequate scrubbing above the elbows (Fig. 7-1, A). The scrub shirttail and pants drawstring should be tucked inside the pants before gowning to prevent contamination by contact with sterile items in the operating room and to decrease the dissemination of bacterial shedding from the thoracic and abdominal skin of the wearer. If it becomes necessary for anyone to leave the operating suite, he should be required to change into a clean scrub suit before reentering the operating room. Furthermore, it is recommended that scrub suits be changed between operations whenever they have become soiled or wet.

It is important that there be adequate locker rooms and facilities for changing clothing and that adequate supplies of clean scrub suits and scrub dresses in good repair be readily available. In hospitals having a great number of dirty and infected cases (such as infected burns), separate locker facilities and gowning areas for the personnel working with these contaminated cases may be desirable.

Traditionally, women have worn one-piece scrub dresses with high necklines, short sleeves, and skirts extending slightly below the knees. Some authorities have recommended that to reduce the possibility of shedding, women also wear scrub suits. Current practice favors their wearing scrub suits to reduce leg and perineal shedding.

For others, such as consultants and technicians who enter the operating room, a one-piece jumpsuit (Fig. 7-2) with snug bands at wrist, neck, and ankles is an appropriate and convenient type of attire. Another type of jumpsuit, which includes attached hood and boots, may be particularly adaptable to consultants and technicians for relatively short visits to the operating room. Visitors of any type should be restricted and should always wear caps, masks, and shoe covers before entering the operating room.

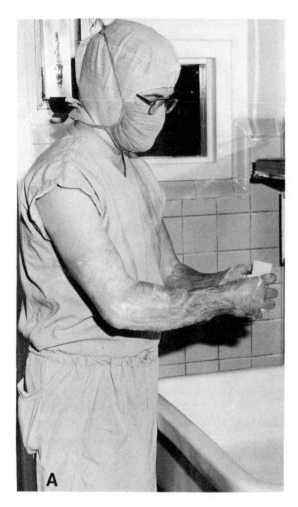

Fig. 7-1. (*A*) Recommended operating room attire and scrubbing techniques for surgical team member. Note that the nose, mouth, and all hair are carefully covered, the shirt and drawstrings are tucked in the trousers, the sleeves are rolled up to the shoulders, and the areas being scrubbed include the forearms, hands, and lower third of the upper arms.

Head Coverings

Hair is a source of bioparticulate matter. All head and facial hair should be covered by a clean operating room cap or, if necessary because of quantity of hair, a cap and hood. In cases of sideburns, beards, or long hair, a hood should be used that exposes only the eyes and ties around the neck.

The Committee on Operating Room Environment of the American College of Surgeons has reported that there is no acceptable standard for testing hoods and masks and that there is a need for further consultation between manufacturer and surgeons, as a joint venture, to design acceptable standard tests. Special aspirating devices now available have not been evaluated by standard methods, and it seems reasonable at the present time to restrict the use of aspirator hoods for specialized purposes.

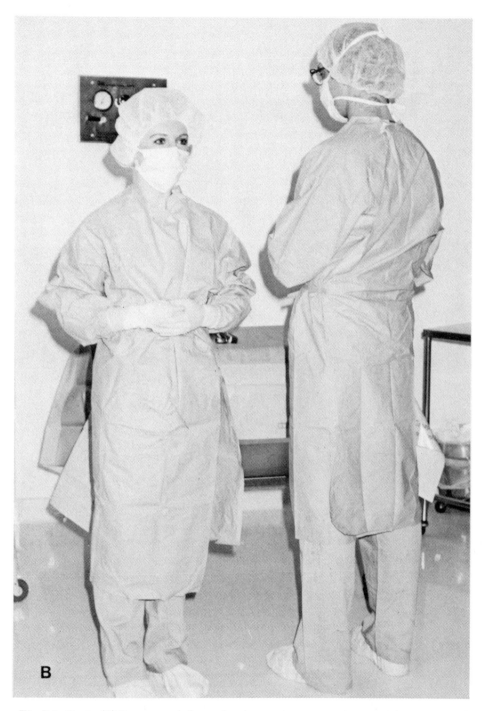

B

Fig. 7-1. Cont. (B) Recommended completed operating room attire. Note the wraparound gowns to provide sterile back surface. (See Fig. 7-5.)

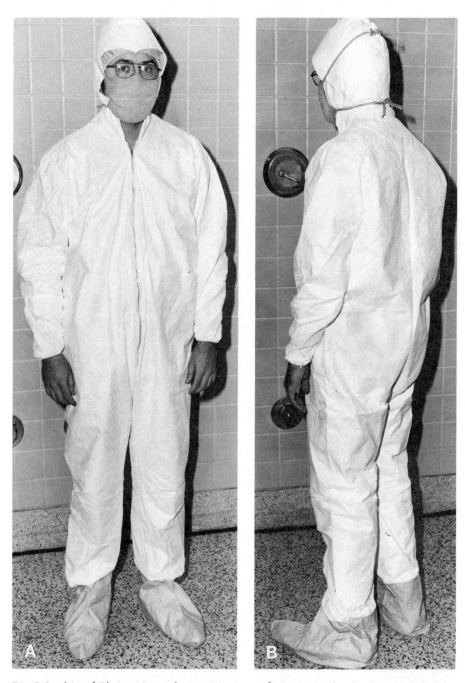

Fig. 7-2. (*A* and *B*) Anterior and posterior views of a jumpsuit that has been developed as acceptable operating room attire for pathologists, consultants, technicians, and others whose presence is required briefly during operations. Note that the hood and boots are attached to the coveralls. The wristlets are elastic. These jumpsuits can be donned over street clothes.

Masks

All personnel in the restricted area of the operating room should wear masks at all times. The type will vary among institutions. A filter type is mandatory and should be constructed to prevent leakage around the edges. Disposable masks are currently popular in many hospitals because of their convenience and the elimination of troublesome laundry problems. Some types have been shown to be highly effective in preventing the passage of oral and nasal bacteria. Reports on their efficiency must be carefully evaluated, because with some masks the expired breath may be prevented from passing through the mask and thus will be exhausted beneath its edges, allowing bacteria to settle on the operative field. It is recommended that a fresh mask be used for each case.

Operating Room Footwear

Some form of protective foot covering should be worn in the operating room area to prevent transmission of bacteria from shoes and to provide electrical grounding of personnel. Specially designed cloth, paper, or plastic shoe covers are available (Fig. 7-3). Disposable, single-use types are in general use in this country. The shoe covers are worn over regular shoes to decrease the number of bacteria that might be transmitted to the operating room from other areas of the hospital. At the same time, they allow the surgeon the comfort of his own footwear. An alternative is to keep special conductive operating room shoes or boots in the operating suite and change

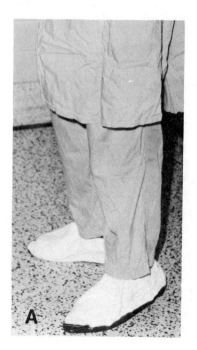

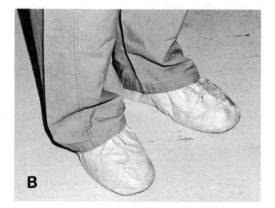

Fig. 7-3. (*A*) One type of reusable canvas shoe covers recommended for shoes of surgical team in the operating room. (*B*) One of various other types of single-use shoe covers now available.

into them in the locker room. This method is less desirable because such shoes must be washed and cleaned regularly to prevent any accumulation of virulent bacteria. Operating room shoe covers or operating room shoes should not be worn outside the operating suite. Conductive shoe covers or conductive shoes must be worn if combustible anesthetic agents are used.

Sterile Gowns

To prevent contamination of the wound or operative field by direct body contact, each member of the scrubbed surgical team must wear a sterile gown extending from the neck to below the knees and to the wrists (Fig. 7-4). The gown should have snug-fitting wristlets that can be overlapped by the cuff of the gloves. The gown is usually tied behind at the neck and waist. The most commonly used gown is one designed to remain sterile in front from the upper chest to the level of the operating table, including the sleeves. Wraparound gowns, designed to provide sterile fields in front and back, are recommended. These have an inside sterile tie in the back at the waist, and a large flap of the gown can be advanced to cover effectively the exposed unsterile back of the scrub suit. These gowns are tied in front by the wearer or the sterile scrub nurse by means of a sterile sash (Fig. 7-5). A vestlike gown back, however, may be used as an alternative to provide a sterile back.

Conventional surgical gowns are made of cotton or muslin and have several thicknesses of cloth in front and over the forearms. These are not impermeable to water and must be changed when they become wet. Several varieties of disposable gowns that meet the above specifications are also available and have come into general use in most hospitals throughout the United States (Fig. 7-6).

Gloves

Many types of gloves are available to the medical profession in plastic, vinyl, and rubber. Plastic and vinyl gloves are useful in preventing the transfer of organisms to or from the wearer. Rubber gloves are the only ones that are suitable for use in the operating room. They may be made of natural latex or synthetic rubber. The light-colored latex gloves are most commonly used. Brown latex gloves are available, and some are slightly thinner than the light-colored ones. Hypoallergenic gloves are also available. The gloves must cover the fingers and hands and extend over the wristlets of the gown in a smooth, unbroken, thin sheet of latex. At the proximal end, a thickened band of rubber discourages the wrist of the glove from rolling back. A flat wide band is more efficient than a small round one.

The majority of gloves currently in use are disposable, but reusable gloves are still available. All gloves are packaged with the cuff turned back so that they can be handled by the exposed part of the inside of the glove (Fig. 7-7). Wet hands will not slip into the glove; therefore, the hands are usually dried (either with a towel or air dried before gloving).

The purpose of scrubbing and disinfection of the hands prior to operation is to reduce the bacterial population to the vanishing point with reasonable assurance that

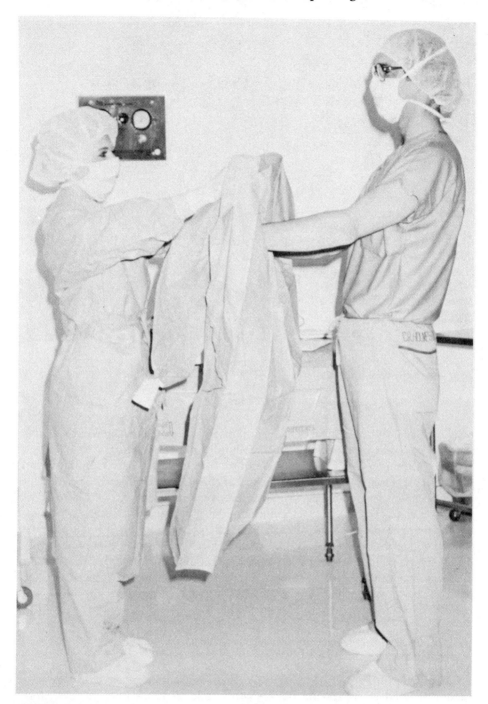

Fig. 7-4. A scrub nurse assisting a surgeon in donning his sterile operating gown to avoid contamination. Note coverage of noses, mouths, and all head and face hair. Nurse's attire includes trousers.

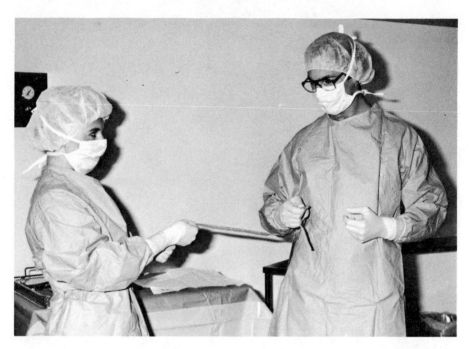

Fig. 7-5. Method of surgeon, with the assistance of the scrub nurse, tying wraparound gown to provide sterility of its back.

it will remain miniscule during the operation. If a hole should develop in the glove, bacterial contamination of the wound should therefore be minimal.

The Committee on Control of Surgical Infections and the Committee on Control of Operating Room Environment have heard evidence that the incidence of puncture holes developing during operations may reach levels of 50% to 70%. Moreover, it was reported that a significant number of gloves have been found with holes when first put on by the surgical team. It has been determined that as many as 40,000 organisms can be liberated through a glove pinhole in a 20-minute period. Better testing methods are needed to eliminate this potential hazard. In addition, it has been recommended that stronger gloves for special operative procedures be developed that would have greater resistance to puncture but retain utility and comfort.

Indications for Change of Attire

Scrub suits, if soiled or wet, shoe covers or operating room shoes, and head coverings should be removed on leaving the operating suite, and new ones put on before returning to the operating room. It is also recommended that masks and head coverings be changed after treating every case.

Fig. 7-6. Completed operating room attire with sterile single-use gown, gloves, cap, and mask. Note that gloves cover gown wristlets.

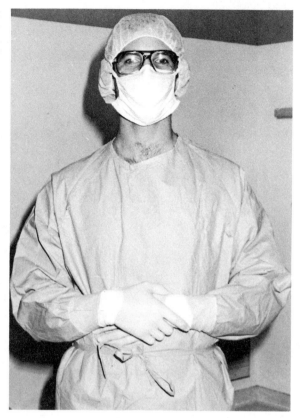

In treating dirty or infected cases, persons wearing special operating room shoes should also put on shoe covers. At the end of the operation, surgical team members should remove the shoe covers in the operating room and step into the hall immediately. Cap and mask should be removed just before leaving through the operating room doorway. Scrub suits (or scrub dresses) should be changed promptly, certainly before entering any clean operating room.

PREOPERATIVE DISINFECTION OR DEGERMING OF THE HANDS: THE SURGICAL SCRUB

As indicated earlier in this chapter, one must be properly attired in scrub suit, cap or hood, mask, and shoe covers prior to preoperative hand scrubbing. Current practice requires the surgeon to scrub his hands, fingernails, and arms meticulously, using an appropriate degerming method, immediately prior to the operative procedure. This aids in the reduction of the possibility of transferring microorganisms from the hands to the wounds. Thereafter, he puts on a sterile gown and sterile gloves in an aseptic manner to complete the bacterial barrier between him and the patient's

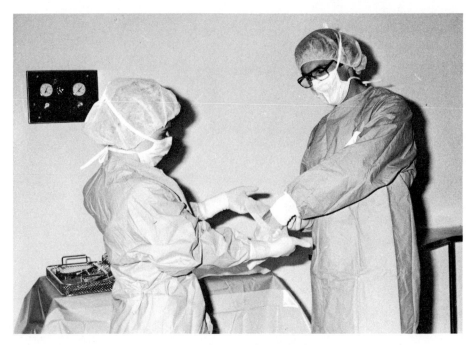

Fig. 7-7. Method recommended for members of a surgical team to prevent contamination when putting on sterile gloves.

operative wound (see Fig. 7-1, *B*). The surgical scrub is practiced to remove or destroy as many bacteria as possible on the skin and under the fingernails of the surgical team members.

The skin flora of the hands and forearms may be divided into "resident" and "transient" populations, as pointed out by Price. Lowbury has reported that the important practical distinction, however, is between superficial organisms, which can be almost completely removed either by washing with soap and water or by disinfection, and the more adherent microorganisms, which are much more effectively removed by disinfection than by washing.

The resident and transient groups of microorganisms represent contamination from the hospital environment and may include the beta-hemolytic *Streptococcus, Staphylococcus aureus, Pseudomonas, Escherichia coli,* and *Klebsiella,* among others. The coagulase-positive *Staphylococcus* is the most common potential pathogen of the deep or resident flora of the skin and fingernails. The gram-negative bacilli have been observed less frequently as part of the resident flora.

Resident bacteria form a comparatively stable flora. Protected skin has, as a rule, a somewhat larger resident flora than exposed skin (Price). After reduction (*e.g.,* by disinfection), reestablishment of the resident flora appears to proceed at a rate represented in general by a sigmoid curve, as is true of bacterial growth in cultures. Hands and arms thoroughly degermed may require a week or more for complete reestablishment of the usual flora. Beneath clothing the generation time is slightly shorter. Under sterile rubber gloves, it is much shorter, the existing flora increasing rapidly until they may exceed by far the ordinary flora.

Transient microorganisms lie free on the surface or are loosely attached along with the dirt by fats; hence, they are removed or killed with comparative ease. Resident bacteria are more firmly attached, and are far more resistant to attack by either detergents or germicides.

The transient flora may contain any number of pathogenic bacteria, the resident flora relatively few as a rule. Certain contaminating organisms, however, seem able to change status slowly and become permanent residents of the skin. Consequently, prolonged or frequent exposure of the skin to contamination may result in a resident flora containing many pathogenic organisms. Such skin is not easily disinfected, and hands may thus become chronic carriers of pathogenic organisms.

Scrubbing with a brush, degerming agent, and water removes the transient flora readily but the resident flora far more slowly. The most effective period of hand scrubbing is still debatable, but is thought to be between 5 and 10 minutes.

As indicated in Chapter 6, there is considerable difference of opinion about the best methods of preparing the skin of the operative area and the most effective types of degerming agents. The same differences of thought exist about the most efficient methods for the preoperative scrubbing and disinfection of the hands and forearms of the surgical team. It has been shown that many antiseptics remain on the skin after the scrub and continue to suppress the growth of bacteria, acting as a "chemical glove." Iodophors, chlorhexidine, and hexachlorophene are the antiseptics most frequently used for the surgical scrub. Such antiseptics, however, are often inactivated by blood, probably by the sulfhydryl groups in the blood cells. This is less evident in iodine solutions. Bernard and Cole have shown that blood from the operative wound may enter the glove through such holes and inactivate residues of antibacterial preparations left on the skin.

Antiseptics Most Frequently Used for the Surgical Scrub
Iodophors
> Iodophors are both good antiseptics with a quick and lasting effect and cleaning agents for the skin. They rarely irritate the skin or cause allergic reactions. They are free from irritating odors, are easily washed off, and do not react with metals. These characteristics have made the iodophors one of the three most commonly used degerming hand-scrubbing agents in use now.

Chlorhexidine
> Antiseptic solutions containing chlorhexidine compounds were used effectively in Great Britain (Lowbury 1972) and in Canada (Cruse 1972). Since its recent approval in the United States by the Food and Drug Administration (Hibiclens, Hibitane), chlorhexidine has been widely used here. It offers a wide range bactericidal activity for the skin, forearms, and hands of the surgical team. Its extensive use in Great Britain indicated that it could be used frequently without causing irritation, dryness, or skin discomfort.

Hexachlorophene
> Hexachlorophene takes time to work. There is less measurable reduction in microbial counts immediately after scrubbing with it, but an appreciable reduction is obtained after 1 hour. Used repeatedly over days, hexachlorophene will markedly reduce the bacterial counts on the hands by 99%, and it is very effective when used properly.

There is evidence that the successive use of two degerming agents can create a state of cleanliness and disinfection in which the hands of about half of those so treated do not transfer any bacteria to a washing fluid. Such specialized disinfection plus the use of two rubber gloves, one on top of the other, may be appropriate for operations on high-risk patients, such as those having immunosuppressive treatment for organ transplantation or for patients having total hip replacement. The Committee has decided to describe two selected effective methods of hand-scrubbing techniques that are in current use. These will provide the surgeon with alternatives to meet different circumstances.

Iodophor Hand Scrub Technique
1. Remove all jewelry and nailpolish.
2. Wash hands, forearms, elbows, and lower one third of upper arms with soap and water, using a sterile brush to remove surface dirt, oils, and other debris. (2 minutes)
3. Discard brush and use nail file or orange stick to thoroughly and meticulously clean the fingernails under running water. Fingernails should be kept short. (1 minute)
4. Using a clean, sterile brush and 2.5 ml of iodophor compound, scrub the entire surface of fingers, hands, forearms, elbows, and distal 2 inches of the upper arms, in that order (3 minutes). Rinse thoroughly with running tap water, always allowing excess water to drip from elbows, with the hands and forearms held higher than the flexed elbows.
5. Repeat #4. (2 minutes)
6. Repeat #5 without brush, and washing fingers, hands, and forearms only, below the elbows. (2 minutes)

A modification of the above iodophor compound scrub also in use is as follows:

1. Same as above
2. Same as above
3. Same as above
4. Using a sterile brush or sponge impregnated with iodophor compound, scrub the entire surface of the fingers, nails, hands, forearms, and distal 2 inches of the upper arms for $2\frac{1}{2}$ minutes. Rinse thoroughly with running tap water, allowing excess water to drip from elbows with hands held higher than the flexed elbows.
5. Repeat #4 for $2\frac{1}{2}$ minutes using the same technique; a 5-minute scrub is recommended between cases.

Chlorhexidine Hand Scrub Technique

There are several modifications in technique that are in active use at this time:

1.
2. } The same as recommended for the iodophor compound scrub
3.
4. Using a sterile brush or sponge impregnated with chlorhexidine compound, methodically scrub the entire surface of the fingers, fingernails, hands, forearms, and distal 2 inches of the upper arms at the elbow for $2\frac{1}{2}$ minutes; follow this by thoroughly rinsing with running tap water. Allow the excess antiseptic and water to drain from the elbows with the hands held higher than the flexed elbows.
5. Repeat #4 for $2\frac{1}{2}$ minutes.

BIBLIOGRAPHY

ALTEMEIER WA: Symposium on hospital-acquired staphylococcal infection. Part III. Recommendations for control of epidemic spread of staphylococcal infections in surgery. Ann Surg 150:774, 1959

ALTEMEIER WA: Control of wound infections. JR Coll Surg Edinb 11:271, 1966

ALTEMEIER WA: Surgical antiseptics. In Block SS (ed): Disinfection, Sterilization, and Preservation, 2nd ed. Philadelphia, Lea & Febiger, 1977

ALTEMEIER WA, BURKE J, PRUITT B, SANDUSKY W: Manual on Control of Surgical Infections in Surgical Patients. Committee on Control of Surgical Infections of the Committee on Pre- and Postoperative Care of the American College of Surgeons. Philadelphia, JB Lippincott, 1976

AMERICAN HOSPITAL ASSOCIATION: Infection Control in the Hospital, pp 100–105. Chicago, American Hospital Association, 1970

ANDERSON K: The contamination of hexachlorophene soap with *Pseudomonas pyocyanea*. Med J Aust 2(12):463, 1962

AYLIFFE GAJ: Surgical scrub and skin disinfection. Infect Control 5:23–27, 1984

BLANK IH, COOLIDGE MH, SOUTTER L, RODKEY GV: A study of the surgical scrub. Surg Gynecol Obstet 91:577, 1950

BRUUN JN, BOE J, SOLBERG CO: Disinfection of the hands of ward personnel. Acta Med Scand 184:417, 1968.

COLE WR, BERNARD HR: Inadequacies of present methods of surgical skin preparation. Arch Surg 89:215–222, 1964

CONNELL JF, ROUSSELOT LM: Povidone iodine: Extensive surgical evaluation of a new antiseptic agent. Am J Surg 108:849, 1964

CROMWELL WH, LEFFLER R: Evaluation of "skin degerming" agents by a modification of the Price method. J Bacteriol 43:51, 1942

CRUSE PJE, FOORD R: A five year prospective study of 23,649 surgical wounds. Arch Surg 107:206, 1973

CRUSE PJE, FOORD R: The epidemiology of wound infection. Surg Clin North Am 60(1):27, 1980

DEWAR NE, GRAVENS DL: Effectiveness of septisol antiseptic foam as a surgical scrub agent. Appl Microbiol 26:544–549, 1973

DINEEN P: An evaluation of the duration of the surgical scrub. Surg Gynecol Obstet 129:1181, 1969

DINEEN P, DRUSIN L: Epidemics of postoperative wound infections associated with hair carriers. Lancet 1:1157, 1973

DINEEN P, HILDICK-SMITH G: Antiseptic care of the hands. In Maibach HI, Hildick-Smith G (eds): Skin Bacteria and Their Role in Infection, p 291. New York, McGraw-Hill, 1965

EDMONDSON EB, PIERCE AK, SANFORD JP: Letter to the editor: *Pseudomonas aeruginosa* cross-infection. Lancet 1:660, 1966

EITZEN HE, RITTER MA, FRENCH ML, GIOE TJ: A microbiological in-use comparison of surgical hand-washing agents. J Bone Joint Surg 61(3):403–406, 1979

FURUHASHI M, MIYAMAE T: Effect of preoperative hand scrubbing and influence of pinholes appearing in surgical rubber gloves during operation. Bull Tokyo Med Dent Univ 26(2):73–80, 1979

GERSHENFELD L: Povidone-iodine as a topical antiseptic. Am J Surg 94:938, 1957

GROSS A, CUTRIGHT DE, DALESSANDRO SM: Effect of surgical scrub on microbial population under the fingernails. Am J Surg 138(3):463–467, 1979

HANDS SPREAD MORE INFECTION THAN AIR. Physicians report in California Modern Hospital 104:174, 1965

HART D: Bactericidal ultraviolet radiation in the operating room: Twenty-nine year study for control of infections. JAMA 172:1019, 1960

LOWBURY EJL, LILLY HA: Disinfection of the hands of surgeons and nurses. Br Med J 1:1445–1450, 1960

LOWBURY EJL, LILLY HA, BULL JP: Methods for disinfection of the hands and operative sites. Br Med J 2:531–536, 1964

LOWBURY EJL, LILLY HA: The effect of blood on disinfection of surgeons' hands. Br J Surg 61:19, 1974

MEERS PD, YEO GA: Shedding of bacteria and skin squames after hand-washing. J Hyg (Lond) 81(1):99–105, 1978

PETERSON AF, ROSENBERG A, ALATARY SD: Comparative evaluation of surgical scrub preparations. Surg Gynecol Obstet 146:63, 1978

PRICE PB: Surgical antiseptics. In Reddish GF (ed): Antiseptics, Disinfectants, Fungicides, and Chemical and Physical Sterilization, p 317. Philadelphia, Lea & Febiger, 1954

REINARZ JA, PIERCE AK, MAYS BB, SANFORD JP: The potential role of inhalation therapy equipment in nosocomial pulmonary infection. J Clin Invest 44:831, 1965

ROTTER ML: Hygienic hand disinfection. Infect Control 5:18–22, 1984

SELK SH, POGANY SA, HIGUCHI T: Comparative antimicrobial activity, in vitro and in vivo, of soft N-chloramine systems and chlorhexidine. Appl Environ Microbiol 43:899–904, 1982

SPRADLIN CT: Bacterial abundance on hands and its implications for clinical trials of surgical scrubs. J Clin Microbiol 11(4):389–393, 1980

WILLIAMS REO: Pathogenic bacteria on the skin. In Maibach HI, Hildick-Smith G (eds): Skin Bacteria and Their Role in Infection, p 49, New York, McGraw-Hill, 1965

8

The hospital is obligated to provide a clean, safe operating room environment for the surgeon and his patients. Unfortunately, there are no hard data that permit significant statements about the architectural design of operating rooms that will ensure a clean and safe environment for surgical practice (Bernard, 1983). However, there are certain routine preparations and maintenance procedures that are necessary to accomplish this end. As surgery has become more complex, prolonged, and extensive, new patterns and practices have become important as means of minimizing or excluding microbial contamination. These are designed to overcome the dynamic propensities of virulent bacteria to breach the barriers of aseptic technique, and to prevent significant contamination of injured or ischemic tissues, denuded bone, or implanted foreign bodies. Specific aseptic practices to prevent bacterial contamination of the operative field may require development in accord with priorities that emerge in given hospitals, and they depend upon the types of surgery practiced and the results of the surveillance of postoperative surgical complications.

It is generally agreed that most infections in postoperative surgical wounds are the result of seeding by endogenous bacteria. The methods of dealing with endogenous infections and their sources are described elsewhere and include dealing with the presence of foreign bodies, preoperative detection and control of associated infection (Chap. 6), careful and defensive surgical technique and avoidance of errors in surgical judgment (Chap. 9), treatment of related diseases and predisposing factors that increase the risk of infection (Chap. 9), and the thoughtful and judicious use of prophylactic antibiotics (Chap. 11). However, it must be kept in mind that microorganisms from exogenous sources are also of etiologic importance. Some areas in the operating room environment can become heavily contaminated by pathogenic microorganisms unless properly cleaned and disinfected. Significant potential exogenous sources to be considered are people; anesthesia equipment; operating room surfaces, such as walls, floors, and furniture; the operating

Preparation and Maintenance of a Safe Operating Room Environment

111

room air and dust; and instruments, supplies, and medications. The frequent contact of operating room personnel with the operating room environment and equipment with the potential of exchange of microorganisms in the hospital reservoir must be kept in mind. In a well-managed operating room, overt contact contamination should be uncommon. Covert contact usually results from unsterile parenteral intravenous setups, urinary catheterization, medication, implants, or anesthesia apparatus.

Disinfection of Operating Room Surfaces. There are many surfaces in the operating room that require daily dust removal and disinfection, including floors, walls, ceilings, furniture, and lights that are fixed or too large to be steam or gas autoclaved. *Disinfection* is defined as the destruction of disease-producing microorganisms (but generally not resistant spores), usually by use of chemical germicides or degerming agents, flowing steam, or ultraviolet radiation.

All surfaces must be thoroughly cleaned before specific methods of disinfection are applied. This is necessary to remove all foreign or organic matter that may preserve bacteria and negate the antimicrobial action of the antiseptic solution. Detergent germicides are available that clean and disinfect simultaneously. These may simplify work.

The *operating room floor,* the largest horizontal surface in the operating room to accumulate settling or floor traffic bacteria, cannot be ignored epidemiologically. A satisfactory floor for the operating room must have a homogenous surface free of cracks and pits in which soil might accumulate. Spalling terrazzo, loose ceramic tile, and deteriorated plastic tiles provide reservoirs of soil from which bacteria-laden particles are pumped into the air. A defective floor *cannot* be effectively disinfected. It may be heavily soiled by organic matter such as blood, pus, urine, or amniotic fluid that preserves bacteria and hinders disinfection as noted above. Activity scuffs flecks of such dried soil into the air to resettle elsewhere, depending upon air currents. To a lesser extent, the same is true of the walls, furniture, and equipment.

Dust and Dust Control. In addition to the operating room floors being clean and bacteriologically safe, they must also be *dust free.* The bacteriological count on the unused surface of the floor 12 hours after cleaning and disinfecting should be less than five organisms per square centimeter. There should be no dust, and airborne counts should not exceed one bacterium per cubic foot (Chap. 12). Dust on the floor is readily demonstrated by walking across it in stocking feet. The accumulation of white fuzz on a black sock indicates that too much dust is present. Airborne dust can be visualized by darkening the room except for the surgical light (Tyndall phenomenon). This permits the dust motes in the beam to be easily seen after activity.

Dust in the operating room is most readily controlled by correcting its source (Bernard). Faulty filtration of air is an obvious but often overlooked source of dust and airborne bacteria. Lint-laden textiles and other supplies used in the operating room may also serve as sources of dust. During washing, the soilage disintegrates and coats textiles. Friction of textile fibers against each other results in fragmentation, particularly of the cotton–synthetic blended materials. The application of a textile lubricant in the final rinse minimizes such linting. Abrasion of mops on ceramic floors results in lint contamination and particulates. Dust or lint settling on an aseptic field carries bacteria and increases contamination as the period of exposure of instruments, supplies, and solutions lengthens. Air contamination by bacteria has been demonstrated on two thirds of instruments, solutions, and supplies after a 4-hour intraoperative exposure. Contamination by dust particles is a factor that must be controlled. Dust particles can be reduced by the use of a wet vacuum and single-use gowns and drapes. Lint on textiles is suppressed by good laundry practices such as sorting trash from soiled laundry.

CLEANING THE OPERATING ROOM SUITE

A representative plan that can be recommended for effectively cleaning and disinfecting the operating room suite includes the following considerations:

I. General Remarks
    A. A phenolic detergent solution is recommended for wet-vacuuming of floors (Fig. 8-1) and all other fomite cleaning chores (one half ounce per gallon of water).
    B. Disposable or launderable cloths should be used with fresh solution for each task. Walls should be cleaned with a mop handle wrapped with a fresh hand towel or bath towel soaked in a phenolic detergent solution. The towel should be discarded immediately following use.

Fig. 8-1. Attendant wet-vacuuming the operating room floor after all equipment has been moved out of the way.

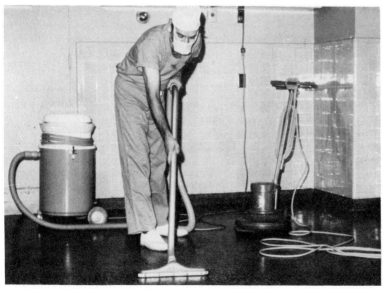

    C.   Clean all operating rooms daily. This includes furniture, lights, equipment, floors, window sills, ledges, scrub rooms, and sinks.

    D.   Clean the entire operating room complex thoroughly once a week.

II.   Daily General Cleaning Procedure

    A.   Before start of first cases (no sooner than one hour)

        1.   Damp-dust all equipment, furniture and lights.

        2.   Rewipe surgical light reflector shields with 70% isopropyl alcohol to remove the film left by the detergent.

    B.   Between cases

        1.   Gather all soiled towels, gloves, drapes, and gowns into a clean laundry bag and send to the laundry. Wrap wet linen or put in a plastic container so that there is no danger of bacteria-laden moisture wetting through.

        2.   Place all soiled instruments and other material in a plastic bag to be sent to the cleaning and preparation area. Terminal sterilizing eliminates occupational hazard.

        3.   Wipe down all used equipment, furniture, and lights.

        4.   Move the operating room table to the periphery of the room and wet vacuum a 3–4-foot perimeter around the operating site. Extend the area of vacuuming as necessary to adjacent areas of spillage or contamination.

        5.   When disposable suction is not available, wash the suction bottle and tubing with a disinfectant solution.

    C.   Terminal daily cleaning of operating rooms and scrub-up areas at the conclusion of scheduled cases

        1.   Remove all portable equipment from the room.

        2.   Wipe down window sills, overhead lights, cabinets, waste receptacles, equipment, and furniture with detergent-disinfectant solution and a cloth.

        3.   Wet-vacuum the total floor area. (Wet-mopping is generally considered a method of second choice.)

        4.   Clean and disinfect all casters. Remove pieces of sutures, wires, *etc.*

        5.   Inspect equipment for safety and proper working order. Unsatisfactory equipment should be removed from the room, marked with a tag noting what is wrong, and designated for repair.

        6.   Restock unsterile supplies.

        7.   Check levels and outdates of sterile supplies; clean cabinets and restock.

        8.   Check the room for all necessary furniture and equipment, and put these in their proper place.

        9.   Remove furniture and equipment not belonging in the room to its proper place.

      10.   Clean the air conditioning vent grills.

      11.   Clean scrub sinks in scrub-up areas with scouring powder applied with a wet sponge.

12. Empty all shelves, wipe them with detergent-disinfectant solution, and dry them before replacing supplies.

III. Weekly General Cleaning Procedure

 A. Remove all portable equipment. Damp-clean lights and fixtures with detergent-disinfectant solution and a cloth.

 B. Clean doors, hinges, facings, and glass inserts and rinse with a cloth wet with solution.

 C. Wipe down the walls with a clean sponge mop or wall-washing device wet with detergent-disinfectant solution.

 D. Scrub the floor with a floor machine using a phenolic detergent-disinfectant solution. Pick up the solution with a wet vacuum.

 E. If baseboards are present, scrub them before rinsing the floor, using a baseboard brush.

 F. Clean stainless steel kick plates and any stainless steel walls with solution. Rinse with clean, warm water.

 G. Replace clean portable equipment. In replacing equipment, clean the wheels and castors by rolling them across toweling or a pad saturated with detergent-disinfectant solution.

 H. Wash and dry all of the furniture and equipment, including
  1. The operating room table
  2. Suction holders
  3. All foot and sitting stools
  4. Mayo stands, IV poles, ring stands
  5. X-ray view boxes
  6. Hamper standards
  7. All tables in the room
  8. Hoses to oxygen tanks
  9. Kick buckets and holder (reline with plastic bags)
  10. Compartments recessed in walls
  11. Shelves of cupboards

The current trend of using sterile disposable single-use equipment eliminates the need for the disinfection of the reusable materials that they replace. *Note:* A clean cloth and detergent-disinfectant solution should be used for each room.

Other Comments and Notes

1. Specific germicide should be selected by the local hospital on the basis of its types of practice, any local problems, and authoritative consultation (see Table 8-1). Wet-vacuuming is the preferred method for cleaning floors.

2. If mops must be used in the operating room, they should be laundered and sterilized by autoclaves. Use a clean autoclaved mop head for each room. Use the two-bucket system. Develop a pattern for flooding, spreading, and picking up that avoids walking in the wet area or wetting the vacuum cleaner. When cleaning the operating room floor, allow the solution to remain on the floor for at least 5 minutes to ensure the destruction of all bacteria.

3. In large operating room suites, the use of a scrubbing machine that automatically dispenses detergent germicide is recommended because it is timesaving, convenient,

Table 8-1. Antiseptic Agents Recommended for Operating Room Floors, Walls, and Hard Surfaces

| Agent | Antibacterial Activity | | | | | Inactivation by Mucus, Proteins, or Organic Material |
	Gram +	Gram −	Proteus or Pseudomonas	Spores	TB	
Ethyl or isopropyl alcohol	+++	+++	+++	0	+	+++
Quaternary ammonium germicidal detergent	+++	+	±	0	0	+
Iodophor germicidal detergent	+++	+++	+++	+	0	++
Phenolic germicidal detergent	+++	+++	+	+	±	+++
Sodium hypochlorite	+	+++	+++	+	+	++++

and efficient. A wet pick-up vacuum cleaner is recommended to remove the slurry of dirt and bacteria loosened from the floor. In this way a clean, dust-free, and bacterially safe floor can be obtained more easily.

4. Cleaners should check with the room nursing supervisor to see which rooms should be cleaned first.
5. Cleaners assigned to the operating room must be attired in cap, scrub clothes, and bootees (conductive shoe covers).
6. If there is any delicate equipment in the operating room, such as a laser, care should be taken not to move or disturb it.
7. Cleaners should make sure when wiping off cabinets that disinfectant solution does not get inside and contaminate sterile supplies. Do not wash inside cabinets.
8. Prior to returning the operating room furniture to the cleaned room, it should be wiped, including the castors, with a germicide-saturated cloth.
9. Furniture should be replaced in rooms according to a diagram furnished by the operating room nursing supervisor.
10. Operating rooms and scrub rooms should never be dry-dusted.

Types of Antiseptic Agents

A large number of agents have been tested as germicidal solutions, and the nonvolatile iodophors or phenolics have been reported to remain active for days when properly applied to a suitable surface.

Chlorine and iodine are extremely rapid in their bacterial killing effect, but their residual activity is less. The quaternary ammonium compounds are bacteriostatic rather than bactericidal, and are lacking in sporicidal and tuberculocidal action. Phenolics are bactericidal for all organisms and possess some residual activity. Used properly, agents of any of these groups can effectively disinfect environmental surfaces. They should be allowed to remain wet on such surfaces for at least 5 to 10 minutes after their application. Hard water, the mop, soil, debris on the floor, and the flooring itself may all deplete the solution of its germicidal or detergent action. Enough of the agent must be used for cleaning to satisfy these affinities and leave a residue for antimicrobial effect.

Pathogenic microorganisms are affected unequally by chemical degerming agents, and there is no disinfectant that is universally effective (see Chap. 7). The effect of all chemical antimicrobial disinfectants can be decreased or neutralized by contact with organic materials such as proteinaceous substances, soaps, and various metals. Incompatibilities that exist must be known to the physician, nurse, or pharmacist and avoided. Some of the other more notable incompatibilities are as follows:

- Hexachlorophene may be neutralized by alcohols.
- The action of quaternary ammonium compounds is impaired by soaps and cotton; be sure to use copious amounts of these compounds.
- Iodine is neutralized by metals such as aluminum.

MAINTAINING A PROPER ENVIRONMENT
Ventilation

Airborne microbial contamination can occur in the operating room, and an effective ventilation system is necessary to minimize contamination from this source. Proper design and maintenance are important in controlling not only the number and types of airborne microorganisms that may be attached to dust particles, lint, or respiratory droplets, but also airstreams that carry and distribute them from one area to another. This matter may be particularly important in surgical operations involving high-risk patients such as the newborn, debilitated, or immunosuppressed. Poor ventilating systems permitting breathing of contaminated air may also predispose to upper respiratory infections or lead to an increase in the carrier state in operating room personnel.

As indicated in the Joint Commission on Accreditation of Hospitals Standards, the ventilation system should provide an effective, controlled, filtered air supply in designated critical areas, including the operating room, recovery room, and surgical intensive care unit. The number of changes per unit of time in any area should be as specified by the authority having jurisdiction in this matter.

Most operating rooms are ventilated by air drawn from outdoors. The air is cleaned, modified in temperature and humidity, and distributed to various rooms. The purpose of the ventilation generally determines the volume of air delivered into each room. Odor control and comfort have been the customary objectives, but the most important consideration is the provision of air as nearly dust-free as possible.

The current minimum requirements of the U.S. Public Health Service and the National Fire Protection Association for operating rooms call for the following: 25 volume changes per hour, positive operating room pressures as compared with surgical corridors, temperatures between 65°F and 75°F, and humidity of 50% to 55% (Laufman). Engineers are now suggesting that air be supplied at a higher rate of flow through ceiling panels directly over the operating table in operating rooms where high risk surgery is to be performed (Chap. 13). A quantity of air proportional to that introduced is exhausted in an attempt to maintain a slight positive pressure of at least 1 cm water within a room with closed doors. At these rates of ventilation, the concentration of a single dispersal of droplet nuclei falls to about 1% of its initial value in 45 minutes. Ventilation in the conventional sense thus contributes little to the control of continuously emitted microbes. The reason is obvious: at such low rates of flow, turbulence redistributes the organisms and insufficient clean air is provided to dilute the continuing cascades of organisms that become airborne. Air flow resulting from the opening of a door between adjoining spaces with different temperatures often moves airborne organisms more rapidly than the ventilating system.

The cleanliness and purity of ventilating air depends upon the design, location, installation, and maintenance of air-handling equipment. Improper location of the air intakes subjects the system to microbial contamination from chimneys, exhaust ducts, sanitary vents, engine exhausts, rookeries, garden litter, or dust from roofs or ledges. Airflow is often restricted by screens choked with leaves or feathers, filters laden with dust, or heat exchangers clogged by deposits of slime and dirt. Where poor location subjects the system to the possibility of such fouling, maintenance becomes a crucial factor, and greater precautions must be taken to filter the air downstream of the conditioning equipment. If pollution and contamination are hazardous in some situations, the air intake should be relocated. The air intake should be the highest point of the hospital structure; a penthouse is best. Unobstructed intake from all directions is essential to avoid the lee effect of wind. The penthouse must be large enough to permit snow or rain to disengage from the airstream. A vertical air intake duct opening above the screened louvers of the enclosing penthouse ensures satisfactory air. Unfortunately, such installations are rare.

Filters are used conventionally to remove trash and dust and are intended to prevent fouling of the heat exchangers. Such filters do not remove microorganisms. Bacteriological filters, such as 90% National Bureau of Standards filters, should be located downstream of the air-processing equipment to ensure trapping of bacteria and fungi. If humidification is effected at the diffuser, steam humidifiers must be used; other types inevitably become colonized with microorganisms that overgrow and contaminate the air.

Thermal gradients cause convection currents that stir the air vertically in the center of the room and militate against settling of bacteria on the aseptic field. Turbulent distribution helps eliminate static islands of air in the lee of personnel, instruments, or fixtures.

In the aseptic field, the use of overhead, wide-source ultraviolet radiation may help in the protection of the wound from airborne contamination by bacteria circulating in the room. Properly installed ultraviolet lamps provide a bactericidal barrier in the air. Ultraviolet radiation of the operating field during surgery has been claimed to reduce postoperative wound infections in special surgical cases. Neurosurgeons, in particular, using ultraviolet irradiation have reported consistently low rates over many years. In a study involving five collaborating hospitals, a reduction in the infection rate related to ultraviolet irradiation was confined to a special category ("refined clean") of operative wounds. In this group of elective, primarily closed, and undrained wounds, the infection rate was 2.9% for irradiated wounds; the control (not irradiated) group had an infection rate of 3.8%. In the total number of wounds surveyed and *in all other categories of wounds,* no benefit was demonstrated (Chap. 13).

If ultraviolet radiation is used, protective cream, goggles, and headgear must be used to prevent irritation and potential damage to the eyes and skin of the operating team. Its intensity on the operating field must also be measured daily with a calibrated meter. Twenty-five $\mu w/cm^2$ at the target (wound) is effective. The ultraviolet output of lamps depends upon the temperature of the lamp and its cleanliness. Since chilling by ventilating air causes low output, lamps must be protected against cold air. The film of grime that collects on the lamp must be removed twice weekly. It should be remembered that the bactericidal effect of ultraviolet radiation declines markedly when the relative humidity exceeds 55%, and that ultraviolet radiation does not disinfect dusty air, penetrate films of mucus, blood, or moisture, or reach areas in the shadow of the radiation.

Laminar Airflow. Laminar airflow (undirectional flow) is a special type of ventilation in which particle-free air is moved over the aseptic field at rates intended to sweep away particulates. Usually this is achieved by recirculating air within the operating room through high-efficiency particle air (HEPA) filters and diffusors that assure undirectional flow. Either downward or horizontal flow is used. Rates of airflow of 30 feet per minute to 600 feet per minute have been advocated, the usual rate being 90 feet. This is the equivalent of 240 air changes per hour in a 22-foot square operating room. In a multicenter randomized study on the incidence of postoperative sepsis after total hip or knee replacement, published in 1982 by Lidwell, Lowbury, and associates, the incidence of joint sepsis confirmed at operation 1 to 4 years later was about half that in those cases operated upon in the operating rooms with ultra-clean air as compared to those operated upon in rooms supplied by conventionally supplied air systems. When whole body exhaust ventilated suits were worn by the surgical team in an operating room ventilated with the ultra-clean air system, the incidence of infection was approximately one fourth that developing in operations performed in an operating room with conventional ventilation. In their series of 4133 operations of this type in the control group (conventional ventilation), the incidence of infection was 1.5%, as compared with the incidence of 0.6% in 3922 cases in which operations were performed under the ultra-clean air conditions. The advantages and the necessity of such systems are still controversial. Some specialty services, such as orthopaedics, have been attracted to their possibilities more than others have. Laminar flow systems are expensive, and it is obvious that more research is necessary to determine their true value and their limitations (Chap. 13).

Traffic Control

The complex and long surgical procedures of today require the close and intense activity of a large team of people and the use of many types of equipment. This situation has made the effective control of traffic in and through the operating room an important consideration in the prevention of wound infection. As indicated earlier, people are the principal sources of contact spread; this applies to both carriers and noncarriers. The chances of infection increase whenever and wherever personnel congregate. Limitation of certain aspects of human contact and separation of functional activities lessen the opportunities for person-to-person contact transfer of pathogenic bacteria.

A basic plan of traffic pattern control should be developed in each hospital for personnel, patients, equipment, soiled linen, and wastes. Architectural design is an important factor in providing a feasible and effective plan for traffic flow that will minimize contact between infected, noninfected, and high-risk patients. Surgical areas should be so designed that all personnel must pass through the dressing rooms before entering the operating rooms proper. In special instances, such as burn hospitals, consideration should be given to plans that completely separate clean or noninfected and infected cases.

Within the surgical suite, Walter has recognized three zones of basic function; outer, intermediate, and inner. The *outer zone,* or *interchange zone,* is the area of admistrative functions, where service, messenger, and sales personnel enter the department and dress in operating room garb, patients are received, and control functions are centered. The *intermediate zone,* or *restricted zone,* is the area of work, preparation, and storage. Outside personnel delivering to this area should not proceed to the inner zone unless they change clothes and put on appropriate operating room attire. The *inner zone,* or *sterile work zone,* is a restricted area; it includes the operating rooms, scrub areas, holding areas, and induction areas. Maximal cleanliness and asepsis should be maintained here, and unauthorized personnel should be excluded (Chaps. 10 and 17).

Waste and Contaminated Substances

All contaminated, soiled, and waste materials in the operating room, intensive care unit, or recovery room should be collected and sealed in plastic bags at the sites of origin and with minimum handling by personnel wearing rubber gloves. Wastes, secretions, excretions, and blood-stained material, particularly from patients in isolation, should be sealed in impervious plastic containers for prompt handling and transport within the hospital.

Storage Area

It has become increasingly apparent during the past 5 years that storage of sterile products on the hospital premises must be carefully managed. Selection of a proper storage area and provision of control measures for inventory and sterility are imperative.

The storage areas must be clean and dry, and must provide ambient temperature and humidity similar to that in the operating room. They must be free of vermin such as rats, mice, cockroaches, and silverfish. Security against tampering must be provided. Few hospitals have adequate facilities for proper storage of sterile supplies. Makeshift accommodations are often used, with corridors, stairwells, basements, garages, and other unused spaces being pressed into service. The need for adequate and safe storage is emphasized.

Control of inventory permits purchasing in economic quantities and ensures continuity of supply. Careful dating of cartons and packages permits sequential use. The use of the oldest supplies first helps to avoid deterioration from aging. Distribution of supplies within the hospital exposes the packages to the possibility of contamination and tampering. Delivery carts, storage cabinets, dressing carts, and bedside tables are possible sources of unknown contamination. The closer the item of supply approaches application to the diseased or injured patient, the more hazardous the contamination may have become.

BIBLIOGRAPHY

ALTEMEIER WA: Surgical Antiseptics. In Block SS (ed): Disinfection, Sterilization, and Preservation, 2nd ed, Chap 32, pp 641–653. Philadelphia, Lea & Febiger, 1977

ALTEMEIER WA, CULBERTSON WR, HUMMEL RP: Surgical considerations of endogenous infections: Sources, types and methods of control. Surg Clin North Am 48:227, 1968

AMERICAN HOSPITAL ASSOCIATION: Infection control in the hospital, 4th ed. Chicago, American Hospital Association, 1979

AYLIFFE GAJ, COLLINS BJ, LOWBURY EJL, WALL M: Protective isolation in single-bed rooms: Studies in a modified hospital ward. J Hyg (Camb) 69:511, 1971

BEALL AC JR: The ideal operating room environment for open heart surgery. Bull Am Coll Surg 55:39, 1970

BECK WC: Air systems requirements are revised by Hill-Burton Program. Bull Am Coll Surg 54:134, 1969

BENNETT JV, BRACHMAN PS (eds): Hospital Infections. Boston, Little, Brown & Co, 1979

BERNARD H: Personal communication, January 1983

BLAKEMORE WS, McVAUGH H, McGARRITY G, WALLACE HW, THURER RJ, CORIELL L: Infection by airborne bacteria with cardiopulmonary bypass. Surgery 70:830, 1971

CASON JS, JACKSON DM, LOWBURY EJL, RICKETTS CR: Antiseptic and aseptic prophylaxis for burns: Use of silver nitrate and of isolators. Br Med J 2:1288, 1966

CENTER FOR DISEASE CONTROL: Isolation Techniques for Use in Hospitals, 2nd ed (DHEW Publication No. [CDC] 78-8314). Washington, D.C., U.S. Government Printing Office, 1975

CENTER FOR DISEASE CONTROL: Guidelines for the Prevention and Control of Nosocomial Infections. Washington, D.C., U.S. Department of Health & Human Services, February, 1981

CHARNLEY J: Low Friction Arthroplasty of the Hip. New York, Springer-Verlag, 1979

CHARNELY JS: A clean-air operating enclosure. Br J Surg 51:202–205, 1964

CORIELL LC, BLAKEMORE WS, McGARRITY GJ: Medical applications of dust-free rooms. II. Elimination of airborne bacteria from an operating theatre. JAMA 203:1038, 1968.

CUNDY KR, BALL W (eds): Infection Control in Health Care Facilities. Baltimore, University Park Press, 1977

FITZGERALD RH, DECLAN RN, ILSTRUP DM, VAN SCOY RE, WASHINGTON JA, COVENTRY MB: Deep wound sepsis following total hip arthroplasty. J Bone Joint Surg (Am) 59:847–855, 1977

GAGE AD, DEAN DC, SCHIMERT G, MINSLEY N: Aspergillus infection after cardiac surgery. Arch Surg 101:384, 1970

GAINSBOROUGH H, GAINSBOROUGH J: Principles of Hospital Design. London, Architectural Press, 1964

GOODRICH EO JR, WHITFIELD WW: Air environment in the operating room. Bull Am Coll Surg 55:7, 1970

HART D: Bactericidal ultraviolet radiation in the operating room: Twenty-nine year study for control of infections. JAMA 172:1019, 1960

HOWARD JM ET AL: Postoperative wound infections: The influence of ultraviolet irradiation of the operating room and of various other factors. Ann Surg 160(Suppl):1–92, 1964

HUME KF: The operating theater designed for the surgeon. Hospital Association Journal (England) 34:14, 1965

IRVINE R, JOHNSON BL, AMSTUTZ HC: The relationship of genitourinary tract procedures and deep sepsis after total hip replacements. Surg Gynecol Obstet 139:701, 1974

JACOBS RH JR: The surgical center: A proposal for the reorganization of the surgical service. American Institute of Architects Journal 38:79–87, 1962

LANGER K: AORN standards for O.R. sanitation. AORN J 21(7):1223–1231, 1975

LAUFMAN H: The surgeon views environmental controls in the operating room. Bull Am Coll Surg (3):129–133; 156, 1969

LAUFMAN H: Operating room systems as seen by a surgeon. Hospitals 44:56, 1970

LAUFMAN H: Pressures for change: The scientific pressures. Hospitals 45:1, 1971

LAUFMAN H: Developments in operating room design and instrumentation. In Ray CS (ed): Medical Engineering, pp 661–681. Chicago, Year Book Medical Publishers, 1973

LAUFMAN H: Report of Inter-Society Commission for Heart Disease. Resources: Surgery Study Group. V. Plant and equipment. Circulation 52:A23–A41, 1975

LAUFMAN H: Section H — The Operating Room. In Bennett JV, Brachman PS (eds): Hospital Infections. Boston, Little, Brown & Co, 1979

LAUFMAN H: Airflow effects in surgery: Perspective of an era. Arch Surg 114:826–830, 1979

LAUFMAN H, LIU D, HARRIS C, VANDERNOOT A: Effects of moisture and pressure on bacterial permeation of operating room apparel. Ann Surg 181:857–862, 1975

LENNETT EH, BALOWS A, HAUSLER WJ, TRUANT JP: Manual of Clinical Microbiology, 3rd ed. Washington, D.C., American Society for Microbiology, 1980

LIDWELL OM: Hospital uses of uni-directional ("laminar") air flow. In Brachman PS, Eickhoff TC (eds): Proceedings of International Conference on Nosocomial Infections, pp 207–215. Chicago, American Hospital Association, 1971

LIDWELL OM (chairman): Report of the Committee on Ventilation in Operating Room Suites. Medical Research Council and Department of Health and Social Security, London, 1972

LIDWELL OM, LOWBURY EJL et al: Effect of ultraclean air in operating rooms on deep sepsis in the joint after total hip or knee replacement: A randomized study. Br Med J 285:10–14, 1982

LOWBURY EJL, BABB JR, FORD PM: Protective isolation in a burns unit: The use of plastic isolators and air curtains. J Hyg (Camb) 69:529, 1971

LOWBURY EJL, LIDWELL OM: Multi-hospital trial on the use of ultraclean air systems in orthopaedic operating rooms to reduce infection. J R Soc Med 71:800–806, 1978

MARKUS FE: Time and motions studies in the operating suite. Mod Hosp 78:83, 1952

MARKUS FE: Time and motions studies in the operating suite: Observations of typical problems. Mod Hosp 78:80, 1952

MARKUS FE: Time and motions studies in the operating suite: Major operating room. Mod Hosp 78:58, 1952

PUTSEP EP: Planning of Surgical Centers. London, Lloyd-Luke, Ltd, 1969

REBER H: Rationale and testing of degerming procedures. Infect Control 5:28–31, 1984

TODD MC: Disinfection of the floor to prevent cross-infection. Hospital Topics 37:80–81, 1959

U.S. DEPARTMENT OF HEALTH, EDUCATION, AND WELFARE: Minimum requirements of construction and equipment for hospitals and medical facilities (DHEW Publication No. [HRA] 79-14500). Washington, D.C., Government Printing Office, 1979

U.S. PUBLIC HEALTH SERVICE: General Standards of Construction and Equipment for Hospital and Medical Facilities. (Publication No. 930-A07). Washington, D.C., U.S. Government Printing Office, 1969

WALTER CW: Control of infection in the operating room calls for good design and safe management. Mod Hosp 78:105, 1952

WALTER CW: Ventilation and air conditioning as bacteriologic engineering. Anesthesiology 31:186, 1969

WALTER CW, KUNDSIN RB: Floor as a reservoir of hospital infections. Surg Gynecol Obstet, 111:412, 1960

WALTER CW, KUNDSIN RB, BRUBAKER MM: The incidence of airborne wound infection during surgery. JAMA 186:908–913, 1963

WILLIAMS REO, BLOWERS R, GARROD LP, SHOOTER RA: Hospital Infections: Causes and Prevention, 2nd ed. Chicago, Year Book Medical Publishers, 1966

9

VARIABLES IN THE OPERATING ROOM

Surgical operative technique is another important factor affecting the occurrence and rate of infection in surgical patients. Although microorganisms are a necessary cause of infections, there are other important factors to be considered. Many of these nonmicrobial factors are related to surgical technique, and a comprehensive knowledge and understanding of them as significant determining factors of wound infection are important to clinical surgeons and other members of the surgical team.

Some degree of bacterial contamination of open wounds, whether produced by accidental injury or induced by surgical operation, usually can be demonstrated by bacteriological cultures of wound surfaces. Clean surgical wounds that heal *per primam* are regularly contaminated by airborne microorganisms; some of these contaminants may be highly virulent, others less so, and still others saprophytic. Fortunately, only a relatively small percentage of such wounds develop actual wound sepsis, and this fact emphasizes the necessity of recognizing the nonmicrobial factors that influence the growth and invasiveness of bacteria in the wound and determine whether or not a septic process develops.

Types, Numbers, and Virulence of Contaminating Bacteria

The types and numbers of contaminating bacteria can increase the probability and the severity of wound infection (Chap. 5). As indicated above, the mere presence of virulent bacteria in a wound does not make infection of that wound a certainty. It is generally conceded that bacterial density of 10^5 of a virulent strain of a pathogen is an important determinant of wound infection. Evidence indicates that the physiological state of tissues within the wound before and after treatment is more important than the mere presence of bacteria. Bacterial synergism or symbiotic activity may also contribute to the phenomenon of infection.

The Influence of Operating Techniques on the Rate of Wound Infection

Presence and Amount of Devitalized Tissue Within the Wound. It should be remembered that healthy, viable tissue possesses considerable resistance to microbial growth and action. In contrast, the presence or development of traumatized, irritated, or dead tissue in wounds may support and enhance the growth of both virulent and nonvirulent bacteria because of the limited power of resistance to their growth and invasive action. Excessive pressure and tension on tissues impair circulation of arterial and venous blood, slow lymph flow, alter the local physiological state of the wound, and predispose to bacterial colonization; therefore, pressure and tension should be minimal. In an operative wound with tissue damage caused by rough handling of tissues, ligatures, or large "bites" of tissues, pressure from retractors, or other factors that impair circulation, the incidence of infection and altered wound healing will be increased. Consequently, such practices should be avoided.

In the surgical management of wounds of trauma and violence, adequate debridement to excise all necrotic and devitalized tissue, preservation of the blood supply, and removal of foreign bodies are important practices. The significance of devitalized tissue and foreign bodies buried in the wound as a determinant of gas gangrene was demonstrated in the experiments of Altemeier and Furste. They showed in experimental animals that the pathogenicity of a virulent strain of *Clostridium perfringens* was enhanced one million times when injected into closed wounds containing lacerated and crushed muscle contaminated with sterile dirt. If the electrocoagulator is used, the production of numerous areas of necrotic tissue should be prevented, since these areas are more susceptible to bacterial growth and infection.

To avoid drying of tissues during long procedures, it is advisable to irrigate them periodically with saline solution and to cover "raw" surfaces with saline-moistened sponges or laparotomy pads or tapes.

Bacterial Barriers. Since numerous studies have shown that the skin of patients cannot be sterilized, various measures may be used for protection of the wound edges from bacteria resident on the skin surface and in the hair follicles and sebaceous glands. Bacterial barriers of uncertain effectiveness have been used on wound edges to minimize bacterial contamination from other sources, both endogenous and exogenous, during surgical procedures. Used for this purpose are wound towels, adhesive skin drapes, moist laparotomy pads over raw surfaces, and laparotomy wound plastic inserts (Cole and Bernard; see also Chap. 6).

Nature, Location, and Duration of the Wound

Wound sepsis is more prone to develop in extensive wounds containing large amounts of devitalized tissues, especially muscle, fascia, and bone (Fig. 9-1). As indicated previously, such wounds furnish excellent cultural material for bacteria. Several pounds of damaged muscle tissue may be present in wounds of the thigh and buttocks, and these large devitalized masses may become infected. Wounds that are

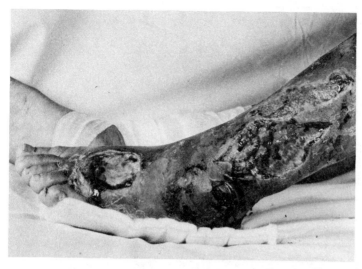

Fig. 9-1. Post-traumatic infection with extensive cellulitis and necrosis of a foot and leg wound of a severe diabetic patient.

produced by crushing or blast injuries and associated with heavy contamination are frequently multiple and characterized by extensive tissue destruction, severe shock, vascular injuries, and early wound sepsis (Fig. 9-2; see also Presence and Types of Foreign Bodies).

The location of the wound is of significance because various tissues in different locations in the body are known to have different powers of local resistance to infection. The amount and condition of tissue vascularity are important determinants of resistance in wounds. Lacerations of the face and neck, for example, are prone to heal neatly unless they communicate with the mouth and the pharynx. Wounds of the perineal area show a greater tendency toward infection.

The multiplicity of severe wounds in one person may compromise his treatment and make adequate debridement of one or more wounds impossible. Because of severe shock, hemorrhage, or associated wounds of the chest and head, the local treatment of wounds may necessarily assume a relatively minor role in relation to the early treatment of the whole patient. Antibiotic therapy, anti-tetanus prophylaxis, and application of sterile wound dressings are important under these circumstances.

Presence and Types of Foreign Bodies

Foreign bodies in wounds frequently harbor large numbers of bacteria and enhance the probability of infection through their local irritative action on tissues. Foreign bodies such as dirt, gravel, cinders, bits of clothing, and fragments of wood, metal, or glass increase the ability of contaminating bacteria to infect the wound. This has

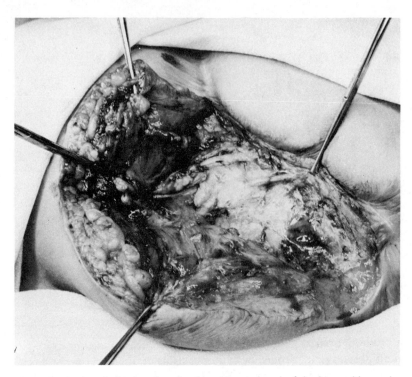

Fig. 9-2. Serious infection that developed in a wound of the hip and buttocks associated with other crushing injuries, which necessitated delayed or incomplete debridement.

been clearly demonstrated experimentally in a study of gas gangrene in animals by Altemeier and Furste, who found that the minimal lethal dose of a highly virulent strain of *Clostridium welchii* was decreased one million times in the presence of crushed muscle and sterile dirt.

It must be kept in mind that although sutures embedded in tissues are foreign bodies, they are necessary for the practice of surgery. The proper technical use of sutures, therefore, becomes important; the surgeons should be particularly attentive to the types of sutures, their spacing, the depth of "bites" taken, and the degree of tension necessary to bring tissues in apposition (Fig. 9-3). Techniques of wound closure are especially important in relation to the incidence of postoperative wound infections. The judgment of whether a wound can be closed primarily with safety and without the threat of developing infection is critical, and such wounds should be differentiated from those wounds that are to be left open and allowed to heal by secondary intention, or subjected to delayed closure in 5 to 8 days.

The choice of suture material and its size must depend on the purpose for which it is intended, as well as on the training, experience, and judgment of the surgeon. Any

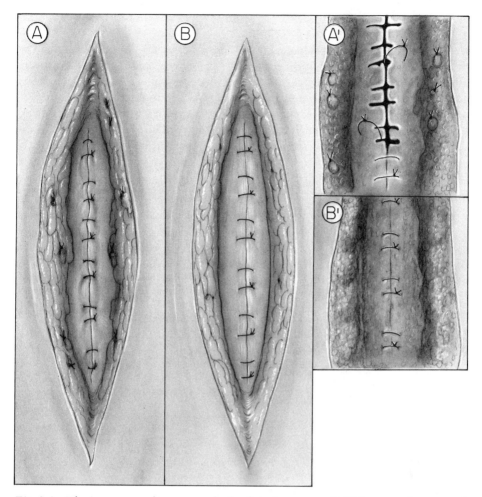

Fig. 9-3. The improper and proper methods of closing a wound. With an equal amount of contamination, wound *A*, which has been traumatized and for which the sutures were tied too tightly, runs a much greater chance of suppuration than does wound *B*, in which the tissues have been properly approximated and no devitalized tissue has been left in the wound. (*A'* and *B'*) The same wounds opened several days later. Neither one was infected, but the drawings tell their own stories. (Redrawn from Reid MR: Some considerations of the problems of wound healing. N Engl J Med 215:753, 1936)

of a variety of sutures may be selected and used effectively in most instances. The suture should excite only minimal reaction in the tissues and not the development of a local situation attractive to microbial growth.

The use of silk, cotton, or other nonabsorbable sutures requires strict aseptic technique and gentleness in handling tissues. Under such circumstances, healing progresses well with minimal induration and a low rate of infection. Within the peritoneal cavity, they may be used in the presence of infection or gross contamination.

In other instances of gross contamination or infection, catgut, steel wire or fasciae, Polyglycol, Dacron, or Teflon may be used, depending upon the circumstances. In penetrating wounds of the abdomen, it may be advisable to close laparotomy wounds with through-and-through wire sutures after the method of Reid, Zinninger, and Merrill (Fig. 9-4), or by using Jones' figure-of-eight suture.

Alexander, Altemeier, and Kaplan (1967) studied the relationship of different suture materials to wound infection. Their investigations indicated that monofilament sutures of any type were superior to multifilament sutures in contaminated wounds, and that multifilamented sutures and plain catgut were less effective for prevention of infection in the closure of contaminated wounds.

Fig. 9-4. Through-and-through wire closure of the abdominal wall. (*A* and *B*) Simple fast closure used for eviscerated or badly contaminated abdominal wounds. The wires are laid with a large hand needle and must be properly spaced. (*C*) A layer closure can be added, if the condition of the patient and of the wound permits. Heavy clamps temporarily applied to the wires at the point of proper tension allow closure of the peritoneal and fascial layers before the wires are twisted. (Redrawn from Altemeier WA, Wulsin JH: Wound healing. In Rothenberg ER [ed]: Reoperative Surgery, p 37. New York, McGraw-Hill, 1964)

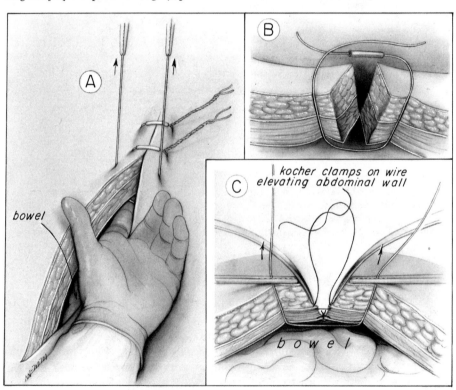

HEMOSTASIS, SEROMA, AND DEAD SPACE

It is generally recognized that careful attention to hemostasis is of great importance in the prevention of postoperative wound infection, yet this principle is too often disregarded. The accumulation of blood or serum among the various levels of the wound results in hematomas, seromas, or "dead spaces," which in turn cause separation of the wound walls, delay wound healing, and predispose toward the development of infection by providing a favorable environment for the growth and invasion of microorganisms. The surgeon is, therefore, reminded that hemostasis should be as complete as the particular operation will allow. Blood vessels should be secured by clamping with as little adjacent tissue as possible and ligation with the finest appropriate material. Under some circumstances, focal electrocoagulation of the vessels *per se* may be done.

TYPE, TIME, AND THOROUGHNESS OF TREATMENT

The development of wound sepsis is influenced by the type, time, and thoroughness of treatment more than many surgeons realize. Of primary importance is the surgical excision and removal of all devitalizing tissue and foreign bodies within the wound, preferably within 6 to 10 hours after injury in order to remove any potential pabulum before invasive bacterial growth can occur. Likewise, care must be exercised to prevent devitalization of tissues during the postoperative state with consequent decrease in the local blood supply. Impairment of the blood supply by thrombosis or damage to large vessels, by the displacement of fractures, by the pressure of hematomas, by tourniquets or ill-applied casts, or by increased tension from swelling or tension by sutures favors the delayed development of devitalized tissue and decreases the local resistance of tissues, which increases the possibility of infection.

Use of Drains

In certain situations, the use of drains is indicated to facilitate the drainage of blood, serum, pus, or secretions that are anticipated postoperatively. There are many types of drains that have been developed for these purposes.

The generally accepted reasons for drainage of wounds, operative areas, and viscera include the following:

1. To drain an abscess cavity so that it can collapse and heal from the deepest portion (Fig. 9-5)
2. For removal of blood, serum, exudates, and foreign material from operative wounds to prevent the development of hematomas, seromas, and dead space conducive to the development of wound infections (Fig. 9-6)
3. Anticipated leakage of bile or digestive enzymes, such as from the gallbladder bed, biliary tract, or pancreas, where small ducts may have been divided by trauma or an operation

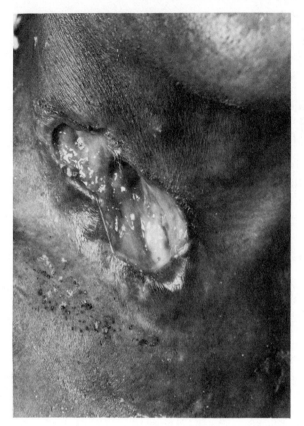

Fig. 9-5. Staphylococcal infection that occurred in an accidental wound. The wound has been reopened throughout its entire length. Some of the remaining thick creamy pus is apparent at the angle of the wound. Granulation tissue has developed near the posterior end of the wound.

4. After severe trauma with extensive soft tissue injury, when debridement may necessarily be incomplete, when foreign bodies may not have been removed, or when extensive contamination is inevitable
5. To effect early adherence of the tissues and surfaces of wounds through the use of suction drainage applied to indwelling catheters (Fig. 9-7)
6. To provide drainage in the vicinity of an insecure closure of a hollow viscus, such as an anastomosis, because of questionable blood supply, tension, infection, integrity of a suture line, or any serious general metabolic abnormalities

Generalized peritonitis *per se* is not always an indication for drainage. Drains are placed in the peritoneal cavity in the presence of thick pus, foul-smelling pus, residual devitalized and infected tissues, or injuries to the pancreas, liver, or biliary tract. It is widely recognized that drainage of the general peritoneal cavity is physically and physiologically impossible.

When oozing of blood or transudation of fluid is expected, the use of tubes with multiple perforations is recommended, attached to a low-pressure suction device and placed in wounds or under skin flaps. This technique is not limited to the

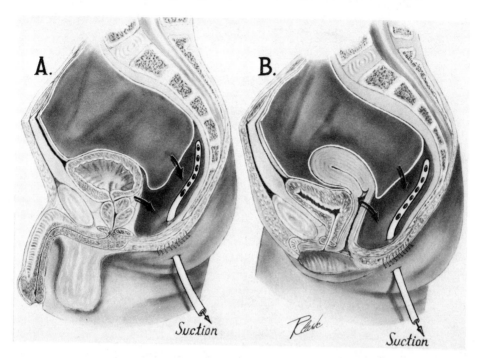

Fig. 9-6. Sagittal drawings of the postoperative use of continuous suction drainage applied to the operative pelvic wound cavity after abdominal perineal resection, (*A*) in the male and (*B*) in the female. Suction prevents the accumulation of serum and blood, and draws the peritoneum and other tissues in apposition to promote healing and help prevent infection.

abdomen, it is also particularly useful after radical mastectomy, radical neck dissection, and primary closure of perineal wounds after abdominoperineal resections for carcinoma of the rectum or rectosigmoid (Figs. 9-7 and 9-8). Drainage of chest wounds under water seal is also important. The use of sump drainage through special tubes is preferred by some surgeons, particularly in cases of pancreatic or duodenal drainage.

OTHER FACTORS PREDISPOSING AND CONTRIBUTING TO WOUND INFECTIONS

There has been an increased awareness that other factors may predispose or contribute to the development of wound infection.

Local and General Immunity Response of the Patient

The relative importance of the immune responses of the individual has become increasingly apparent. This subject is considered in detail in Chapters 5, 11, and 12.

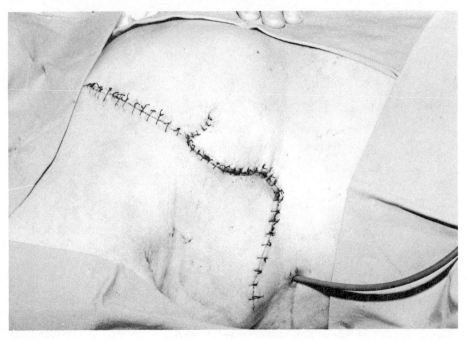

Fig. 9-7. Use of sterile suction catheter drainage of radical mastectomy wound five days postoperative for carcinoma. The catheter had been introduced through a lower axillary stab wound. Total serosanguinous drainage 110 ml. Wound healed per primam.

General Physical Condition of the Patient

Dehydration, shock, malnutrition, uremia, uncontrolled diabetes, anemia, and various associated diseases listed in Table 9-1 may lower the patient's resistance sufficiently to enhance the chances for bacterial growth and wound sepsis. Other contributing factors include advanced age of the patient, marked obesity, the presence of active remote areas of infection, and debilitating injuries (Howard and associates, and Altemeier).

Diabetes. In the collaborative five-university Ultraviolet Collaborative Study, the incidence of surgical wound infection in 356 diabetic patients was 10.4%, significantly higher than the overall infection rate. This higher rate may have been related in part to the large number of elderly patients constituting the diabetic group. It should be kept in mind that diabetes may be a senescent change that impairs the elderly patient's resistance to infection.

Obesity. Severe obesity was found to be associated with an infection rate of 18.1%, confirming the belief of experienced surgeons. In this collaborative study,

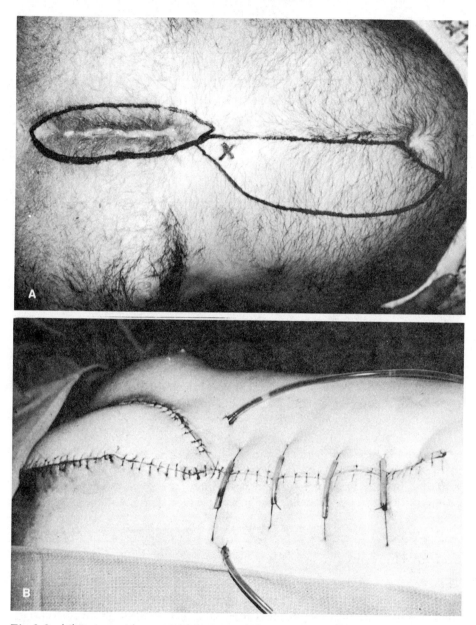

Fig. 9-8. (*A*) Patient with sternal dehiscence and chronic infected wound showing surgeon's mapped plan for its excision and replacement by a rectus myocutaneous flap. (*B*) Appearance of operative wound 5 days later after closure of the operative wound and the use of two suction catheters for drainage. Wound healed per primam. (Courtesy of Henry Neale, M.D.)

Table 9-1.   Effect of Metabolic and Nutritional Conditions on Incidence of Infection: USPH/NRC Ultraviolet Collaborative Study

Factors	Number of Wounds	Infection (%)
None	14,800	7.1
Diabetes	356	10.4
Steroid therapy	119	16.0
Severe obesity	166	18.1
Severe malnutrition	67	22.4
Unknown	129	9.3
Total*	15,613	7.4

* Since a few patients had more than one of the specific factors listed, the sums of the wounds and infections exceed the totals.

the operative procedures on these patients tended to be longer than the average, but adjustment for the duration of operation appeared to reduce the rate only slightly, to 16.5%.

Malnourishment.   Of the 67 severely malnourished patients who underwent surgery in this same study, 15 developed wound infection, an incidence of 22.4%, suggesting that this group of patients represents a population of high risk. Many of these patients, however, were older, had longer operations, or had operations more likely to be associated with greater contamination than the average.

Remote Infection.   Patients who harbor infection remote from the operative incision have been found to be at higher risk for the development of wound infection. In the Ultraviolet Collaborative Study, there was an infection rate of 18.4% in this group of patients, but it was 6.7% in those without such remote infection.

Steroid Therapy

The infection rate for 119 patients receiving steroid therapy was 16%, more than twice the rate for all patients. The patients receiving steroid therapy, however, tended to be older, had longer procedures, and had been in the hospital longer preoperatively than had the average patient. It should be remembered that the symptomatic relief often observed after the use of adrenocorticosteroids should be weighed against the potential danger of suppressing the host's response to infection. Weakening of host defenses may involve the depression of antibody formation, alteration of vascular reactivity, diminished phagocytic capacity, and suppression of the reparative process through new capillary formation and fibrogenesis (Chap. 5).

Table 9-2. Incidence of Infection Related the Hour Operation Began:
USPH/NRC Ultraviolet Collaborative Study

Time Operation Began*	Number of Wounds	Number of Infections	Infection Rate (%)
0730–0929	5,921	382	6.5
0930–1229	4,542	332	7.3
1230–1529	3,152	245	7.8
1530–2359	1,280	140	10.9
0000–0729	564	46	8.2
Unknown	154	12	7.8
Totals	15,613	1,157	7.4

* Military time

Time of Operation

It has also been interesting to note the relationship of the incidence of postoperative infections to the scheduled time of operation, the duration of operation, the use of prophylactic antibiotic therapy, and the presence of active remote infection.

Higher infection rates have been encountered in the later hours of the day, and these appear to be explainable almost entirely by the type of operative procedure performed. The data in the Collaborative Ultraviolet Study, however, indicated that the time of day at which an operation begins could not be considered a primary determinant of the rate of wound infection (Table 9-2).

Table 9-3. Incidence of Infection Related to Duration of Operation:
USPH/NRC Ultraviolet Collaborative Study

Duration of Operation (min)	Number of Wounds	Number of Infections	Infection Rate (%)
0–29	1,340	48	3.6
30–59	3,055	181	5.9
60–119	5,671	363	6.4
120–179	2,806	253	9.0
180–239	1,295	129	10.0
240–299	651	71	10.9
300–359	337	52	15.4
360 or more	267	47	17.6
Unknown	191	13	6.8
Total	15,613	1,157	7.4

Duration of Operation

As the duration of operation increases, a progressive increase in the infection rate generally can be expected, although exceptions to this may occur. It was of interest to note that this relationship was demonstrated rather consistently in the experience of each of the five hospitals in the Ultraviolet Collaborative Study (Table 9-3).

SUMMARY

It must be concluded that surgical sepsis is a complex phenomenon that is real, significant, continuing, and changing. The discovery and application of the germ theory of infection, antiseptic and aseptic techniques, and antibiotic therapy during the past 100 years have produced revolutionary effects on the one hand, but failure in reducing the overall incidence of infection in surgery on the other. Although we have been successful in preventing or controlling some types of infections, others have taken their places, and the overall incidence has continued to be a serious problem of worldwide scope.

The relative importance of nonbacterial factors have become more and more apparent as determinants of wound infection. A better understanding of these factors and a thoughtful incorporation of this understanding in surgical practice should be valuable assets in the prevention and control of surgical infections.

BIBLIOGRAPHY

ALEXANDER JW, ALTEMEIER WA, KAPLAN JZ: Role of suture materials in the development of wound infection. Ann Surg 165:192, 1967

ALEXANDER JW, KORELITZ J, ALEXANDER NS: Prevention of wound infections: A case for closed suction drainage to remove wound fluids deficient in opsonic proteins. Am J Surg 132:59–63, 1976

ALEXANDER JW, MONCRIEF JA: Alterations of the immune response following severe thermal injury. Arch Surg 93:75, 1966

ALTEMEIER WA: The significance of infection in trauma (Scudder oration). Bull Am Coll Surg 57(2):7, 1972

ALTEMEIER WA, FURSTE WL: Gas gangrene. Surg Gynecol Obstet 84:507, 1947

BERNARD HR, COLE WR: Wound isolation in prevention of postoperative wound infections. Surg Gynecol Obstet 125:257–260, 1967

CRUSE PJE, FOORD R: A five year prospective study of 23,649 surgical wounds. Arch Surg 107:206, 1973

CRUSE PJE, FOORD R: The epidemiology of wound infection. Surg Clin North Am 60(1):27, 1980

DAVIDSON AI, CLARK C, SMITH G: Postoperative wound infection: A computer analysis. Br J Surg 8:47–48, 1970

ELEK SD, CONEN PE: The virulence of *Staphylococcus pyogenes* for man: A study of the problems of wound infection. Br J Exp Pathol 38:573–586, 1957

HOWARD JM ET AL: Postoperative wound infections: The influence of ultraviolet irradiation of the operating room and of various other factors. Ann Surg (Suppl) 160:1–192, 1964

MELENEY FL: The study of the prevention of infection in contaminated accidental wounds, compound fractures, and burns. Ann Surg 118:171, 1943

MELENEY FL, WHIPPLE AO: A statistical analysis of a study of the prevention of infections in soft part wounds, compound fractures, and burns with special reference to the sulfonamides. Surg Gynecol Obstet 80:263, 1945

MILES AA, MILES EM, BURKE J: The value and duration of defense reactions of the skin to the primary lodgement of bacteria. Br J Exp Pathol 38:79–96, 1957

NICHOLS RL: Techniques known to prevent postoperative wound infection. Infect Control 3(1):34–37, 1982

PRUITT BA JR, FOLEY FD, MONCRIEF JA: Curling's ulcer: A clinical-pathological study of 323 cases. Ann Surg 172:523, 1970

REID MR: Some considerations of the problem of wound healing. N Engl J Med 215:753, 1936

REID MR, STEVENSON J: The treatment of fresh wounds. Surg Gynecol Obstet 66:313–319, 1938

WRIGHT RL: Septic Complications of Neurosurgical Spinal Procedures. Springfield, IL, Charles C Thomas, 1970

ZINNINGER MM, REID MR, MERRILL P: Closure of the abdomen with through-and-through silver wire sutures in cases of acute abdominal emergencies. Ann Surg 98:890, 1933

10

In-Hospital
(Nosocomial)
Infections
Other Than
Surgical
Wound
Infections

SOURCES

The hospitalized surgical patient has many opportunities to acquire infections. A nosocomial infection is one that is caused by microorganisms acquired during a patient's hospitalization. Infections that were incubating at the time of admission are *not* nosocomial infections. A nosocomial infection can occur in any anatomical location, and may assume any of a variety of clinical patterns ranging in intensity from that of scarcely recognizable symptoms and signs to that of life-threatening alterations of organ function.

Many diagnostic and therapeutic techniques carry with them a certain risk of infection for hospitalized patients and personnel. The most frequent sites for these nosocomial infections are the urinary tract, the respiratory tract and pleural cavity, the bloodstream, and the alimentary tract and peritoneal cavity. Estimates of the incidence of hospital-acquired surgical infections may vary between 2.5% and 15%, with an average of 7%.

Microorganisms enter the hospital in or on people and inanimate objects, air currents, and occasionally lower animals and insects. Within the hospital they are harbored in or on a variety of reservoirs, including patients with infections, healthy carriers, inanimate surfaces, particles capable of being airborne (*e.g.,* dust, lint, or shed epidermal squames), unsterile solutions, food, lower animals, and insects. In these reservoirs the pathogens may acquire higher virulence and greater antimicrobial resistance. From the reservoirs, they may be disseminated by contact or by air to hospital personnel or patients. Many patients are especially vulnerable to infection because of underlying disorders, host-compromising therapy, trauma, invasive procedures, or surgical operations (Fig. 10-1).

Measures to reduce or control nosocomial infections include sterilization of supplies and equipment, aseptic treatment techniques, isolation practices, the judicious use of antimicrobial agents, frequent disinfection of hands, prompt disposal of trash, and, in selected cases, special techniques and procedures of preoperative and postoperative care.

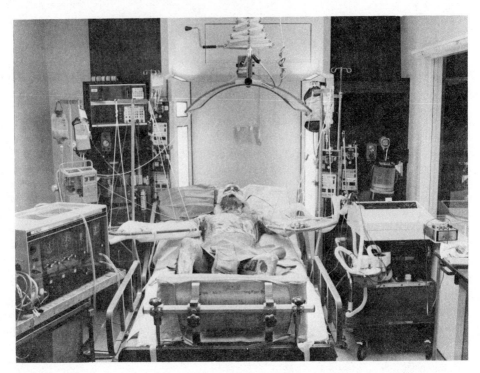

Fig. 10-1. A severely injured or, as shown here, an extensively burned patient requires support of numerous organ systems. Each of the monitoring and treatment devices represents a potential portal of entry for microorganisms, and mandates meticulous aseptic technique and assiduous patient surveillance for the prevention and early diagnosis of treatment-related infection.

These measures must be applied with particular care in the three distinct areas of the operating room recognized by Walter as being important sites for introduction and spread of bacteria within the hospital environment, that is, (1) the interchange area open to personnel generally; (2) the restricted area in which only authorized personnel properly attired are admitted; and (3) the sterile work area in the center of the operating room occupied by the surgical team.

During the past 15 to 20 years, the pattern of hospital-acquired or nosocomial infection has shifted from one in which the gram-positive staphylococcus was the major offender to one in which the aerobic gram-negative bacilli predominate. Between 1942 and 1956, studies of microbial etiology of surgical infections showed that approximately two thirds of the surgical infections were caused by the gram-positive cocci, particularly *Staphylococcus aureus,* the beta-hemolytic *Streptococcus,* and *Pneumococcus.* Since 1956, however, and particularly since 1965, there have been significant changes in the types of infections seen in surgical practice. These changes have included an increase in the incidence of gram-negative infections; the development of superimposed or secondary infections during antibiotic therapy; an increasing incidence of gram-negative infections by bacteria formerly recognized as having little or no virulence; the association of an increasing number of infections with atypical microbial variants such as L-forms; and a greater incidence of infections by fungi and viruses (Fig. 10-2).

There exist certain common factors that are important determinants in the occurrence of nosocomial infection. First, such infections occur within an environment in which antibiotic-resistant bacteria predominate, including hospitals, animal feed mills, and antibiotic processing plants. Second, nosocomial infections may develop in persons with anatomical or physiological defects in their antibacterial defenses — a feature of the hospital patient. Within the framework of these determinants, a variety of bacteria currently may be incriminated. The bacteria most often involved in nosocomial infections have been *Escherichia coli, Staphylococcus aureus, Proteus, Pseudomonas aeruginosa,* and *Serratia.* Altemeier and co-workers have observed that approximately 80% of serious infections by these bacteria developed while patients were on antibiotic prophylaxis or therapy for other infections. These

Fig. 10-2. Invasive fungal infection (phycomycosis) produced the black discoloration of the burn wounds of the chest wall and posterolateral aspect of the right arm of this patient. The hemorrhagic discoloration of the subcutaneous tissue in the infraclavicular biopsy site (*arrow*) is a characteristic change. At operation the fungi were found to be invading the intercostal muscles. (U.S. Army Institute of Surgical Research, Brooke Army Medical Center, Fort Sam Houston, Texas)

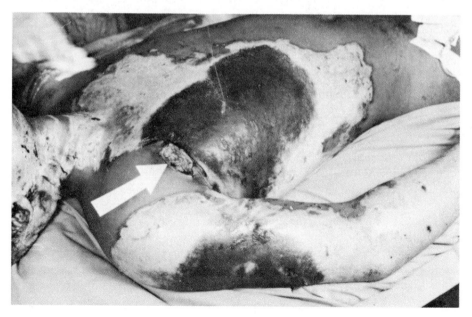

infections have been designated as *secondary* or *superimposed infections.* It should be noted that in secondary infections there has been a sharp increase in the number of cases caused by invasive gram-negative bacteria previously considered to have little or no virulence.

The bacteria associated with nosocomial infections have certain characteristics in common, such as the propensity to acquire resistance to a variety of antibiotics, ubiquity in distribution, and, in those with a major environmental reservoir, the ability to survive at room temperature or even under refrigeration. It is also important to realize that virtually all microbial agents, from viruses to fungi and protozoa, have the potential for causing nosocomial infections. The growing significance of nosocomial infections has focused attention upon the prevention and control of those occurring most commonly.

URINARY TRACT INFECTION

The urinary tract has been shown to be the most frequent source of nosocomial infections. Approximately 53% to 55% of gram-negative septicemias in hospitalized patients studied by Altemeier and his associates had their source of origin in the urinary tract. Indwelling urethral catheters and urinary tract instrumentation are important causative factors. The occurrence of urinary tract infection in the surgical patient, especially in the postoperative period, may be lessened, however, by adequate fluid intake, complete emptying of the bladder, early postoperative walking, and especially discretion, gentleness, and asepsis in the use of the catheter and closed urinary drainage system. The incidence of hospital-acquired urinary tract infections was reported to be approximately 40% of all nosocomial infections in the National Nosocomial Infection Study (1971–1974).

Urethral catheterization is not recommended as a routine method for collecting urine specimens for culture. In most instances a specimen obtained by clean-catch is satisfactory for bacteriological examination. Urethral catheterization is the only reliable means of obtaining a valid specimen, however, if the patient is unable to void or has difficulty even after suitable hydration; if a woman has marked obesity or redundant labia; if a patient is too ill or weak to pass a reliable specimen; and during the course of definitive urologic evaluation (*e.g.,* during assessment of urethral caliber or residual urine, or prior to other urethral instrumentation). In the collection of specimens from infants and young children for culture, it is customary to use some type of strap-on device. A negative culture thus obtained is assumed to reflect accurate information; however, owing to the possibility of contamination during collection, a positive culture may be misleading. In this event a suprapubic needle aspiration of the bladder may be required to obtain an uncontaminated specimen.

The need to place a catheter into the urinary tract is common in the care of the surgical patient. Not only is a catheter required occasionally to obtain a specimen for culture, but also it may be needed to observe and measure urinary output, to drain the bladder of the patient unable to void, and to prevent wetting and sacral cutaneous maceration in the incontinent patient. It is well known that with each invasion of the urinary tract by catheter, the opportunity for infection occurs. Moreover, when an indwelling catheter is left in place, the incidence of infection increases with the duration of indwelling catheterization.

Major emphasis is put on catheter management not only because of catheter-induced urinary tract infection *per se,* but also because catheter-induced urinary tract infection is the most common cause of gram-negative septicemia. In a recent study of over 400 cases of gram-negative sepsis, Altemeier and his associates noted that the urinary tract was the source in 53%. In order to lessen the chances of catheter-induced contamination, certain procedures must be carefully followed:

1. The use of sterile equipment
2. The use of aseptic technique at the time of catheter insertion
3. Preparation and maintenance of the catheter site
4. *Possibly* the local use of an antimicrobial agent

If a situation necessitates catheterization, aseptic technique is of utmost importance. The procedure in Table 10-1, as modified from recommendations by Kunin, outlines the important steps and key points.

The conventional route for an indwelling catheter is by way of the urethra as described in Table 10-1. There are two other techniques for urine collection: suprapubic bladder drainage and condom drainage.

Suprapubic bladder drainage is being used with increasing frequency when Foley catheters cannot be inserted safely through the urethra into the bladder. The methods most commonly employed are trocar cystostomy with a mushroom-type catheter and needle cystostomy with small plastic tubes. Suprapubic drainage appears not to interfere with reestablishment of normal voiding patterns, and it is associated with a lower incidence of epididymitis or prostatitis since it does not obstruct the urethra. However, it does afford an opportunity for introduction of microorganisms, as does the transurethral method, and the possibility of infection or bleeding at the cystostomy site. There is not sufficient evidence either to recommend or categorically to condemn any form of suprapubic drainage in the surgical patient, and it is generally conceded that controlled studies comparing transurethral and suprapubic drainage need to be done. When suprapubic drainage is employed, a closed collecting system is indicated.

Condom drainage offers protection against urinary soilage in the unconscious or incontinent patient without the risk of infection associated with the indwelling urethral catheter. Its use is limited to the male in whom there is no interference with normal emptying of the bladder. Maceration of penile skin restricts its usefulness, and daily changing and thorough cleansing are mandatory. The use of silicone ointment may be helpful. There are several well-made condom catheters available commercially, but entirely satisfactory devices can be fashioned using a condom and rubber tubing.

Table 10-1.   Urethral Catheterization

Equipment and Materials

Sterile tray containing the following:

Waterproof pad	Urethral catheter
Fenestrated drape	Lubricant
Gloves	Specimen cup with cover
Sponges (5 to 8)	Collecting basin for urine (not neces-
Antiseptic solution	sary if drainage bag is connected to
Forceps	catheter)

Label
Laboratory slip
*If an indwelling catheter is used, the sterile tray should also include the following:
Foley catheter
Syringe of sterile water
Drainage bag and tubing

Important Steps	Key Points
Place patient in supine position with legs spread apart.	
Drape patient with draw sheet.	
Wash hands.	
Open tray.	Use aseptic technique.
Expose perineal area.	
Place waterproof pad under buttocks.	Touch only the corners of the pad.
Don gloves.	
Place fenestrated drape so the meatal region is visible.	
Saturate sponges with antiseptic solution.	
Open lubricant and place in accessible area.	
In the female:	
Separate labia with thumb and index finger. Continue to separate labia until catheter is inserted.	Do not use this hand on sterile tray hereafter.
Cleanse labia with sponges.	Cleanse slowly from front to back, using a clean sponge with each stroke.
In the male:	
Hold penis with one hand.	Cleanse glans with sponge in opposite
Retract foreskin in uncircumcised males.	hand. Cleanse meatus.

(Continued)

Table 10-1 (*continued*)

Important Steps	Key Points
Lubricate approximately 4 inches of catheter.	
Place distal end of catheter in receptacle to collect urine.	
Gently insert catheter into meatus.	Insert until urine flows—approximately 3 inches in the female, 6 inches in the male. NEVER FORCIBLY INSERT A CATHETER
Catch some urine in specimen cup.	
Collect remaining urine in basin.	Do not contaminate distal end of catheter.
	If amount of urine exceeds 1 liter, stop flow for 1 hour, then resume emptying. (This procedure will guard against rapid decompression of the bladder.)
*If an indwelling catheter is used,	
1. Insert Foley catheter 1 or 2 inches beyond point at which urine began to flow.	
2. Inflate balloon with amount of sterile water designated on the catheter.	
3. Connect catheter to drainage bag.	
4. Tape catheter to lower abdominal wall or to inner aspect of leg. Allow some slack to guard against trauma to the urethra.	
5. To prevent kinking, attach tubing to bottom sheet by pinning sheet around tube, by placing rubber band around tube and pinning, or by using a plastic clamp (included in some insertion kits).	

Closed Urinary Drainage Systems

Once an indwelling catheter has been inserted, prevention of infection is a major consideration. The best preventive method is a closed drainage system. The convenience of an "open" system for the collection of samples and the measurement of timed urinary volumes is popular with those caring for the patient, but an open

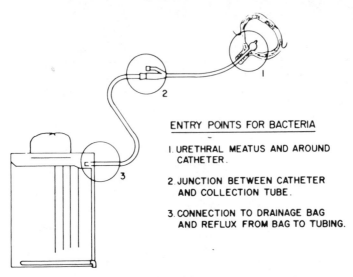

ENTRY POINTS FOR BACTERIA

1. URETHRAL MEATUS AND AROUND CATHETER.

2. JUNCTION BETWEEN CATHETER AND COLLECTION TUBE.

3. CONNECTION TO DRAINAGE BAG AND REFLUX FROM BAG TO TUBING.

Fig. 10-3. A urinary bag and the sites at which microorganisms may enter a closed urinary drainage system. (Kunin CM: Detection, Prevention and Management of Urinary Tract Infections, 2nd ed. Philadelphia, Lea & Febiger, 1974)

system provides sites for potential contamination and must be condemned. Many excellent closed urinary drainage systems are available, and one should be chosen that is safe and accepted by the hospital personnel.

The entry of bacteria into the urinary tract of a patient with an indwelling catheter connected to a closed drainage system may occur in several ways: through pericatheter ascent of bacteria; through a break in the connection between the catheter and the collecting system; or through reflux of urine from the collecting system up into the bladder (Fig. 10-3). In the care of a closed drainage system it is essential that good flow without reflux be maintained and that obstruction and contamination of the system be prevented.

Intermittent Single Catheterizations

In some patients who have protracted urinary bladder distention and paresis, intermittent single catheterizations may be used every 6 to 8 hours. If employed, strict aseptic technique is advisable.

Maintaining Good Flow

The importance of the following precautions must be strongly emphasized to all personnel caring for patients with an indwelling catheter:

1. The bag must *always* be kept below the level of the bladder. Urine reflux into the urethra and bladder must be avoided (Fig. 10-4).

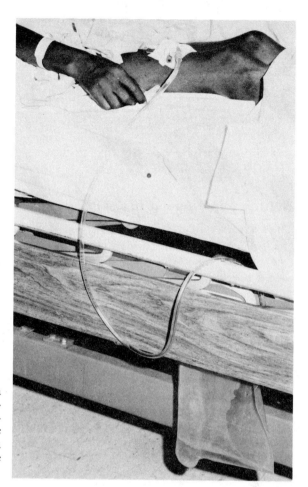

Fig. 10-4. Care must be taken to see that the plastic bag connected to the continuous drainage urinary catheter is *always kept below the level of the bladder* in order to avoid reflux of urine into the urethra and bladder.

2. Care must be taken while turning or moving the patient in bed, sitting him up in a chair, or preparing him to ambulate, to see that good descending flow is maintained and that the tubing is arranged so that there are no kinks to obstruct flow.
3. The bag must *never* be allowed to touch the floor.
4. The bag should not be held upside down while emptying.
5. Urine should flow well from the drainage tube. Obstruction should be suspected if the entire tube is filled with urine.
6. Irrigations are not recommended unless the physician suspects obstruction, because the chance of infection is great.
7. When it is necessary to irrigate, a sterile, large volume syringe must be used for *each* irrigation, employing sterile solution.
8. The use of catheter plugs is not recommended.
9. Leg bags should not be employed for short-term use in acutely ill patients. If the patient is ambulatory, the catheter bag may be carried or pinned to the robe.
10. It is suggested that all catheters be monitored for evidence of infection by sending a culture specimen from the catheter to the bacteriology laboratory at frequent or regular intervals. (Drainage bags may become contaminated even though catheter urine remains sterile.)

Catheters should be monitored by culture when there is reason to suspect infection on clinical grounds. When a urine sample is required with a closed catheter drainage system, it should be drawn by inserting a needle through the catheter wall at an acute angle to the long axis of the catheter. Catheters are self-sealing following withdrawal of the needle. It is important to recognize that drainage bags may become contaminated while the catheter urine remains sterile. A urine culture should be obtained immediately prior to withdrawal of an indwelling catheter (Fig. 10-5).

The recommended daily care for patients with indwelling catheters is outlined in Table 10-2.

Antimicrobial Agents in the Prevention of Urinary Tract Infection

There is no proof that either local or systemic antimicrobial agents reduce the incidence of postoperative urinary tract infection. Systemic agents are generally not recommended unless there is infection present in the urinary tract. Limited topical use of prophylactic antibacterial agents may be prudent in patients requiring instrumentation or catherization. Prior to the single catheterization or instrumentation of the urinary tract, an ointment containing a combination of bactericidal agents (*e.g.,* neomycin, polymyxin, and bacitracin) may be instilled in the urethra for lubrication as well as for antibacterial action. When prolonged urinary drainage is required, a closed system is mandatory and, at the interface between meatus and

Fig. 10-5. A method using needle and syringe to obtain a specimen of urine from the catheter. (Kunin CM: Detection, Prevention and Management of Urinary Tract Infections, 2nd ed. Philadelphia, Lea & Febiger, 1974)

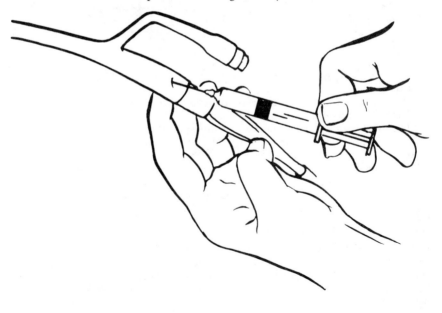

Table 10-2.   Recommended Daily Care for Patients with Indwelling Catheters

Equipment and Materials	Important Steps	Key Points
Soap and water Washcloth	Wash perineal area and genitalia with soap and water.	At least *twice* daily
	Arrange the tubing to eliminate kinks.	
	Observe the output.	Note amount, color, *etc.*
	Observe the bag.	Bag must *never* touch floor.
		Bag must *always* be kept below level of bladder.
	Empty the bag every 8 hours.	Empty more often if bag fills rapidly.
	DO NOT HOLD BAG UPSIDE DOWN WHEN EMPTYING.	

(Kunin CM: Detection, Prevention and Management of Urinary Tract Infections, 2nd ed. Philadelphia, Lea & Febiger, 1974)

catheter, daily application of the same antibacterial ointment is recommended for both bactericidal effect and reduction of trauma. Catheters impregnated with antimicrobial agents have demonstrated no more effectiveness than nonimpregnated catheters (Butler and Kunin). Following catheterization or instrumentation, the instillation of 30 ml of 1% neomycin solution into the bladder has been recommended by some urologists.

Antimicrobial solutions have been used for irrigation by Martin and co-workers and by Thornton and co-workers; they reported excellent results in lowering catheter-induced infections. A polymyxin–neomycin solution administered through a three-way catheter was used as an irrigating solution. Figure 10-6 is a representation of such a system. It is safe, practical, and entirely compatible with a closed drainage system.

RESPIRATORY TRACT INFECTIONS

There are numerous and varied factors that contribute to the development of respiratory tract infections. Many of these factors are related to the functions of surgeons, anesthetists, internists, and nurses, whose close collaboration is necessary for prevention and control of pulmonary infections (Fig. 10-7). In addition, impaired host defense mechanisms, prolonged intubation, coma, and tracheostomy are intimately related to the development of respiratory nosocomial infections.

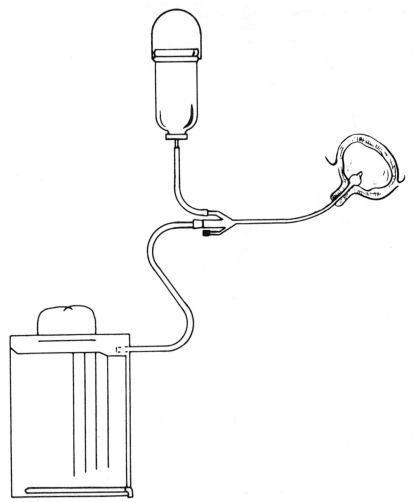

Fig. 10-6. Example of a closed three-way urinary drainage system suitable for irrigation. (Kunin CM: Detection, Prevention and Management of Urinary Tract Infections, 2nd ed. Philadelphia, Lea & Febiger, 1974)

Atelectasis and aspiration are significant occurrences predisposing to the development of postoperative pulmonary infection. The incidence of atelectasis can be reduced by relief of pain, deep breathing, coughing, changes in position, activity, suction (by means of nasotracheal catheter, endotracheal tube, or bronchoscopy), humidification of the atmosphere, bronchodilators, intermittent positive-pressure breathing, respiratory exercises, avoidance of drugs that increase viscosity of secretions, and abstention from smoking prior to operation. Relief of pain needs to be balanced against the avoidance of heavy sedation, and on rare occasions intercostal

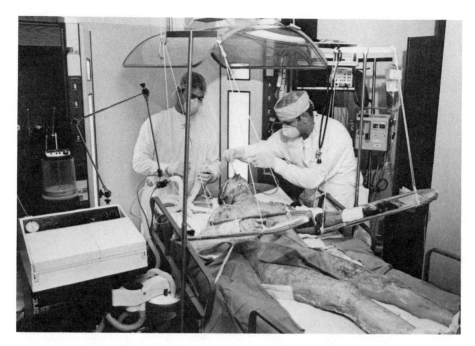

Fig. 10-7. Endobronchial toilet in critically ill patients is carried out using a new sterile catheter for each aspiration procedure. Note use of sterile gloves to introduce and manipulate catheter, which is passed through the nasotracheal tube. Periods of suction aspiration must be brief to avoid hypoxia. A second attendant can assist, as shown here, to prevent contact contamination of ventilatory tubing and connectors and to reinstitute mechanical ventilatory support promptly if such is required.

nerve block may be required. If atelectasis occurs, the obstruction causing it may be relieved by suction, followed by the maintenance of adequate pulmonary function (Fig. 10-8, *A* and *B*).

The aspiration of blood or gastric contents may lead to pulmonary sepsis. Such mishaps can be prevented by emptying the stomach before operation, maintaining the head-down position during periods of unconsciousness, and using a cuffed endotracheal tube. Unless aspiration is recognized and relieved quickly, serious pulmonary disease commonly results.

Anesthesiology Considerations

The influence of anesthesia on the occurrence of postoperative pulmonary and other infections is an important consideration for the anesthesiologist as well as the surgeon. To provide optimal safety for the patient, the physiological alterations produced by the infection and the potential infectious hazards to which he may be exposed must be recognized.

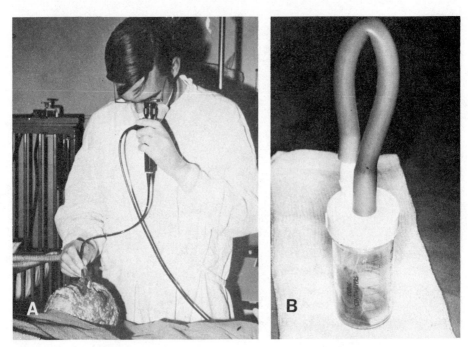

Fig. 10-8. (*A*) A physician with mask, sterile gown, and gloves introduces a fiberoptic bronchoscope through a nostril in a burn patient with tracheobronchial inflammation. (*B*) The microbial content of endobronchial secretions may be reliably determined by the use of Luken's tube aspiration cultures. Note blood-stained endobronchial secretions adherent to the wall of the Luken's tube. (U.S. Army Institute of Surgical Research, Brooke Army Medical Center, Fort Sam Houston, Texas)

Bridenbaugh, in his report to the Committee on Control of Surgical Infections, emphasized the current concept that the modern anesthesiologist is committed to providing the surgeon with optimal operating conditions compatible with the safety of his patient. Improvements in background knowledge of the present-day practitioners and the development of sophisticated monitoring systems have failed to cause any dramatic decline in the overall anesthetic and surgical morbidity and mortality. This failure is due in part to a change in attitude toward case acceptance. Rejecting a patient on grounds of his "being unfit for anesthesia" is now virtually unheard of. When the anesthesiologist and surgeon consider whether or not the patient is fit for operation, their main concern is usually with the effect of the anesthesia and the operation on his cardiorespiratory system. However, some consideration must also be given to his susceptibility to infection. Assessment of patient "risk" of infection is difficult because so many factors influence it (*i.e.,* the surgical procedure, the hospital and operating room environment, length of the preoperative stay, the patient's physical status, operating time, the abilities of the anesthetist, surgeon, nurse, *etc.*).

Specific Infectious Diseases

The location and nature of the infectious process may be even more significant to the anesthesiologist than the general effects of acute febrile disease. Two infections in which anesthesia is a risk are acute upper respiratory infection and acute parenchymal liver disease.

The presence of an acute upper respiratory infection is a traditional contraindication to an elective surgical procedure because of the clinical impression that postoperative pulmonary complications frequently ensue. The administration of a volatile anesthetic may increase the susceptibility of the respiratory tract to infection caused by inhaling pathogenic microbes. Viral infection of the respiratory tract produces changes in the epithelial lining varying from no perceptible alteration to complete necrosis, depending on the host reaction and the infecting species. With severe involvement, the ciliated and mucus-secreting cells may be damaged and patchy areas totally destroyed within the airway. Less severe damage may upset the delicate balance between mucus secretion and ciliary action. Clinical experience with influenza has amply demonstrated the reduced capacity of the damaged lung to resist secondary infection.

In the patient with chronic obstructive pulmonary disease, it may be difficult to differentiate active infection from a nonspecific exacerbation of bronchitis. The effect upon the respiratory tract of the inhalation of anesthetics is not favorable for the patient with excessive mucus production. Although about 50% of the water content must be removed from sputum before measurable increases in viscosity occur, preanesthetic medication and the inhalation of relatively dry gas may lead to this degree of dehydration of the respiratory secretions, particularly if a nonrebreathing circuit is employed. The increased viscosity of secretions, mechanical obstruction by the endotracheal tube, and depressing effects of lowered temperature and humidity on ciliary action impair mucus transport and lead to accumulation of secretions.

Atelectasis is initiated by bronchial obstructions, but bacterial multiplication in the distal airways occurs rapidly, and the resultant clinical picture of fever, tachycardia, and tachypnea is due in large part to the secondary infection. Thus, as Bridenbaugh has emphasized, the effective prevention of postoperative respiratory infection in patients with either acute or chronic inflammatory disease of the respiratory tract requires meticulous respiratory care before, during, and after anesthesia.

The choice of anesthetic technique may influence the patient's risk of infection. A general anesthetic administered to a patient with a systemic disease and fever can further lower systemic resistance to infection. Under such circumstances, a regional block anesthetic, avoiding endotracheal manipulation, would certainly decrease the risk of pulmonary complications of surgical procedures on the extremities.

Anesthesia has the potential for causing cross-infection and nosocomial infections, and for increasing the risk of postoperative surgical infections, but there are means available to minimize or prevent these hazards. The problem is how to transfer these means into practical measures that every anesthesiologist can apply.

The numerous articles about and intense interest in the sterilization of anesthesia and inhalation therapy equipment, the correct usage of sterilizing gases and solutions, such as ethylene oxide and Cidex, and the newly introduced disposable accessories are indicative of interest in this area of surgical care.

Ventilatory Assistance

Many surgical patients require some type of ventilatory assistance during hospitalization. This may range from occasional endotracheal suction or intermittent positive-pressure breathing to ventilation by way of an endotracheal tube or tracheostomy. The equipment used and the techniques employed in ventilatory assistance should minimize the risk of infection. A variety of acceptable techniques have been described for endotracheal suction by way of nostril, endotracheal tube, or tracheostomy. From the standpoint of infection control, it is mandatory that a sterile catheter and sterile lubricant be used each time suction is applied and that the catheter be manipulated by a washed and gloved dominant hand (see Fig. 10-7). Absolute sterility of air is impossible, but at the very least the gas or air delivered by the ventilatory equipment should be as clean as the surrounding room air.

Humidifiers and Nebulizers

It is appropriate to distinguish humidifiers from nebulizers because of differences between the two in their frequency of contamination (Sanford). In a humidifier, the tension of water vapor in the air or a gas is increased by bubbling the air or gas through the water. Bacteria in water will not be transmitted unless the water is sprayed into the air. Although the water in the humidifier reservoir may be contaminated, particulate water containing bacteria is not delivered into the effluent stream of gas going to the patient. Thus, the humidifier could actually act as a bacterial trap (see Chap. 16).

In contrast to a humidifier, a nebulizer is designed to deliver particulate water into the effluent gas system. The most common design used in nebulizers involves the Venturi principle. There are two other types of nebulizers: in one, water is dropped onto a rapidly spinning disc; the other is the ultrasonic nebulizer involving a vibrating crystal that produces particulate water. In contrast to humidifiers, all three of these nebulizers deliver particulate water, which may be contaminated. Medication nebulizers, as contrasted with reservoir nebulizers, seem to pose little or no contamination problem unless contaminated fluids are placed into them.

Endotracheal Intubation and Tracheostomy

Except in cases of extreme emergency, endotracheal intubation should be done under aseptic conditions, using sterile tubes and gloved hands while masked. Elective tracheostomy should be performed in the operating room as an aseptic surgical procedure. The skin of the patient's neck is degermed and draped as for any other operation (see Chap. 6). Sterile instruments and supplies must be used, and the surgical team should be appropriately clothed and prepared for the operation. For either endotracheal intubation or tracheostomy, facilities for assisted ventilation must be available.

The introduction of new strains of microorganisms into these patients may lead to tracheobronchial or pulmonary superinfection, or both, with adverse consequences. Therefore, aspiration and manipulation should be done using strict asepsis, gloved hands, and separate sterile catheters for each aspiration, as indicated below (see also Fig. 10-7):

1. Thoroughly wash hands before and after aspiration, toilet, or other attention to tracheostomies.
2. All personnel must use sterile gloves.
3. Place sterile towel or small apertured drape about the tracheostomy.
4. Use sterile catheter connected to a Y-tube adapted to permit delivery of intermittent suction and instillation of sterile solutions. A sterile disposable catheter setup is satisfactory.
5. Remove inner cannula of tracheostomy tube and have an attendant start suction machine.
6. Turn patient's head to one side and instill 3 or 4 drops of sterile normal saline solution to aid in the toilet of the trachea and bronchi.
7. Cautiously and aseptically insert sterile catheter attached to Y-tube suction into the tracheostomy tube and pass it to the tracheal bifurcation. Rotate catheter while suction is continued. Apply suction for only brief, 3- to 5-second periods to prevent induction of hypoxia.
8. Place thumb on Y-tube opening and remove catheter. Take care to avoid trauma to mucous membranes during introduction of catheter and aspiration of secretions.
9. Repeat the procedure, turning the patient's head to the other side.
10. Clear catheter of any purulent or mucous plugs by aspirating sterile saline through its lumen.
11. Once each shift, using sterile pipe cleaners, thoroughly clean the inner tracheostomy cannula that has been removed. Wash it in glutaraldehyde or a phenolic compound and rinse in sterile water.
12. Again wash hands with degerming soap or detergent at the completion of procedure and before attending next patient. Hand-washing and hand-washing with disinfection of hands are of great importance in preventing transfer of nosocomial infections.
13. Perform aerobic and anaerobic cultures, and antibiotic sensitivity testing of the tracheal secretions at frequent intervals, as indicated by the patient's course.
14. Examination of gram-stained smears of tracheal secretions may be helpful in suggesting antibiotic therapy pending culture and sensitivity reports.

Serious infections may occur in patients with tracheostomies, including those caused by *Pseudomonas*, *Klebsiella*, *Staphylococcus aureus*, *Streptococcus hemolyticus*, *Candida*, and *Herpes simplex*.

Prophylactic Antibiotics

There is no convincing evidence that antimicrobial agents administered either systemically or locally reduce the incidence of postoperative pulmonary infection, or that their use will prevent colonization or invasive infection of the tracheobronchial tree in patients with an endotracheal tube or a tracheostomy. Moreover, it is likely that the empiric use of an antimicrobial agent may serve only to hasten colonization with resistant bacteria, yeasts, or fungi.

BLOODSTREAM INFECTION

The intravenous introduction of microorganisms is an important source of hospital-acquired infection. Septicemia may be caused by the introduction of microorganisms from contaminated fluids, infected venesection sites, or foci of septic thrombophlebitis as a complication of indwelling intravenous catheters.

Recent experience has indicated that prolonged intravenous therapy with indwelling needles or catheters is associated with a surprisingly high incidence of postoperative infections. This has been observed more frequently in high-risk, debilitated, and aged patients, and in patients receiving steroid or immunosuppressive therapy. Surveys at the University of Cincinnati Medical Center showed that over 70% of patients with indwelling intravenous catheters for 72 or more hours developed significant areas of thrombophlebitis or active cellulitis, along with their resultant discomfort, fever, and increased morbidity. A new syndrome, called "third day surgical fever," has been described; it is a gram-negative septicemia occurring 3 days postoperatively in trauma and other high-risk patients (Fig. 10-9). This type of

Fig. 10-9. "Third day surgical fever" with *Enterobacter* sp. septicemia and septic shock, which developed in association with acute thrombophlebitis 3 days postoperatively during penicillin and continuous intravenous therapy. (Altemeier WA, Hummel RP, Hill EO, Lewis S: Changing patterns in surgical infections. Ann Surg 178:436, 1973)

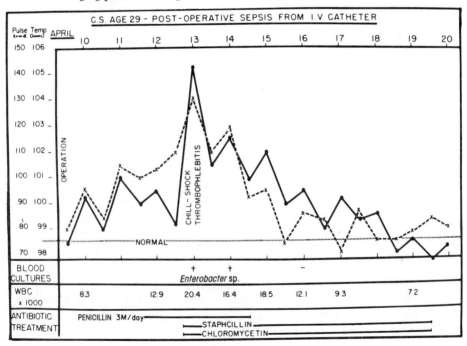

hospital-acquired infection is indicative of contamination of the intravenous solution or catheter and of the need to provide safer methods of continuous intravenous therapy. A contaminated intravenous system may produce little or no general systemic infection, yet may seed a site of lowered resistance such as the operative wound, the catheterized urinary tract, or the respiratory system following inhalation anesthetics. Except in unusual circumstances, intravenous equipment and supplies delivered for patient use may be considered sterile. Currently, bloodstream bacterial invasion in conjunction with intravenous therapy usually results from other types of contamination.

Prior to insertion of an intravenous needle, catheter, or cannula, the skin of the patient should be degermed using an accepted method (see Chap. 6). During the course of inserting the needle and catheter, gentleness and strict attention to aseptic detail is mandatory. After the needle hub is connected to the intravenous tubing, the interface of needle and skin should be dressed to minimize contamination. The topical application of antimicrobial agents at the interface between cannula and skin is widely practiced. However, evidence of its effectiveness against cannula-related sepsis is conflicting and is under question; moreover, there is a possibility of resistant bacterial, yeast, or fungal superinfection. The use of an iodophor ointment applied at the interface of intravenous catheter and skin has been recommended by some authorities. The entire device, including needle hub and adjacent tubing, should be covered by an occlusive dressing, which should be kept dry and changed daily. The needle and indwelling line must be secured so that their position on the skin and in the underlying vein is not disturbed by movement. If such movement does occur, contamination of the skin may be carried into the subcutaneous tissues, to the vein, or even within the vein.

Multiple lines (tandem, "piggyback") are not encouraged; however, they are frequently necessary. When used, extreme care should be taken to prevent contamination at the point of entrance of one line into the other. If any medication is to be administered with intravenous solutions by direct injection into the line, great care should be taken at the time the needle is inserted. It is recommended that all intravenous tubing and solutions proximal to the catheter or needle hub be changed every 24 hours (also, see Intravenous Hyperalimentation, below).

Prolonged catheterization of a central vein is frequently necessary to monitor central venous pressure for a variety of clinical conditions. Such lines should be inserted and maintained with the same attention to asepsis as with other intravenous lines, and they should not be used to administer medications or to obtain blood specimens, except under demanding or dire circumstances. Transvenous pacemakers and heparin locks require the identical meticulous care for insertion and maintenance as any other intravenous line.

Contamination of the intravenous system should be considered in the differential diagnosis of fever. If local signs of inflammation or thrombosis appear, the administration of fluid at that site should be discontinued. Contaminated catheters may be responsible for seeding the bloodstream with microorganisms, even when local signs of inflammation are absent. Therefore, if sepsis is suspected in the patient with an indwelling intravenous line for whatever purpose, the line should be withdrawn, and the catheter tip and intravenous solution cultured aerobically and anaerobically; if positive, antibiotic sensitivities must be obtained and appropriate treatment instituted.

Wherever practical, it may be of value from the standpoint of both efficiency and infection control to have a special intravenous team that is proficient in the task of establishing and maintaining intravenous lines and equipment.

Intravenous Hyperalimentation

The insertion of a catheter into a central vein for the purpose of parenteral nutrition carries a definite risk of sepsis as well as other complications, including pneumothorax, hemothorax, or perforation of the regional great vessels. Such misadventures can be minimized by increased care and experience. A number of studies have now clearly demonstrated that the prevention of infection in patients with hyperalimentation is a direct consequence of catheter care. It must be kept in mind that these patients are also at risk for nosocomial infections because of their debilitated and malnourished state, and as a result of steroid and multiple antibiotic therapy. However, Fischer and his associates have reported that, in a busy ICU environment, a rate of approximately 2% can be obtained with good technique and restriction of the catheter for purposes of parenteral nutrition.

Solutions used for parenteral nutrition contain a high concentration of protein and sugar, media favorable for microbial growth. Asepsis in mixing and handling of these solutions is mandatory, and preparation in a laminar flow hood is desirable. It is recommended that the fluid be used immediately and, if it must be stored, that it be kept at 4°C and used as soon as possible (Goldmann and Maki; see Fig. 10-10). In high-risk patients, such as those with extensive burn injuries, the line should be changed every 2 to 3 days.

Insertion of the catheter should be treated as a surgical procedure requiring aseptic technique and avoidance of trauma. The patient's skin should be degermed, using an accepted method (see Chap. 6). The operator and assistants should dress, mask, wash, gown, and glove as for any operation. Upon completion of the procedure, securing the line and dressing should be carried out as described above. Intravenous tubing, in-line filter (if one is used), and the solution bottle proximal to the needle hub should be changed frequently, every 24 hours if the solution is prepared with synthetic amino acids, every 12 hours if prepared with casein hydrolysates (Goldmann and Maki). Changes should be done by clean, gloved hands and with strict attention to aseptic detail. No controlled studies have been performed to determine how frequently catheters being used for parenteral alimentation should be changed, but it is advisable that dressings be changed every other day with a sterile prep. The patient should be masked and the person changing the patient gowned and masked according to procedures that are now well established. Bower, Bjornson, and co-workers have suggested that colonization of the site of catheter entry by a bacterial density of greater than 10^3/ml is associated with a higher incidence of sepsis. Studies continue in an effort to demonstrate whether

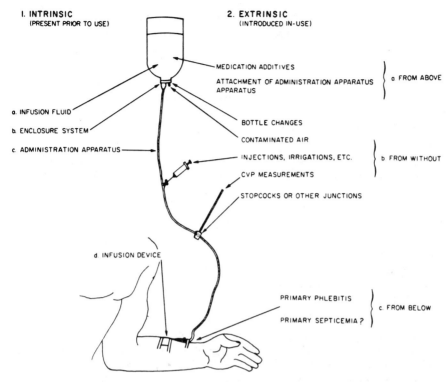

Fig. 10-10. Potential mechanisms for microbial contamination of intravenous infusion fluids. (Maki DG, Rhame FS, Goldmann DA, Mandell GL: The infection hazard posed by contaminated intravenous infusion fluid. In Sonnenwirth AC (ed): Bacteremia — Laboratory and Clinical Aspects. Springfield, IL, Charles C Thomas, 1973)

removal of such catheters when colony counts exceed this will result in a lower rate of infection.

Micropore filters have been inserted into hyperalimentation systems for the purpose of blocking the passage of microorganisms. This should reduce the hazard of infection from a contaminated solution; however, there are few hard data to indicate that this is indeed the case.

The risk of infection clearly dictates that parenteral hyperalimentation be employed only when definitely indicated by the patient's nutritional requirements. Moreover, infection control must be a paramount consideration in every step of its use. Hyperalimentation infusion lines should not be used to administer medications, to obtain blood samples, or to measure venous pressure, in order that contamination from these manipulations may be avoided.

Minimizing Complications: The Team Approach.   Many centers that specialize in the treatment of severely ill patients have arrived at the concept that this important therapeutic modality should be controlled and administered by a team of individuals interested in parenteral nutrition. This team usually is headed by a physician, but may be headed by a pharmacist or another interested party. The team generally includes nurses (for the education of staff nurses or those who may change dressings), pharmacists, dieticians, etc. Such a team is generally available for consultation and, although the team members may accept patients for primary care, it probably works better when they are available for consultations with the patient remaining under the care of his primary physician.

Interest in the field of nutritional support is increasing, and a number of developments are taking place in the constituents of the solutions as well as modes of administration. The greatest activity exists in the area of the so-called second generation solutions. Modifications of various amino acid mixtures for patients with different disease states have been the primary method by which such new solutions have evolved. Thus, solutions consisting of essential amino acids for patients with renal failure, 35% branched-chain enriched solutions low in aromatic amino acids for patients with hepatic failure, and 45% branched-chain amino acid solutions for patients with sepsis or severe trauma have been developed. Undoubtedly, additional solutions will be forthcoming. An important thing to recognize is that this is also a potentially dangerous therapeutic modality, and careful control and attention to the details of its use will result in the maximum benefit to patients with the least number of complications.

Fig. 10-11. Course of patient who developed popliteal arterial thrombosis and gas gangrene following femoral arteriography.

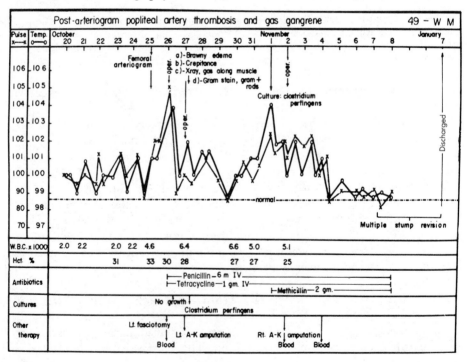

Intra-arterial Lines

The recommendations made for intravenous lines apply equally to intra-arterial lines, including arteriovenous shunts. Several additional factors are important in intra-arterial lines. First, they may be needed for longer periods than are intravenous lines. For example, arteriovenous shunts required for hemodialysis frequently must be maintained for weeks or even months. Second, intra-arterial lines are placed by means of an incision, thus increasing the vulnerability to subsequent infection. Third, intra-arterial lines may reduce the viability of tissue because of the infringement upon arterial blood flow. The resulting distal ischemia may predispose the involved tissue to infection (Fig. 10-11). The intra-arterial site should be inspected at least once a day and the catheter removed if there is any sign of inflammation at the point of insertion. The patient in whom an intra-arterial line is to remain for a long time must be trained to maintain meticulous care of the arterial puncture site, particularly if he is to leave the hospital.

Banked Blood and Blood Products

Banked blood is one of the most significant advances in clinical medicine in this century. Unfortunately, its use may be associated with hazards because of preexisting conditions within the donor.* Before blood is obtained, an accurate medical history must be taken, and the donation should be rejected under the following circumstances:

1. If fever is present
2. If the donor has any acute illness
3. If the donor has had dental surgery within the previous 72 hours
4. If the donor has a history of viral hepatitis or jaundice, or has received hepatitis B immune globulin within the past 12 months
5. If the donor has had close contact with hepatitis patients within the past 6 months
6. If the donor is a narcotic drug addict or an alcoholic
7. If there is infectious skin disease at the venipuncture site
8. If the donor has been vaccinated within the previous 2 weeks with live virus (*e.g.,* measles, mumps, yellow fever, oral poliomyelitis). Donors vaccinated against smallpox are acceptable after separation of the scab, or 2 weeks after immune reaction; donors vaccinated against rubella are acceptable 4 weeks after their last injection.
9. If there is evidence of malaria; if the donor has traveled in malarial endemic areas within the past 6 months or has lived in an endemic area within the past 3 years; or if he has taken antimalarial drugs within the past 3 years
10. If there is evidence of symptoms or signs of acquired immune deficiency syndrome (AIDS), or if the donor has indicated that he is at high risk of AIDS (see Chap. 12).
11. If there is evidence of recent infection caused by cytomegaloviruses and Epstein-Barr viruses, which have been implicated in the "postperfusion syndrome," an infectious mononucleosis-like illness appearing 3 to 5 weeks after transfusion

---

* For details on selection of donors to minimize transmission of disease, refer to the American Association of Blood Banks' publications, *Technical Methods and Procedures,* 8th edition, 1981, and *Standards for Blood Banks and Transfusion Services,* 10th edition, 1981.

The decision to administer human blood to a patient requires careful clinical judgment. In addition to the well-known problems of proper cross-matching, satisfactory preservation methods, and adverse reactions, bacteria introduced at the time of collection or during subsequent processing may be present. Therefore, blood should not be administered if its potential advantages do not outweigh the risk of acquiring transmissible disease, of which hepatitis is by far the most important. The use of noncommercial donors is advisable.

Liquid plasma also carries risk and should not be used if plasma protein fraction or albumin is available. Irradiation of liquid plasma with ultraviolet light is *not* an effective method of inactivating the virus of serum hepatitis. Recent results using betapropiolactone in conjunction with ultraviolet irradiation are encouraging but are still indefinite. Current investigation of ethylene oxide sterilization is at an early stage and cannot be considered to be a clinical success at this time.

Other blood products, such as antihemophilic globulin, thrombin, and platelet concentrates, also carry the risk of transmission of serum hepatitis. Fibrinogen concentrate and Factors 2, 7, 9, and 10 complex carry a very high risk of hepatitis and should be given only on specific indications.

Records of the origin, distribution, and administration of blood and blood products should be maintained if control of their hazards is to be satisfactory. Such records include identifying data for donors contributing to each product; batch numbers of products issued to hospitals and of all data relating to various batches; and accurate notation in patient's records of the batch numbers of the products used with the date of administration, as well as the recording of the recipient's names and the hospital record of products received and issued.

Securing blood from donors or administering it to patients requires the same careful technique as that used for any venipuncture. If a vented system is used, it must have a suitable antibacterial air filter. The production of plasma or packed red cells should be done using a closed system. All blood should be inspected before use and discarded if color and appearance are in any way abnormal or if it appears to be hemolyzed.

Viral Hepatitis

Blood from all human beings should be considered a potential source of hepatitis A or B, or non-A, non-B hepatitis virus. Any wound caused by a needle, scalpel, broken glass, or other object that has been in contact with the blood of another person should be considered a potential site for inoculation with hepatitis virus; thus, hospital personnel are especially vulnerable.

It has been estimated by the Centers for Disease Control that approximately 200,000 people, primarily young adults, develop hepatitis B virus (HBV) infection each year. One fourth of these become ill with jaundice, and more than 10,000 patients are hospitalized with this type of hepatitis each year. Of particular concern are the 6% to 10% of young adults with this infection who become carriers, with an estimated pool of 400,000 to 800,000 carriers existing currently in the United

States. Carriers can be recognized as individuals who are HB_sAg positive on at least two occasions, 6 or more months apart. However, it should be remembered that any person with positive test results for HB_sAg should probably be considered as infectious.

Carriers and individuals with acute infections have a high concentration of hepatitis B virus in their blood and serous fluids, and lesser concentrations in saliva, semen, and other body fluids. Thus, its transmission is possible by way of percutaneous or permucosal routes, by the introduction of infective blood or other fluids through contaminated needles, or by sexual contact. Close personal contacts can also spread the infection. The use of routine screening with highly sensitive tests for HB_sAg, however, has reduced the danger of transmission of infection by transfusion of contaminated blood or blood products.

Serologic surveys have demonstrated that the prevalence of hepatitis B viral infection is high in certain groups of the general population. These include the following:

1. Immigrants or refugees from areas with high incidence of endemic disease
2. Homosexually active males
3. Users of illegal parenteral drugs
4. Patients in hemodialysis units
5. Individuals having intimate sexual or household contacts with hepatitis B virus carriers
6. Inmates of prisons
7. Patients and staff in custodial institutions for the mentally retarded
8. Certain medical, dental, and related laboratory and support personnel who have frequent contact with blood from infective patients

Gamma globulin provides passive protection against hepatitis A virus. It is recommended that hospital personnel who suffer skin-breaking injury from an object contaminated with a patient's blood, or who are in direct contact with patients who have type A viral hepatitis, should receive 2 ml of gamma globulin intramuscularly. This will provide passive protection for approximately 6 weeks. Gamma globulin produces poor protection against hepatitis B virus. However, the recent introduction of inactivated hepatitis B virus vaccine has provided a means of preventing or reducing the incidence of this type of hepatitis. The cost of this vaccine is high, and its cost effectiveness must be considered.

Field trials of the United States-manufactured vaccine have shown that a series of three intramuscular doses of HBV vaccine produced 80% to 95% efficacy in preventing this type of hepatitis among susceptible persons, protection against illness being complete for persons who developed antibodies after vaccination but before exposure. The duration of the period of protection and the requirements for booster doses are unknown, although protective antibody titers have persisted for 3 years. Serologic screening before vaccination to detect carriers or persons having antibody from previous infection may or may not be cost effective. Screening of persons in groups having the highest risk of HBV infection should be cost effective. Individuals who are at substantial risk of HBV infection and who are judged likely to be susceptible should be vaccinated. These include those groups with frequent exposure to blood or needles, as follows:

1. *Hospital personnel,* including surgeons, residents, interns, operating room staff, phlebotomists and intravenous therapy nurses, medical technologists, and oncology and dialysis unit staffs. Other groups to be considered in some hospitals include the emergency room staff, physicians, and nursing personnel.
2. *Health-care workers* such as medical, dental, laboratory, and other support groups also have risk of exposure to HBV depending on their functions. Vaccination for these workers is recommended as soon as possible after starting employment in a high-risk environment.
3. *Hemodialysis patients.* A number of investigators have established the high risk of HBV virus transmission in hemodialysis units, and vaccination is recommended for susceptible patients and personnel.
4. *Susceptible patients and staff of institutions for the mentally retarded* should be vaccinated. The risk for the staff in this institutional environment is related not only to blood exposure but also to bites and unusual contact with skin lesions, saliva, and other infective secretions.
5. *Homosexually active males.* It is important to vaccinate homosexually active males as soon as possible after their homosexual activity begins, regardless of their age or duration of their practices. Homosexually active females apparently are not at increased risk of sexually transmitted HBV infection.
6. *Illicit injectable drug users* who are susceptible to HBV should be vaccinated as soon as possible after their drug use begins.
7. *Recipients of certain blood products.* Patients with clotting disorders receiving factor VIII or IX concentrates have an increased risk of HBV infection. Vaccination is, therefore, recommended for these persons, and should be started early when their clotting disorder is identified. For those patients who have already received multiple infusions of these products, screening is recommended.
8. *Household contacts of HBV carriers* are at high risk of HBV infection, and their vaccination is recommended.
9. *Other contacts of HBV carriers.* Persons in contact with carriers at schools, offices, and so forth are at minimal risk of contracting HBV, and their vaccination is not routinely recommended.
10. *Special high-risk populations.* Alaskan Eskimos, and immigrants and refugees from areas with highly endemic disease (particularly eastern Asia and Africa) have high HBV infection rates and deserve special attention, and more extensive vaccination programs may be warranted. *Inmates of long-term correctional facilities* may benefit from screening and vaccination programs because of their greater risk of acquiring hepatitis B virus, owing to their higher rates of use of illicit injectable drugs and homosexual practices.

HBV Vaccination.   Adult HBV vaccination requires three intramuscular doses of 1 ml of vaccine (20 μg/1 ml) each, with the second and third doses being given at 1 and 6 months after the first. For patients undergoing hemodialysis and for other immunosuppressed patients, three 2-ml doses (40 μg) should be used. For children under 10 years of age, three similarly spaced doses of 0.5 ml (10 μg) are sufficient. Vaccine doses administered at longer intervals than those stipulated apparently provide equally satisfactory protection, but optimal protection is not obtained before the third dose.

COMMUNICABLE DISEASES

Unrecognized or inapparent communicable disease in patients or personnel may be the source of hospital-acquired infection in other patients. Control of this potential source of sepsis is by surveillance and detection, and, when indicated, by isolation (see Chap. 14), as well as by appropriate methods of housekeeping, food handling, and disposal of feces and materials contaminated by feces, saliva, sweat, and so forth. For example, the obtaining of chest films of all patients admitted to the hospital is a helpful method of surveillance for pulmonary tuberculosis; periodic examinations of hospital personnel may detect carriers or those with inapparent disease. Methods to promote voluntary reporting of disease in personnel should be encouraged so that those with communicable disorders may be excluded from patient contact. The employee who loses time from work for this reason should be compensated.

BIBLIOGRAPHY

Albert RK, Condie F: Hand-washing patterns on medical intensive-care units. N Engl J Med 304:1465–1466, 1981

Altemeier WA: Bodily response to infectious agents. JAMA 202:1085, 1967

Altemeier WA: Bacteriology of surgical infections. Clinical and experimental considerations, pp 53–70. Presented at Vingt-quatrieme Congres de la Societe Internationale de Chirurgie, Moscow, 1971

Altemeier WA, Barnes BJ, Pulaski EJ, Sandusky WR, Burke JF, Clowes GA Jr: Infections: Prophylaxis and management — A symposium. Surgery 67:369, 1970

Altemeier WA, Culbertson WR, Fullen WD, McDonough JJ: Serratia marcescens septicemia: A new threat in surgery. Arch Surg 99:232, 1969

Altemeier WA, Hummel RP, Hill EO, Lewis S: Changing patterns in surgical infections. Ann Surg 178(4):436–445, 1973

Altemeier WA, McDonough JJ, Fullen WD: Third-day surgical fever. Arch Surg 103:158, 1971

Altemeier WA, Todd JC, Inge WW: Gram-negative septicemia: A growing threat. Ann Surg 166:530, 1967

Arnold TR, Hepler CD: Bacterial contamination of intravenous fluids opened in unsterile air. Am J Hosp Pharm 28:614, 1971

Barrett FF, Casey JI, Finland M: Infections and antibiotic use among patients at Boston City Hospital, February, 1967. N Engl J Med 278:5, 1968

Baskin TW, Rosenthal AA, Pruitt BA Jr: Acute bacterial endocarditis: A silent source of sepsis in the burn patient. Ann Surg 184:618–621, 1976

Bennett JV, Brachman PS (eds): Hospital Infections. Boston, Little, Brown & Co, 1979

Bennett JV, Scheckler WE, Maki DG et al: Current national patterns — United States. In Center for Disease Control: Proceedings of the International Conference on Nosocomial Infections, pp 42–49. Chicago, American Hospital Association, 1971

Bentley DW, Lepper MH: Septicemia related to indwelling venous catheter. JAMA 206:1749, 1968

Brachman PS: Nosocomial infection control: An overview. Rev Infect Dis 3(4):640–648, 1981

Brachman PS, Dan BB, Haley RW, Hooton TM, Garner JS, Allen JP: Nosocomial surgical infections: Incidence and cost. Surg Clin North Am 60(1):15–25, 1980

Brennan MF, Goldman MH, O'Connell RC, Kundsin RB, Moore FD: Prolonged parenteral alimentation: Candida growth and the prevention of candidemia by amphotericin instillation. Ann Surg 176:265, 1972

BUTLER HK, KUNIN CM: Evaluation of polymyxin catheter lubricant and impregnated catheters. J Urol 100:560, 1968

CENTER FOR DISEASE CONTROL: Nosocomial bacteremias associated with intravenous fluid therapy. MMWR 20(Suppl 9), 1971

CENTER FOR DISEASE CONTROL: National Nosocomial Infections Study. Report No. 8, Aug 1970 through Mar 1971, Vol 11, p 22. Atlanta, Center for Disease Control, 1972

CENTER FOR DISEASE CONTROL: Septicemias associated with contaminated intravenous fluids. MMWR 22(11):99, 1973

CENTER FOR DISEASE CONTROL: National Nosocomial Infections Study Quarterly Report, 1st and 2nd Quarters, 1973, pp 20–27. Atlanta, Center for Disease Control, July, 1974

CENTER FOR DISEASE CONTROL: Immune globulins for protection against viral hepatitis. MMWR 30:423–435, 1981

CENTER FOR DISEASE CONTROL: ACIP Recommendation: Inactivated hepatitis B virus vaccine. MMWR 31(24):317, 1982

CRAVEN DE, CONNOLLY MG JR, LICHTENBERG DA et al: Contamination of mechanical ventilators with tubing changes every 24 or 48 hours. N Engl J Med 306:1505–1509, 1982

DEEB EN, NATSIOS CA: Contamination of intravenous fluids by bacteria and fungi during preparation and administration. Am J Hosp Pharm 28:764, 1971

DESAUTELS RE: Proper use of the catheter. Hospital Medicine 2(8):97, 1966

DESAUTELS RE, WALTER CW, GRAVES RC, HARRISON JH: Technical advances in the prevention of urinary tract infection. Trans Am Assoc Genitourin Surg 53:184, 1961

DIENSTAG JL, RYAN DM: Occupational exposure to hepatitis B virus in hospital personnel: Infection or immunization. Am J Epidemiol 115:26–39, 1982

EICHOFF TC, BRACHMAN PS, BENNETT JV, BROWN JF: Surveillance of nosocomial infections in community hospitals. I. Surveillance methods, effectiveness, and initial results. J Infect Dis 120:305, 1969

FINEGOLD SM, SMOLENS B, COHEN AA, HEWITT WL, MILLER AB, DAVIS A: Necrotizing pneumonitis and empyema due to microaerophilic streptococci. N Engl J Med 273:462, 1965

FINLAND M, JONES WF, BARNES MW: Occurrence of serious bacterial infections since introduction of antibacterial agents. JAMA 170:2188, 1959

FISCHER JE (ed): Surgical Nutrition. Boston, Little, Brown & Co, 1983

FITZGERALD RH JR, NOLAN DR, ILSTRUP DM, VAN SCOY RE, WASHINGTON JA II, COVENTRY MB: Deep wound sepsis following total hip arthroplasty. J Bone Joint Surg (Am) 59(7):847–855, 1977

FOLEY FD, GREENAWALD KA, NASH G, PRUITT BA JR: Herpesvirus infection in burned patients. N Engl J Med 282:652, 1970

FOLEY FD, SHUCK JM: Burn wound infection with Phycomycetes requiring amputation of the hand. JAMA 203:596, 1968

FRANCIS DP, HADLER SC, THOMPSON SE et al: The prevention of hepatitis B with vaccine: Report of the CDC multi-center efficacy trial among homosexual men. Ann Intern Med 97:362, 1982

GOLDMANN DA, MAKI DG: Infection control in total parenteral nutrition. JAMA 223:1360, 1973

GOLDMANN DA, MAKI DG, RHAME FS, KAISER AB, TENNEY JH, BENNETT JV: Guidelines for infection control in intravenous therapy. Ann Intern Med 79:848, 1973

GOLDMANN DA, MARTIN WT, WORTHINGTON JW: Growth of bacteria and fungi in total parenteral nutrition solutions. Am J Surg 126:314, 1973

GREENWALT TJ, JAMIESON GA (eds): Transmissible Disease and Blood Transfusion. New York, Grune & Stratton, 1974

HAMMARSTEN J, HOLM J, SCHERSTEN T: Infections in vascular surgery. J Cardiovasc Surg (Torino) 18(6):543–545, 1977

JOHANSON WG JR, PIERCE AK, SANFORD JP, THOMAS GD: Nosocomial respiratory infections with gram-negative bacilli: The significance of colonization of the respiratory tract. Ann Intern Med 77:701, 1972

JOHANSON WG JR, SANFORD JP: Problem of infection and antimicrobials relating to anesthesia and inhalation therapy. Clinical Anesthesia 3:299, 1968

JUDD PA, TOMLIN PJ, WHITBY JL, INGLIS TCM, ROBINSON JS: Disinfection of ventilators by ultrasonic nebulization. Lancet 2:1019, 1968

KRUGMAN S, HOLLEY HP JR, DAVIDSON M et al: Immunogenic effect of inactivated hepatitis B vaccine: Comparison of 20 μg and 40 μg doses. J Med Virol 8:119–121, 1981

KUNDSIN RB, WALTER CW, SCOTT JA: In-use testing of sterility of intravenous solutions in plastic containers. Surgery 73:778, 1973

KUNIN CM: Urinary tract infections: Flow charts (algorithms) for detection and treatment. JAMA 233:458, 1975

LERNER AM, FEDERMAN MJ: Gram-negative bacillary pneumonia. J Infect Dis 124:425, 1971

LONG JM III, PRUITT BA JR: Suppurative thrombophlebitis. In Rutherford RB (ed): Vascular Surgery, pp 299–325. Philadelphia, WB Saunders, 1977

LOWBURY EJL, AYLIFFE GAJ, GEDDES AM, WILLIAMS JD: Control of Hospital Infection, 2nd edition. Philadelphia, JB Lippincott, 1981

MAKI DG, ANDERSON RL, SHULMAN JA: In-use contamination of intravenous infusion fluid. Appl Microbiol 28:778, 1974

MAKI DG, GOLDMANN DA, RHAME FS: Infection control in intravenous therapy. Ann Intern Med 79:867, 1973

MAKI DG, MARTIN WT: Nationwide epidemic of septicemia caused by contaminated infusion products. IV. Growth of microbial pathogens in fluids for intravenous infusion. J Infect Dis 131:267, 1975

MAKI DG, RHAME FS, GOLDMANN DA, MANDELL GL: The infection hazard posed by contaminated intravenous infusion fluid. In Sonnenwirth AC (ed): Bacteremia: Laboratory and Clinical Aspects, Chap 6. Springfield, IL, Charles C Thomas, 1973

MAKI DG, RHAME FS, MACKEL DC, BENNETT JV: Nationwide epidemic of septicemia caused by contaminated intravenous products. I. Epidemiologic and clinical features. Am J Med 60:471, 1976

MARTIN CM, VAQUER F, MEYERS MS, EL-DADAH A: Prevention of gram-negative rod bacteremia associated with indwelling urinary tract catheterization. In Antimicrobial Agents and Chemotherapy, p 617. Ann Arbor, Braun-Brumfeld, 1963

MAYNARD JE: Viral hepatitis as an occupational hazard in the health care profession. In Vyas GN, Cohen SN, Schmid R (eds): Viral hepatitis, pp 321–331. Philadelphia, Franklin Institute Press, 1978

MEEKS CH, PEMBLETON WE, HENCH ME: Sterilization of anesthesia apparatus. JAMA 199:276, 1967

MILLER DR, SETHI G: Tracheal stenosis following prolonged cuff intubation: Cause and prevention. Ann Surg 171:283, 1970

MOFFETT HL, ALLAN D: Colonization of infants exposed to bacterially contaminated mists. Am J Dis Child 114:21, 1967

NASH G, FOLEY FD, PRUITT BA JR: Candida burn wound invasion: A cause of systemic candidiasis. Arch Pathol 90:75, 1970

NOBLE WC: *Staphylococcus aureus* on the hair. J Clin Pathol 19:570, 1966

PATTISON CP, MAYNARD JE, BERQUIST KR, WEBSTER HM: Epidemiology of hepatitis B in hospital personnel. Am J Epidemiol 101:59–64, 1975

PHILLIPS I: *Pseudomonas aeruginosa* respiratory tract infections in patients receiving mechanical ventilation. J Hyg (Camb) 65:229, 1967

PHILLIPS I, EYKYN S, LAKER M: Outbreak of hospital infection caused by contaminated autoclaved fluids. Lancet 1:1258, 1972

PIERCE AK, SANFORD JP, THOMAS GD, LEONARD JS: Long-term evaluation of decontamination of inhalation-therapy equipment and the occurrence of necrotizing pneumonia. N Engl J Med 282:528, 1970

PRUITT BA JR: Infections caused by *Pseudomonas* sp. in patients with burns and other surgical patients. J Infect Dis 130:S8–S13, 1974

PRUITT BA JR, FLEMMA RJ, DIVINCENTI FG, FOLEY FD, MASON AD JR: Pulmonary complications in burned patients: A comparative study of 697 patients. J Thorac Cardiovasc Surg 59:7–20, 1970

PRUITT BA JR, MCMANUS WF, KIM SH et al: Diagnosis and treatment of cannula-related sepsis in burn patients. Ann Surg 191:546–554, 1980

PRUITT BA JR, O'NEILL JA, MONCRIEF JA, LINDBERG RB: Successful control of burn-wound sepsis. JAMA 203:1054, 1968

REINARZ JA, PIERCE AK, MAYS BB, SANFORD JP: The potential role of inhalation therapy equipment in nosocomial pulmonary infection. J Clin Invest 44:831, 1965

RENDELL-BAKER L, ROBERTS RB: The hazards of ethylene oxide sterilization. Anesthesiology 30:349, 1969

RHOADES E, RINGROSE R, MOHR JA, BROOKS L, MCKOWN BA, FELTON F: Contamination of ultrasonic nebulization equipment with gram-negative bacteria. Arch Intern Med 127:228, 1971

ROBERTS RB: Disposables in anesthesiology and respiratory care—infections and sterilization problems. Int Anesthesiol Clin 10:157, 1972

ROBERTSON KB: Fungi in fluids—a hazard of intravenous therapy. J Med Microbiol 3:99, 1970

ROGERS DE: A changing pattern of life-threatening microbial disease. N Engl J Med 261:677, 1959

ROGERS KB, GITTENS B: Proceedings: An epidemic due to *Serratia marcescens* in a neurosurgical unit. J Clin Pathol 27:930, 1974

RYAN PB, RAPP RP, LELUCA PP: In-line final filtration—a method of minimizing contamination in intravenous therapy. Bulletin of the Parenteral Drug Association 27:1, 1973

SACK RA: Epidemic of gram-negative organism septicemia subsequent to elective operation. Am J Obstet Gynecol 107:394, 1970

SANDERS CV JR, LUBY JP, JOHANSON WG, BARNETT JA, SANFORD JP: *Serratia marcescens* infections from inhalation therapy medications: Nosocomial outbreak. Ann Intern Med 73:15, 1970

SANDUSKY WR: Spread of infection in hospitals. Surgery 67:372, 1970

SANFORD JP, PIERCE AK: Current infection problems—respiratory. In Center for Disease Control: Proceedings of the International Conference on Nosocomial Infections, pp 77–81. Chicago, American Hospital Association, 1971

SCHIMMELBUSCH C: Die Durchfuhrung der Aseptis in der Klinik des Herrn Geheimrath von Bergmann, in Berlin. Arch f Klin Chir 42:123, 1891

SCHIMMELBUSCH C: Aseptic Treatment of Wounds. New York, GP Putnam's Sons, 1895

SMITH PW, RUSNAK PG: Aminoglycoside-resistant *Pseudomonas aeruginosa* urinary tract infection: Study of an outbreak. J Hosp Infect 2(1):71–75, 1981

SOUTHAMPTON INFECTION CONTROL TEAM: Evaluation of aseptic techniques and chlorhexidine on the rate of catheter-associated urinary tract infection. Lancet 1:89–91, 1982

STAMM WE: Guidelines for prevention of catheter-associated urinary tract infections. Ann Intern Med 82:386, 1975

STAMM WE, MARTIN SM, BENNETT JV: Epidemiology of nosocomial infection due to gram-negative bacilli: Aspects relevant to development and use of vaccines. J Infect Dis 136(Suppl P):S151–S160, 1977

SZMUNESS W, STEVENS CE, HARLEY EJ et al: Hepatitis B vaccine: Demonstration of efficacy in a controlled clinical trial in a high-risk population in the United States. N Engl J Med 303:833–841, 1980

SZMUNESS W, STEVENS CE, OLESZKO WR ET AL: Passive-active immunization against hepatitis B: Immunogenicity studies in adult Americans. Lancet 1:575–577, 1981

THORNTON GF, LYTTON B, ANDRIOLE VT: Bacteriuria during indwelling catheter drainage. JAMA 195:179, 1966

TILLOTSON JR, FINLAND M: Bacterial colonization and clinical super-infection of the respiratory tract complicating antibiotic treatment of pneumonia. J Infect Dis 119:597, 1969

WALTER CW: Cross-infection and the anesthesiologist. Anesth Analg (Cleve) 53:631, 1974

WEYRAUCH HM, BASSETT JB: Ascending infection in an artificial urinary tract: An experimental study. Stanford Medical Bulletin 9:25, 1951

11

The successful control of infection in surgical patients requires the use of many measures, including the direct attack on microorganisms by antimicrobial agents.* These drugs are of enormous value, yet they are but one means available for infection control in the surgical patient. They must neither be omitted when indicated nor relied on to the exclusion of other methods.

CRITERIA FOR ANTIMICROBIAL EFFECTIVENESS

Certain criteria must be met if antimicrobial agents are to be effective in the treatment of established infection or in the prevention of potential infection:

1. The pathogen must be sensitive to the antimicrobial agent
2. The agent must make contact with the pathogen
3. There should be nothing at the site of microbial activity that interferes with the action of the antimicrobial agent
4. Untoward consequences of drug therapy should be anticipated, recognized, and treated promptly
5. Unsatisfactory response during treatment must be evaluated

The Pathogen Must Be Sensitive to the Antibiotic Agent. A microorganism is considered sensitive to an antimicrobial agent if its growth *in vitro* is inhibited in a concentration of that agent usually obtainable in tissue fluid or blood following the customary dose. Ideally, selection of an antimicrobial agent involves identification of the offending microbe and, with exceptions to be noted, the determination of the agent or agents to which it is susceptible (its antibiogram). This is accomplished by the collection and culture of pathological material (*e.g.,* pus, urine, blood, exudate, secretions) under anaerobic as well as aerobic conditions, and by *in vitro* testing for sensitivity to commonly used drugs, measured by standardized laboratory techniques.

The Use of Antimicrobial Agents

* Agents and methods used in the preoperative preparation of the skin of the patient and the hands and forearms of the surgeon, and for environmental disinfection are considered in Chapters 6, 7, 14, and 17.

Specimens should be obtained before starting the administration of an antimicrobial agent; it is important that a representative specimen in appropriate transport media be sent to the laboratory for culture and processing. Susceptibility testing of microbial isolates to antimicrobial drugs is generally done with disk diffusion tests, which have been designed for most of the common bacterial pathogens such as staphylococci and the rapidly growing aerobic gram-negative rods.

The terms *susceptible* or *resistant* are based on the zones of inhibition produced by concentrations of the antimicrobial agent usually obtainable in blood levels with the usual doses of a particular drug. It should be kept in mind, also, that antimicrobial blood and tissue levels may vary among different patients on the same dosage schedule, and that many different schedules are used.

Disk susceptibility tests with *Hemophilus influenzae* and enterococci may be misleading. Standard disk testing is not suggested for gonococci, tubercle bacilli, or *Nocardia;* it is recommended that these pathogens be tested by other methods (Barry and Thornsberry). Currently, no procedure is universally accepted for testing the antimicrobial susceptibility of anaerobes. In certain infections, such as those due to the *Streptococcus pneumoniae* and the Group A beta-hemolytic streptococcus, the identification of the organism is sufficient without testing for sensitivity, since these bacteria have remained highly sensitive to penicillin and related agents. Conversely, in some clinical circumstances it may be more important to determine the drug sensitivity of the microorganism than to identify it completely (Table 11-1).

Although the laboratory is essential for definitive diagnosis, there are other considerations that the clinician should keep in mind in order to arrive at an early and correct etiologic diagnosis:

1. Some infections have characteristics that permit the early prediction of the most probable causative organism before the results of culture techniques become available (see Table 11-3).
2. The microscopic examination of the gram-stained direct smear of the material to be cultured is a simple and inexpensive test that often gives immediate information that may be very valuable as an early guide to therapy, or clues to the type of organism causing the infection.
3. The possibility may exist that positive results of culture and sensitivity tests may relate to nonpathogenic or commensal microorganisms and not the primary etiologic agent. In such instances, special cultures, biopsies, or other tests may be necessary to establish the correct diagnosis before effective antimicrobial therapy can be initiated.
4. The lesion may be viral with other commensal bacteria.
5. Anaerobes causing infections may be missed and associated aerobes, more easily cultured, may be mistaken as the etiologic agents.

Antimicrobial agents abet the usual defense mechanisms of the host against infection. Some drugs are bactericidal; others are bacteriostatic (they inhibit multiplication without destroying bacteria). When bacteriostatic agents are used, the final resolution of the infection depends on the natural defenses of the body, and it follows that if maximum effectiveness of drug therapy is to be expected, the usual host defense mechanisms should be intact. When dealing with life-threatening infections or infection in the host whose natural microbial defense mechanisms are impaired, bactericidal agents are preferable to those that are bacteriostatic.

(Text continues on p 180)

Table 11-1. A Guide to the Selection of Antimicrobial Agents Pending the Results of Specific Sensitivity Determinations

Microorganism	Agent or Agents of First Choice	Alternative Agents
Gram-positive cocci		
Staphylococcus aureus		
Non-penicillinase producing	Penicillin G or V	A cephalosporin; clindamycin; vancomycin
Penicillinase producing	A penicillinase-resistant penicillin	A cephalosporin; vancomycin; clindamycin
Streptococcus pyogenes Groups A, C, and G	Penicillin G or V	An erythromycin; a cephalosporin; vancomycin
Group B streptococci	Penicillin G or ampicillin	Vancomycin; an erythromycin; a cephalosporin
Streptococcus viridans group	Penicillin G with or without streptomycin	A cephalosporin; vancomycin
Streptococcus bovis	Penicillin G	A cephalosporin; vancomycin
Streptococcus, Enterococcus group		
Endocarditis or other severe infection	Ampicillin or penicillin G with gentamicin or streptomycin	Vancomycin with gentamicin or streptomycin
Uncomplicated urinary tract infection	Ampicillin or amoxicillin	Nitrofurantoin
Streptococcus, anaerobic	Penicillin G	Clindamycin; an erythromycin; a cephalosporin
Streptococcus pneumoniae	Penicillin G or V	An erythromycin; a cephalosporin; chloramphenicol; vancomycin
Gram-positive bacilli		
Bacillus anthracis	Penicillin G	An erythromycin, a tetracycline
Clostridium welchii	Penicillin G	Chloramphenicol, clindamycin; metronidazole; a tetracycline
Clostridium tetani	Penicillin G	A tetracycline
Clostridium difficile	Vancomycin	Metronidazole
Corynebacterium diptheriae	An erythromycin	Penicillin G

(Continued)

Table 11-1 *(Continued)*

Microorganism	Agent or Agents of First Choice	Alternative Agents
Gram-negative cocci		
Neisseria gonorrhoeae	Amoxicillin followed by a tetracycline; or penicillin G	A tetracycline; ampicillin; spectinomycin; cefoxitin; cefotaxime; cefuroxime; ceftizoxime
Neisseria meningitidis	Penicillin G	Chloramphenicol; a sulfonamide
Gram-negative bacilli		
Bacteroides		
Oropharyngeal strains	Penicillin G	Clindamycin; cefoxitin; metronidazole
Gastrointestinal strains	Clindamycin or metronidazole	Cefoxitin; chloramphenicol; mezlocillin, ticarcillin, or piperacillin
Enterobacter	Gentamicin, tobramycin, or netilmicin	Amikacin; cefotaxime or ceftizoxime; carbenicillin, ticarcillin, mezlocillin, piperacillin, or azlocillin; chloramphenicol; trimethoprim-sulfamethoxazole
Escherichia coli	Gentamicin, tobramycin, or netilmicin	Amikacin; ampicillin; carbenicillin, ticarcillin, mezlocillin, azlocillin, or piperacillin; a cephalosporin; trimethoprim-sulfamethoxazole; chloramphenicol
Francisella tularensis	Streptomycin, gentamicin, tobramicin, or amikacin	A tetracycline; chloramphenicol
Fusobacterium	Penicillin G	Metronidazole; clindamycin; chloramphenicol
Gardnerella (Hemophilus) vaginalis	Metronidazole	Ampicillin

Table 11-1 (*Continued*)

Microorganism	Agent or Agents of First Choice	Alternative Agents
Hemophilus ducreyi	Trimethoprim-sulfamethoxazole or erythromycin	A tetracycline; streptomycin
Hemophilus influenzae		
Meningitis, epiglottitis, arthritis, and other serious infections	Chloramphenicol plus ampicillin initially	Cefuroxime; cefotaxime; trimethoprim-sulfamethoxazole
Other infections	Ampicillin or amoxicillin	Trimethoprim-sulfamethoxazole; cefuroxime; a sulfonamide; cefaclor; cefamandole; cefotaxime; cefizoxime; a tetracycline
Klebsiella pneumoniae	Gentamicin or tobramycin; or netilmicin	Amikacin; a cephalosporin; amikacin; trimethoprim-sulfamethoxazole; a tetracycline; chloramphenicol; mezlocillin or piperacillin
Leptothrix buccalis (Vincent's infection)	Penicillin G	A tetracycline; clindamycin
Pasteurella multocida	Penicillin G	A tetracycline; a cephalosporin
Pseudomonas aeruginosa		
Urinary tract infection	Carbenicillin or ticarcillin	Piperacillin, mezlocillin, or azlocillin; gentamicin; tobramycin; amikacin; a polymyxin
Other infections	Tobramycin, gentamicin, or netilmicin with carbenicillin; ticarcillin; mezlocillin; pipercillin; azlocillin	Amikacin with carbenicillin; ticarcillin; mezlocillin; piperacillin
Proteus mirabilis	Ampicillin	A cephalosporin; gentamicin, tobramycin, or netilmicin; amikacin; carbenicillin, ticarcillin, mezlocillin, or piperacillin; trimethoprim-sulfamethoxazole; chloramphenicol

(*Continued*)

Table 11-1 *(Continued)*

Microorganism	Agent or Agents of First Choice	Alternative Agents
Proteus (other species)	Gentamicin, tobramycin, or netilmicin	Amikacin, cefotaxime, or ceftizoxime; carbenicillin, ticarcillin, mezlocillin or piperacillin; amikacin; a tetracycline; trimethoprim-sulfamethoxazole; chloramphenicol; cefoxitin
Providencia stuartii	Amikacin	Cefotaxime or ceftizoxime; gentamicin, tobramycin, or netilmicin; carbenicillin, ticarcillin, mezlocillin, piperacillin, or azlocillin; trimethoprim-sulfamethoxazole; chloramphenicol, cefoxitin, or cefamandole
Salmonella typhosa	Chloramphenicol	Ampicillin; amoxicillin; trimethoprim-sulfamethoxazole
Other *Salmonella*	Ampicillin or amoxicillin	Chloramphenicol; trimethoprim-sulfamethoxazole
Serratia	Gentamicin or amikacin	Cefotaxime or ceftizoxime; trimethoprim-sulfamethoxazole; carbenicillin, ticarcillin, mezlocillin, piperacillin, or azlocillin; cefoxitin
Shigella	Trimethoprim-sulfamethoxazole	Chloramphenicol; a tetracycline; ampicillin
Acid-fast bacilli		
Mycobacterium tuberculosis	Isoniazid with rifampin	Ethambutol; streptomycin; pyrazinamide; para-aminosalicylic acid; cycloserine; ethionamide; kanamycin; capreomycin

Table 11-1 (*Continued*)

Microorganism	Agent or Agents of First Choice	Alternative Agents
Actinomycetes		
Actinomyces israelii (actinomycosis)	Penicillin G	A tetracycline
Nocardia	Trisulfapyrimidines	Trimethoprim-sulfamethoxazole; minocycline; trisulfapyrimidines with minocycline, ampicillin, or erythromycin; amikacin; cycloserine
Fungi		
Aspergillus	Amphotericin B	No dependable alternative
Blastomyces dermatitidis	Amphotericin B	Ketoconazole
Candida species	Amphotericin B with or without flucytosine	Ketoconazole
Chromomycosis	Flucytosine	Ketoconazole
Coccidioides immitis	Amphotericin B	Ketoconazole; miconazole
Cryptococcus neoformans	Amphotericin B with or without flucytosine	Ketoconazole; miconazole
Dermatophytes (tinea)	Clotrimazole (topical) or miconazole (topical)	Tolnaftate (topical); haloprogin (topical); griseofulvin; ketoconazole
Histoplasma capsulatum	Amphotericin B	Ketoconazole
Mucor	Amphotericin B	No dependable alternative
Paracoccidioides brasiliensis	Amphotericin B or ketoconazole	Ketoconazole; a sulfonamide; miconazole
Sporothrix schenckii	An iodide	Amphotericin B

The microorganisms listed are ones that may be etiologic agents of infection in the surgical patient. Each agent that appears above is recommended as the agent of first choice or as an alternative until the results of sensitivity determinations are available.

(Modified from Medical Letter on Drugs and Therapeutics 26:19–26, 36–38, 1984)

The Agent Must Make Contact with the Pathogen. One of the cardinal tenets in achieving effective antimicrobial therapy requires contact between microorganisms and an adequate amount of drug. (Tables 11-2 and 11-3 list the recommended dosages for adults and children.) The method of administration and the route whereby the agent travels to make this contact are of importance. Oral administration is the route of choice when there is no urgency, but this route is not possible in many surgical patients, particularly in the perioperative period. Intravenous administration provides more rapid perfusion of tissue by drug than is accomplished by other routes. In some infections it is probable that intermittent administration by intravenous bolus, resulting in intermittent yet very high tissue levels of drug, is preferable to continuous infusion. Subcutaneous and intramuscular administration result in slower absorption; in the presence of shock, these routes are unreliable and not recommended.

When an antibacterial agent is used systemically, blood flow to the area of infection must be adequate to permit delivery of an effective concentration to the site of microbial activity. In acute unlocalized infection without tissue necrosis, such as lymphangitis or cellulitis, blood flow into the area of infection usually is abundant, and drugs introduced by systemic routes can be expected to reach the area of inflammation. Conversely, some lesions, such as pyogenic abscesses, may be penetrated poorly or not at all.

Open wounds and accessible body cavities (*e.g.,* thorax, joints, peritoneum) present the surgeon with unique opportunities to supplement systemic administration. Although the peritoneal cavity, when exposed at operation, is an attractive

Table 11-2. Recommended Antibiotic Dosage for Adults*

Drug	Oral Dosage	Intramuscular Dosage
Aminoglycosides		
Amikacin		15 mg/kg/day ÷ 2–3
Gentamicin		3–5 mg/kg/day ÷ 3
Kanamycin		1–1.5 g/day ÷ 2
Neomycin	Poorly absorbed from GI tract	Not recommended
Netilmicin		3–5 mg/kg/day ÷ 2–3
Streptomycin		2–4 g/day ÷ 2–4
Tobramycin		3–5 mg/kg/day ÷ 3
Cephalosporins		
Cefamandole		4–12 g/day ÷ 4–6
Cefazolin	750 mg–4 g/day ÷ 4	
Cefotaxime		2–12 g/day ÷ 3–4
Cefoxitin		4–12 g/day ÷ 4–6
Cephalexin	1–4 g/day ÷ 4	
Cephaloridine		
Cephalothin		2–6 g/day ÷ 4–6

* Doses recommended are for adults who have normal renal function.
† See text for recommendations for bowel preparation.

target for topical application of an antimicrobial agent, it is not recommended for common use. In the presence of peritonitis, a probable benefit is an immediate high concentration of drug at the site of microbial activity. However, when the peritoneal circulation is intact, and especially when its vascularity is increased by the inflammatory reaction, diffusion and absorption of drug are rapid, and the high concentration, initially so important, is soon dissipated; thus, direct topical application in this area has no advantage over intravenous administration, which is the preferable route under ordinary circumstances.

Fatalities have occurred following intraperitoneal administration of aminoglycoside antibiotics in the anesthetized patient. This is said to be due to a curare-like action caused by neuromuscular blockage, which is potentiated by nondepolarizing muscle relaxants and volatile anesthetics. Protection against this very serious complication is accomplished by effective ventilation, monitoring neuromuscular transmission, and the administration of calcium and neostigmine.

Topical instillation as an adjunct to systemic administration has been used in pleural and joint cavities. As is the case with the peritoneum, the membranes lining these cavities absorb antibiotics avidly. Therefore, the dosage of such agents must be monitored to avoid undesirable levels. Table 11-4 outlines the characteristics of a number of topical agents.

In neurosurgery, the local use of antibacterial agents is often a necessity, because many agents are virtually excluded by the blood–cerebrospinal fluid barrier. Other conditions in which topical instillation has proved useful are ophthalmic infections and inner ear infections.

(*Text continues on p 188*)

Intravenous Dosage	Comments
15 mg/kg/day ÷ 2–3	
3–5 mg/kg/day ÷ 3	
1–1.5 g/kg/day ÷ 2	
Not recommended	Recommended for bowel preparation only†
3–5 mg/kg/day ÷ 2–3	
Not recommended	
3–5 mg/kg/day ÷ 3	
4–12 g/day ÷ 4–6	
2–6 g/day ÷ 4–6	
2–12 g/day ÷ 3–4	Should not exceed 12 g/day
4–12 g/day ÷ 4–6	
	Not recommended — nephrotoxic
2–6 g/day ÷ 4–6	Should not exceed 12 g/day

(Continued)

Table 11-2 (*Continued*)

Drug	Oral Dosage	Intramuscular Dosage
Cephalosporins *(cont'd.)*		
Cephapirin		2–6 g/day ÷ 4–6
Cephradine	1–4 g/day ÷ 4	2–8 g/day ÷ 4–6
Moxalactam		2–6 g/day ÷ 2–3
Penicillins		
Amoxicillin	750–1500 mg/day ÷ 3	
Ampicillin	1–2 g/day ÷ 4	1–2 g/day ÷ 4
Azlocillin		4–8 g/day ÷ 4
Carbenicillin		20–40 g/day ÷ 4–6
Cloxacillin	1–2 g/day ÷ 4	
Dicloxacillin	0.5–1 g/day ÷ 4	
Methicillin		4–6 g/day ÷ 4–6
Mezlocillin		16–18 g/day ÷ 4–6
Nafcillin	1–6 g/day ÷ 4–6	2–6 g/day ÷ 4–6
Oxacillin	2–6 g/day ÷ 4–6	2–6 g/day ÷ 4–6
Penicillin G		2–30 million units/ day ÷ 4–6 depending upon severity of infection
Phenoxyethyl penicillin	375 mg–1.5 g/day ÷ 3	
Phenoxymethyl penicillin	375 mg–1.5 g/day ÷ 3	
Piperacillin		12–18 g ÷ 4–6
Ticarcillin		4–24 g/day ÷ 4–6
Polymyxins		
Colistimethate		2.5–5 mg/kg/day ÷ 2–4
Polymyxin B		1.5–2.5 mg/kg/day ÷ 4
Tetracyclines		
Demeclocycline	600 mg/day ÷ 2–4	
Doxycycline	100–200 mg/kg/day ÷ 1–2	
Methacycline	600 mg/day ÷ 2–4	
Minocycline	200 mg/day ÷ 2	
Oxytetracycline	1–2 g/day ÷ 4	200–600 mg/day ÷ 2–4
Tetracycline	1–2 g/day ÷ 4–6	200–600 mg/day ÷ 2–6
Other Antibiotics		
Chloramphenicol	50–100 mg/kg/day ÷ 4	Not recommended
Clindamycin	600–1800 mg/day ÷ 4	600–2700 mg/day ÷ 2–4
Erythromycin	1–2 g/day ÷ 4	200–6000 mg/day ÷ 2–6
Lincomycin	1.5–2 g/day ÷ 3–4	600 mg–1.2 g/day ÷ 1–2
Vancomycin		Not recommended

Intravenous Dosage	Comments
2–6 g/day ÷ 4–6 2–8 g/day ÷ 4–6 2–6 g/day ÷ 2–3	Up to 12 g for severe infection
1–2 g/day ÷ 4 200–300 mg/kg/day ÷ 4–6 20–40 g/day ÷ 4–6	Up to 12 g/day for severe infections Should not exceed 24 g/day For urinary tract infection: 8 g/day ÷ 4 Should not exceed 6 g/day

4–6 g/day ÷ 4–6
16–18 g/day ÷ 4–6
2–6 g/day ÷ 4–6
2–6 g/day ÷ 4–6
2–30 million units/
   day ÷ 4–6 depending
   upon severity of infection
	Should not exceed 12 g/day
	
	Should not exceed 6 g/day
	Should not exceed 6 g/day
	
	Should not exceed 12 g/day
	
	Should not exceed 23 g/day

12–18 g/day ÷ 4–6 4–24 g/day ÷ 4–6	
2.5–5 mg/kg/day ÷ 2–4 2.5 mg/kg/day ÷ 2–3	
	The use of tetracyclines is not recommended during pregnancy.
	Should not exceed 400 mg/day
0.5–2 g/day ÷ 2 1–2 g/day ÷ 2–4	
50–100 mg/kg/day ÷ 4 600–2700 mg/day ÷ 2–4 1–4 g/day ÷ 4–6 600 mg–1.8 g/day ÷ 2–3 2–3 g/day ÷ 2–3	

Table 11-3. Recommended Antibiotic Dosage for Children*

Drug	Oral Dose	Intramuscular Dose
Aminoglycosides		
Amikacin		15–22 mg/kg/day ÷ 3
Gentamicin		3–5 mg/kg/day ÷ 3
Kanamycin		15 mg/kg/day ÷ 2
Neomycin	Not absorbed from GI tract†	Not recommended
Netilmicin		3–5 mg/kg/day ÷ 3
Streptomycin		20–40 mg/kg/day ÷ 2–3
Tobramycin		3–5 mg/kg/day ÷ 3
Cephalosporins		
Cefamandole		
Cefazolin	25–50 mg/kg/day ÷ 3–4	
Cefotaxime		50–180 mg/kg/day ÷ 4–6
Cefoxitin		80–160 mg/kg/day ÷ 4–6
Cephalexin	25–50 mg/kg/day ÷ 4	
Cephaloridine		
Cephalothin		40–80 mg/kg/day ÷ 4
Cephapirin		40–80 mg/kg/day ÷ 4–6
Cephradine	250 mg–1 g ÷ 4	
Moxalactam		50 mg/kg/day ÷ 3–4
Penicillins		
Amoxicillin	20–40 mg/kg/day ÷ 3	
Ampicillin	50–200 mg/kg/day ÷ 4	50–200 mg/kg/day ÷ 4–6
Azlocillin		450 mg/kg/day ÷ 6
Carbenicillin		50–500 mg/kg/day ÷ 4–6
Cloxacillin	50 mg/kg/day ÷ 4	
Dicloxacillin	25 mg/kg/day ÷ 4	
Methicillin		25 mg/kg/day ÷ 4
Mezlocillin		150–300 mg/kg/day ÷ 2–4
Nafcillin	50–100 mg/kg/day ÷ 4	50–100 mg/kg/day ÷ 4
Oxacillin	50–100 mg/kg/day ÷ 4–6	50–100 mg/kg/day ÷ 4
Penicillin G		20,000–50,000 units/kg/day ÷ 2–4 depending upon severity of infection
Phenethicillin	25–40 mg/kg/day ÷ 4	
Phenoxymethyl penicillin	25–50 mg/kg/day ÷ 4	
Piperacillin		
Ticarcillin		100–300 mg/kg/day ÷ 4–6
Polymyxins		
Colistimethate		2.5–5 mg/kg/day ÷ 2–4
Polymyxin B		2.5 mg/kg/day ÷ 4
Tetracyclines		
Demeclocycline	6–12 mg/kg/day ÷ 2–4	
Doxycycline	2–4 mg/kg/day ÷ 2	

* Doses recommended are for children who have normal renal function.
† See text for recommendations for bowel preparation.

Intravenous Dose	Comments
15 – 22 mg/kg/day ÷ 3	
Not recommended	
Not recommended	
Not recommended	Recommended for bowel preparation only†
3 – 5 mg/kg/day ÷ 3	
Not recommended	
3 – 5 mg/kg/day ÷ 3	
25 – 100 mg/kg/day ÷ 4	
50 – 180 mg/kg/day ÷ 4 – 6	Children over 50 kg use adult dosage
80 – 160 mg/kg/day ÷ 4 – 6	
	Not recommended — nephrotoxic
40 – 80 mg/kg/day ÷ 4	
40 – 80 mg/kg/day ÷ 4 – 6	
50 mg/kg/day ÷ 3 – 4	
50 – 200 mg/kg/day ÷ 4 – 6	
450 mg/kg/day ÷ 6	Should not be used in newborns
50 – 500 mg/kg/day ÷ 4 – 6	
25 mg/kg/day ÷ 4	
150 – 300 mg/kg/day ÷ 2 – 4	
50 – 100 mg/kg/day ÷ 4	
50 – 100 mg/kg/day ÷ 4	
	Dosage for children not established
100 – 300 mg/kg/day ÷ 4 – 6	
2.5 – 5 mg/kg/day ÷ 2 – 4	
2.5 mg/kg/day ÷ 4	
	The use of tetracyclines in infants or children during tooth development may cause permanent discoloration of teeth.

(Continued)

Table 11-3 (*Continued*)

Drug	Oral Dose	Intramuscular Dose
Methacycline	6–12 mg/kg/day ÷ 2–4	
Minocycline	4 mg/kg/day ÷ 2	
Oxytetracycline	25–50 mg/kg/day ÷ 4	6 mg/kg/day ÷ 2
Tetracycline	20–40 mg/kg/day ÷ 4	12 mg/kg/day ÷ 2
Other Antibiotics		
Chloramphenicol	50–100 mg/kg/day ÷ 4	Not recommended
Clindamycin	8–20 mg/kg/day ÷ 3–4	15–40 mg/kg/day ÷ 3–4
Erythromycin	25–40 mg/kg/day ÷ 4	10–20 mg/kg/day ÷ 3–4
Lincomycin	30–60 mg/kg/day ÷ 3–4	10–20 mg/kg/day ÷ 2–3
Vancomycin		Not recommended

Table 11-4. Characteristics of Topical Antibacterial Agents

Agent	Antibacterial Spectrum	Penetration Nonviable Tissue
AgNO^3 soaks, 0.5%	Gram-negative and gram-positive	Extremely limited: precipitated by protein
Mafenide (Sulfamylon) acetate cream, 10%	Gram-negative and gram-positive	Excellent: freely diffuses
Silver sulfadiazine cream, 1%	Gram-negative and gram-positive, but some *Pseudomonas* are resistant	Limited
Nitrofurazone	Gram-positive and gram-negative	Limited
Povidone iodine	Gram-positive and gram-negative	Limited

Intravenous Dose	Comments
10–20 mg/kg/day ÷ 2	
10–15 mg/kg/day ÷ 2	
50–100 mg/kg/day ÷ 4	
15–40 mg/kg/day ÷ 3–4	
40–70 mg/kg/day ÷ 4	
10–12 mg/kg/day ÷ 2–3	
20 mg/kg/day ÷ 2–3	

Technique of Wound Care	Advantages	Disadvantages
Occlusive dressings: moistened q2h and changed b.i.d.	Painless No bacterial resistance No hypersensitivity	Electrolyte deficits Methemoglobinemia Impairs joint motion Discolors environment
Exposure with application to wound b.i.d.	Wound visible Easy to use No bacterial resistance Joint motion maintained Biologically and chemically stable	Pain on application to 2° Carbonic anhydrase inhibition Hypersensitivity in 7%
Either light dressing or exposure applied b.i.d.	Painless Wound can be visible Easy to use With open treatment, joint motion maintained	Hypersensitivity (rare) Crystalluria (rare) Leukopenia Selection of strains resistant to sulfonamides
Light dressing Occlusive dressing Light dressing b.i.d.	Painless Easy to use Wide spectrum	Rare hypersensitivity Rare nephrotoxicity Pain on application Rare acidosis

The burn wound is frequently the site for the use of topical antimicrobial agents. Agents such as silver nitrate, silver sulfadiazine, or Sulfamylon (mafenide) can be used with benefit at concentrations not possible systemically. Only when invasive infection is present or threatened should antibiotics be delivered systemically. Experience, however, has shown that antibiotics applied topically can lead to development of microbial resistance without eliminating surface colonization.

Although the method and route of drug administration are important, these alone cannot ensure contact between drug and pathogen if a foreign body has placed the organism beyond the reach of the agent. In addition, for greatest effect, contact between the drug and the pathogen must be made at an appropriate time in the metabolic cycle of the microorganism. Some antimicrobial agents have their greatest effect on actively reproducing organisms.

There Should Be Nothing at the Site of Microbial Activity that Interferes with the Action of the Antimicrobial Agent.   The penicillins are inhibited by penicillinase, a specific enzyme produced by certain staphylococci and coliform bacilli; the cephalosporins are inhibited by cephalosporinase and the sulfonamides by para-aminobenzoic acid. Another example of interference with antibacterial activity is the presence of dirt or of a coagulum that develops in some open wounds. In addition, drug incompatibilities also limit antibiotic effectiveness (Drug incompatibilities and other characteristics of antibiotic agents are listed in Tables 11-5 through 11-10.)

Untoward Consequences of Drug Therapy Should Be Anticipated, Recognized, and Treated Promptly.   None of the available effective chemotherapeutic or antibiotic agents is free of potentially unfavorable effects. Therefore, the surgeon who prescribes such agents should be familiar with possible adverse consequences and should monitor the patient for their appearance. Examples of untoward manifestations include a toxic action of the drug, hypersensitivity of the patient, changes in microbial flora resulting in the development of a superinfection, and patient idiosyncrasy. Such effects may range from drug fever, mild skin rashes, or troublesome gastrointestinal symptoms to deafness, renal damage, blood dyscrasia, or anaphylactoid shock (Table 11-11).

Undesirable manifestations preclude the common use of certain drugs. Nonetheless, for the patient with life-threatening infection, the probable benefit of effective therapy with a potentially toxic agent may override the risk of an adverse reaction. This conflict must be weighed carefully and settled on an individual basis.

Unsatisfactory Response During Treatment Must Be Evaluated.   If a patient does not improve during drug therapy, diagnostic reevaluation is imperative. This evaluation may include wound inspection, physical examination, and laboratory tests including blood culture, diagnostic x-ray films, isotopic studies, or ultrasonography, all in search of sites of new or continuing sepsis, such as undrained collections of pus, metastatic foci, or contaminated intravenous lines.

Therapeutic failure may be traced to one or more of the following: the initial diagnosis was in error; the organism that was initially susceptible has become resistant; a new organism has been introduced; or organisms initially present in small numbers and insensitive to the agent being employed have overgrown and become the predominant flora (superinfection). When any of these circumstances is suspected, one should obtain, when possible, specimens for culture and sensitivity testing so that drug therapy can be tailored to the changing needs of the individual patient.

For most acute surgical infections, it is unusual to prescribe antibiotic therapy for more than 10 days. However, chronic infections, such as osteomyelitis, subacute bacterial endocarditis, and tuberculosis, usually require prolonged antimicrobial therapy.

PHARMACOKINETICS AND ANTIBIOTIC DOSING

Pharmacokinetic characteristics of antimicrobial agents in a given patient will have a profound influence on the effectiveness of the drug. For an antibiotic to be effective, its concentration at the site of infection must exceed the minimal concentration of antibiotic required to inhibit or kill the bacteria involved in the infection. Factors that determine the concentration of antibiotic within the body include absorption, interactions with plasma proteins (protein binding), distribution, biological transformations, and excretion. Differences in antibiotic levels in various body compartments can be caused by active concentration (*e.g.,* in urine or bile); by the presence of a physiological barrier (*e.g.,* the blood–cerebrospinal fluid barrier); or by the diffusion characteristics of semipermeable membranes.

Under pathologic conditions, pharmacokinetic parameters may be dramatically altered by changes in absorption, volume of distribution, biological transformation, and excretion. In disorders of the gastrointestinal tract, absorption of an orally administered antibiotic is erratic. In shock, absorption from intramuscular sites is markedly delayed; in addition, patients in shock often have significant amounts of "third spaced" fluid and therefore an increased volume of distribution. The elimination of antibiotics through excretion in the urine or metabolism by the liver is impaired by disturbed renal or hepatic function; consequently, in such situations, antibiotic dosage must be adjusted according to the half-life of the drug. In meningitis, the blood–brain barrier becomes more permeable, and therapeutic concentrations of some antibiotics can reach the spinal fluid.

Technological advances that allow the rapid, accurate measurement of antibiotic concentrations in blood have made it possible to apply our knowledge of pharmacokinetics to antibiotic dosing. This is particularly important in managing the dosage of aminoglycoside antibiotics, due to their narrow toxic/therapeutic ratio, and the wide interpatient variation in elimination rate and dosage requirements of these antibiotics. This variability is accentuated in critically ill patients who have superimposed infection. These patients are frequently in a hyperdynamic state with increased intravascular volume, increased cardiac output, and increased glomerular

(*Text continues on p 212*)

Table 11-5. The Aminoglycosides: Action, Spectrum, Distribution, Excretion, Half-Life, and Incompatibilities

Agent	Mode of Action	Antibacterial Spectrum of Clinical Importance
Amikacin	Bactericidal (interferes with bacterial protein synthesis)	*Pseudomonas* species, *E. coli, Proteus* species, *Providentia, Klebsiella, Enterobacter, Serratia, Acinetobacter fremodii, Staphylococcus aureus* (lower activity against *Streptococcus pyogenes, Enterococcus, Streptococcus pneumoniae*)
Gentamicin	Same as above	*Klebsiella, Aerobacter, P. aeruginosa, Serratia,* indole-positive *Proteus,* some methicillin-resistant *Staphylococcus* species
Kanamycin	Same as above	*E. coli, Aerobacter, Proteus, Klebsiella,* some methicillin-resistant *Staphylococcus* species, *Salmonella, Shigella, Enterobacter, Serratia, Acinetobacter*
Neomycin	Same as above	*E. coli, Aerobacter, K. pneumoniae, Salmonella, Shigella, V. coma, S. faecalis*
Streptomycin	Same as above	*M. tuberculosis* and *P. pestis, F. tularensis, Enterococcus, E. coli, H. influenzae, Klebsiella, Streptococcus viridans*
Tobramycin	Same as above	*P. aeruginosa,* Enterobacteriaceae, some methicillin-resistant *Staphylococcus* species, *E. coli, Proteus* species, *Klebsiella, Citrobacter* species, *Providentia* species

* Important incompatibilities are also listed in Tables 11-6, 11-7, 11-8, 11-9, and 11-10. Each antibiotic may be incompatible with other agents including antibiotics, and the reader is referred to pharmacology texts and review articles for specific details on such incompatibilities.

Distribution	Excretion (Principal Route)	Biologic Half-Life	Important Incompatibilities*
Extracellular fluid; cerebral spinal fluid; peritoneal fluid; amniotic fluid	Renal	2+ hr	Should not be premixed with other drugs
Extracellular fluid; 30% protein bound	Renal	2 hr	Heparin; vitamin B complex
Extracellular and most body fluid; no protein binding	Renal	4 hr	Calcium salts, chlorpromazine, Dilantin, heparin, some steroids, barbiturates, phenothiazines, protein hydrolysates, sodium bicarbonate, vitamin B complex
Extracellular fluid	Renal	3.2–4.2 hr	
Extracellular fluid, 33% protein bound	Renal	2.2–3.2 hr	Calcium salts, chlorpromazine, Dilantin, heparin, some steroids, barbiturates, phenothiazines, protein hydrolysates, sodium bicarbonate, vitamin B complex
Extracellular fluid (no protein binding); amniotic fluid	Renal	2 hr	Inactivation by beta-lactam type antibiotics (*in vitro*), potent diuretics

Table 11-6. The Cephalosporins: Action, Spectrum, Distribution, Excretion, Half-Life, and Incompatibilities

Agent	Mode of Action	Spectrum of Clinical Importance
Cephalosporins in general	Bactericidal (interfere with bacterial cell wall synthesis)	Broad-spectrum activity: *Staphylococcus aureus*, streptococci (aerobic and anaerobic), pneumococci, clostridia, *E. coli*, *Klebsiella*, *Proteus mirabilis*, *Hemophilus influenzae* (additional activity listed below)
First Generation Cephalothin Cephapirin Cephradine Cefazolin		Spectrum is the same for all drugs in this group. Cefazolin produces higher serum concentrations and the biological half-life is longer; it is now used frequently when surgical prophylaxis is indicated.
Second Generation Cefamandole Cefoxitin		There is broader activity against gram-negative bacilli than with first-generation drugs. Cefoxitin is active against *Bacteroides fragilis*, cefamandole against *Enterobacter* sp.
Third Generation Cefotaxime Moxalactam Cefoperazone		Cefotaxime and moxalactam are active against Enterobacteriaceae. Moxalactam and cefoperazone are active against *Pseudomonas aeruginosa* and *B. fragilis,* and have an extended half-life compared with other cephalosporins. Moxalactam shows improved penetration of CNS.
Oral† Cephalexin Cephradine Cefaclor Cefadroxil		Cephalexin and cephradine are similar to first-generation parenteral agents. Cefaclor is active against *Hemophilus influenzae*. Cefadroxil has a longer half-life than the earlier agents.

* Important incompatibilities are also listed in Tables 11-5, 11-7, 11-8, 11-9, and 11-10. Each antibiotic may be incompatible with other agents including antibiotics, and the reader is referred to pharmacology texts for specific details on such incompatibilities.

† These agents are for oral administration; others listed are for parenteral use.

Distribution	Excretion (Principal Route)	Biologic Half-Life	Important Incompatibilities*
Body fluids; low concentration in CSF; protein binding is variable: 15% to 75%	Renal	Variable: 40–120 min	Calcium salts, Dilantin, chlor-promazine, barbiturates, protein hydrolysates, magnesium salts, parabenes, sympathomimetic agents, vitamin B complex

Table 11-7. The Penicillins: Action, Spectrum, Distribution, Excretion, Half-Life, and Incompatibilities

Agent	Mode of Action	Antibacterial Spectrum of Clinical Importance
Penicillin G (sodium salt available for patients with renal failure)	Bactericidal (interferes with bacterial cell wall synthesis)	*Streptococcus,* pneumococci, *Clostridium, Neisseria, Corynebacterium, P. multocida, Actinomyces, Treponema, Listeria*
Phenoxymethyl penicillin, phenethicillin	Bactericidal (same as above)	Same as above
Methicillin	Bactericidal (same as above)	Penicillinase-producing *Staphylococcus* species
Oxacillin	Bactericidal (same as above)	Penicillinase-producing *Staphylococcus* species
Cloxacillin, dicloxacillin	Bactericidal (same as above)	Penicillinase-producing *Staphylococcus* species
Nafcillin	Bactericidal (same as above)	Penicillinase-producing *Staphylococcus* species; useful against methicillin-resistant staphylococci
Ampicillin	Bactericidal (same as above)	*H. influenzae, Proteus mirabilis, Salmonella, Shigella,* some *E. coli,* gram-positive (same as with penicillin G)

* Important incompatibilities are also listed in Tables 11-5, 11-6, 11-8, 11-9, and 11-10. Each antibiotic may be incompatible with other agents including antibiotics, and the reader is referred to pharmacology texts for specific details on such incompatibilities.

Distribution	Excretion (Principal Route)	Biologic Half-Life	Important Incompatibilities*
All body fluids, but little in CSF and anterior chamber of eye; 65% protein bound	Renal, delayed by probenacid	0.5 – 1 hr	Ascorbic acid, Dilantin, heparin hydroxyzine, phenylephrine, phenothiazines, sodium bicarbonate, protein hydrolysates, vitamin B complex
Same as above; 75% protein bound	Renal, same as above		
Same as above; 38% protein bound	Renal and hepatic	0.5 – 1 hr	Aminophylline, barbiturates, calcium salts, some steroids, sympathomimetic agents, codeine, phenothiazines, narcotics, protein hydrolysate, sodium bicarbonate, vitamin B complex
Same as above; 80% protein bound	Renal and hepatic	0.7 hr	
Same as above; 95% protein bound	Renal and hepatic	25 min for cloxacillin; 43 min for dicloxacillin	
Same as above; 70% protein bound	Hepatic and renal	43 min	
Same as above; 25% protein bound	Renal and hepatic	1 – 2 hr	Aminophylline, barbiturates, calcium salts, some steroids, sympathomimetic agents, codeine, protein hydrolysate, sodium bicorbonate, vitamin B complex, succinylcholine

(Continued)

Table 11-7 (*Continued*)

Agent	Mode of Action	Antibacterial Spectrum of Clinical Importance
Carbenicillin, ticarcillin, hetacillin, amoxicillin	Bactericidal (same as above)	*P. aeruginosa*, indole-producing *Proteus, Enterobacter*, some strains of *Bacteroides fragilis*
Mezlocillin, azlocillin, pipericillin	Generally bactericidal	Wide spectrum: *P. aeruginosa, E. coli, Klebsiella, Serratia, Proteus, Enterobacter, Citrobacter, H. influenzae, N. gonorrhoeae, Streptococcus*, enterococci, *B. fragilis*

Table 11-8. The Tetracyclines: Action, Spectrum, Distribution, Excretion, Half-Life, and Incompatibilities

Agent	Mode of Action	Antimicrobial Spectrum of Clinical Importance
Chlortetracycline	Bacteriostatic (interference with bacterial ribosome)	Clostridia, pneumococci, Group A streptococci, salmonellae, *F. tularensis, Borrelia, Leptospira icterohaemorrhagiae*, some rickettsiae, *Entamoeba histolytica*
Oxytetracycline	Same as above	Same as above
Tetracycline hydrochloride	Same as above	Same as above plus *Pseudomonas pseudomallei*
Minocycline	Same as above	Same as above plus some "resistant" staphylococci
Methacycline	Same as above	Same as chlortetracycline
Demeclocycline	Same as above	Same as above
Doxycycline	Same as above	Same as above

* Important incompatibilities are also listed in Tables 11-5, 11-6, 11-7, 11-9, and 11-10. Each antibiotic may be incompatible with other agents including antibiotics, and the reader is referred to pharmacology texts for specific details on such incompatibilities.

Distribution	Excretion (Principal Route)	Biologic Half-Life	Important Incompatibilities*
Same as above; 50% protein bound	Renal and hepatic	1–1.9 hr	Dilantin, sympathomimetic agents
Body fluids, bile	Renal and hepatic		

Distribution	Excretion (Principal Route)	Biologic Half-Life	Important Incompatibilities*
Total body; 50%–70% protein bound	Renal and hepatic	2.3–5.6 hr	
"Total body water"; 20%–25% protein bound	Renal		Aminophylline, barbiturates, calcium salts, Dilantin, heparin, some steroids, sympathomimetic agents, phenothiazines, protein hydrolysate, vitamins, thiazide, diuretics, warfarin
"Total body water"; 20%–30% protein bound	Renal	8.5 hr	
"Total body water" with tissue levels commonly exceeding serum levels; 70%–75% protein bound	Renal and hepatic	18.6 hr	
90% protein bound	Renal	14 hr	
91% protein bound	Renal	12 hr	
93% protein bound	Renal	18 hr	

Table 11-9. Miscellaneous Antimicrobial Agents: Action, Spectrum, Distribution, Excretion, Half-Life, and Incompatibilities

Agent	Mode of Action	Antimicrobial Spectrum of Clinical Importance
Bacitracin	Bactericidal (inhibits cell wall synthesis)	*Staphylococcus, Streptococcus, Neisseria*
Chloramphenicol	Bacteriostatic; inhibits protein synthesis	*K. pneumoniae, A. aerogenes, B. pertussis, E. coli, Salmonella, Pasteurella, Brucella,* some *Rickettsiae*
Clindamycin	Bactericidal and bacteriostatic; inhibits protein synthesis	Same as above plus anaerobic bacteria
Colistimethate	Bactericidal; alters cytoplasmic membrane, allowing leakage of nucleosides	*Pseudomonas, E. coli, A. aerogenes, K. pneumoniae, H. influenzae*
Erythromycin	Bacteriostatic and bactericidal; inhibits protein synthesis	*S. aureus*, pneumococci, enterococci, *Neisseria, T. palidum, P. multocida,* streptococci, *B. pertussis*
Lincomycin	Bactericidal and bacteriostatic; inhibits protein synthesis	*S. aureus*, streptococci, pneumococci
Metronidazole	Bactericidal	*B. fragilis*, other anaerobes except non-spore-forming gram-positive cocci and bacilli; *Gardnerella vaginalis*
Polymyxin B	Bactericidal; alters bacterial lipoprotein membrane permeability	*Pseudomonas, Shigella, Vibrio, Aerobacter, E. coli, Hemophilus, Klebsiella, Salmonella, Shigella*
Vancomycin	Bactericidal; inhibits bacterial cell wall synthesis	*S. aureus, C. diphtheriae,* streptococci, *N. gonorrhoeae,* clostridia

* Important incompatibilities are also listed in Tables 11-5, 11-6, 11-7, 11-8, and 11-10. Each antibiotic may be incompatible with other agents including antibiotics, and the reader is referred to pharmacology texts for specific details on such incompatibilities.

Distribution	Excretion (Principal Route)	Biologic Half-Life	Important Incompatibilities*
Extracellular fluid	Renal	1.3 hr	
Body fluids; 50% protein bound	Renal and hepatic	3.5–5 hr	Ascorbic acid, Dilantin, heparin, some steroids, phenothiazines, protein hydrolysate, vitamin B complex
Total body water except CSF	Hepatic	2.4 hr	Hydrocortisone, vitamin B complex
Body fluids	Renal	1.5–2 hr	Hydrocortisone, hydroxyzine
All body fluids	Hepatic	1.5 hr	Dilantin, heparin, some barbiturates, protein hydrolysate, vitamin B complex
Total body water except CSF	Hepatic	4.4 hr	Dilantin, hydrocortisone, vitamin B complex
Body fluids	Renal	6–8 hr	Alcohol, warfarin
Body fluids	Renal		Dilantin, protein hydrolysate, heparin, some steroids
Body fluids except spinal fluid; 10% protein bound	Renal	2–4 hr	Aminophylline, some steroids, Dilantin, heparin, phenothiazines

Table 11-10. Antifungal Agents: Action, Spectrum, Distribution, Excretion, Dosage, Half-Life, and Incompatibilities

Agent	Mode of Action	Antimicrobial Spectrum of Clinical Importance	Distribution
Nystatin	Fungicidal and fungistatic; alters cell wall permeability	*Candida, Cryptococcus, Histoplasma, Blastomyces, Trichophyton, Epidermophyton, M. audouini*	Minimal absorption of oral dose
Amphotericin	Fungicidal and fungistatic; alters cell wall permeability	*Histoplasma, Cryptococcus, Coccidioides immitis, Candida, Blastomyces, Sporotrichum*	Extracellular fluid
Flucytosine	Fungicidal and fungistatic	*Candida, Torulopsis Cryptococcus*	Total body water
Hamycin	Fungicidal and fungistatic; alters cell wall permeability	*Candida, Aspergillus, Blastomyces*	Extracellular fluid
Miconazole	Interferes with ergosterol synthesis	*Coccidioides immitis, Candida albicans, Cryptococcus neoformans, Paracoccidioides brasiliensis*	CSF penetration is poor
Ketoconazole	Interferes with ergosterol synthesis	Same as above plus *Histoplasma capsulatum, Phialophora* sp.	To most organs

* Important incompatibilities are also listed in Tables 11-5, 11-6, 11-7, 11-8, and 11-9. Each antibiotic may be incompatible with other agents including antibiotics, and the reader is referred to pharmacology texts for specific details on such incompatibilities.

Excretion (Principal Route)	Adult Dose for Severe Infection	Pediatric Dose	Biologic Half-Life	Important Incompatibilities*
Feces with absorbed fraction via kidney	600,000 U 4× daily, orally	200,000 U 4× daily, orally		
Renal	1 mg/kg/day	Test dose 0.1 mg/kg/day IV over 6 hr (maximum dose: 1 mg/kg/day	18–24 hr	Antihistaminics, calcium salts, chlorpromazine, corticosteroids, diphenhydramine, metaraminol, sodium chloride, vitamins, water for injection with preservatives
Renal	150 mg/kg/ day	1.5–4.5 g/m²/day for <50 kg	2.89 hr	Other bone marrow depressants
Renal				
Renal	200–300 mg/day÷3 (IV)	20–40 mg/kg/ day÷3	0.4–24 hr	Coumadin (anticoagulant affect)
Bile	Oral: 200–400 mg/day	20 kg or less: 50 mg daily; 20–40 kg: 100 mg daily; over 40 kg: 200 mg daily	2–8 hr	No significant interaction with oral anticoagulant or oral hypoglycemic agents

Table 11-11. Adverse Side-Effects of Common Antibiotics

	Hypersensitivity	Nephrotoxicity	Ototoxicity
Aminoglycosides			
Amikacin	Occasional skin rash, fever	Renal damage with azotemia, proteinuria; increased nephrotoxicity with poly-myxins, cephalosporins	Vestibular damage, rarely auditory damage
Gentamicin	Occasional skin reaction, rash	Renal impair-ment, azotemia, proteinuria	Vestibular, auditory
Kanamycin	Rarely rash	Azotemia, proteinuria	Auditory, vestibu-lar
Neomycin	Occasional skin reaction, contact derma-titis	Occasional renal damage, increased nephrotoxicity with other nephrotoxic drugs	Eighth nerve damage, auditory, vesti-bular
Streptomycin	Rash, toxic erythema, fever, anaphy-laxis (rare)	Occasionally renal failure may develop; increased nephrotoxicity with cephalo-sporins, polymyxins	Vestibular (frequent), auditory
Tobramycin	Occasionally skin rash	Azotemia, proteinuria, renal impair-ment	Vestibular, auditory

Central Nervous System Toxicity	Gastrointestinal Disturbances	Hematologic Toxicity	Other Adverse Effects
Rarely CNS reactions, neuromuscular blockade, paresthesias, headache, tremor	Rarely nausea and vomiting, numbness, tingling, muscle twitchings, convulsions	Eosinophilia, anemia, leukopenia, granulocytopenia, thrombocytopenia	Rarely superinfection, arthralgia, hypotension, increased SGOT and SGPT
Neuromuscular blockade			Rarely superinfection, disturbed mental function, polyneuropathy, anaphylaxis
Neuromuscular blockade, headache			Rarely superinfection, fever, peripheral neuritis
Neuromuscular blockade (frequent)	Malabsorption syndrome with oral use, GI		Superinfection, pseudomembranous enterocolitis, possible decreased digoxin effect
Neuromuscular blockade, rare central scotomata, optic neuritis, vertigo, paresthesias		Blood dyscrasia (rare), eosinophilia	Superinfection, paresthesias, occasional pruritis, myocarditis, hepatic necrosis
Neuromuscular blockade, headache, lethargy, mental confusion, disorientation	Nausea, vomiting	Anemia, granulocytopenia, thrombocytopenia, leukopenia, eosinophilia	Rarely superinfection, disturbed mental function, polyneuropathy, anaphylaxis, decrease in serum calcium, magnesium, sodium

(Continued)

Table 11-11 (*Continued*)

	Hypersensitivity	Nephrotoxicity	Ototoxicity
Cephalosporins (considered as a group in regard to adverse side-effects)			
For parenteral administration (relatively nontoxic)			
First generation Cephalothin Cephapirin Cephradine Cefazolin Second generation Cefamandole Cefoxitin Third generation Cefotaxime Moxalactam For oral administration Cephalexin Cephradine Cefadroxil Cefaclor Cephaloridine	Maculopapular rash, urticaria, angioedema, drug fever, anaphylaxis	Interstitial nephritis, proteinuria, azotemia	
Polymyxins	Rarely	Renal damage with azotemia, proteinuria, hematuria	Vestibular
The tetracyclines Tetracycline Oxytetracycline Chlortetracycline Demeclocycline Methacycline Minocycline	Skin rash, drug fever	Increased BUN, Fanconi's syndrome from outdated drug	

Central Nervous System Toxicity	Gastrointestinal Disturbances	Hematologic Toxicity	Other Adverse Effects
	Nausea, vomiting, diarrhea	Eosinophilia, neutropenia, hemolytic anemia, thrombocyto- penia, elevated prothrombin time (moxalac- tam), abnormal platelet, adherence (moxalactam), disulfiram-like reaction with alcohol inhibit- ing (moxalac- tam)	Relatively frequent super- infection, hepatocellular damage; *Clostridium difficile* enterocolitis, clinical hemor- rhage; nephro- toxic
Neuromuscular blockade with parenteral administration	Nausea, vomiting		Superinfection, peripheral neuropathy, thrombophle- bitis
	GI irritation with nausea, anorexia, vomiting, diarrhea	Prolonged prothrombin time, atypical lymphocytoses, thrombocytopenia	Pseudomem- branous colitis, staphylococcus enterocolitis

(Continued)

Table 11-11   (*Continued*)

	Hypersensitivity	Nephrotoxicity	Ototoxicity
Other Antimicrobials			
Bacitracin	Atropy	Proteinuria, hematuria, azotemia, nephrotoxicity	
Chloramphenicol	Rash, atrophic glossitis, drug fever		Optic neuritis, digital paresthesias
Clindamycin	Skin rash, drug fever, anaphylactoid reactions		Neuromuscular blockade (rare)
Erythromycin	Skin rash, drug fever, eosinophilia (all rare)		
Lincomycin	Allergic reactions, rarely anaphylactic, serum sickness		Vestibular
Rifampin	Rare	Occasionally nephrotoxic	

Central Nervous System Toxicity	Gastrointestinal Disturbances	Hematologic Toxicity	Other Adverse Effects
	Nausea, vomiting		Pain at site of injection
	Nausea, vomiting	Bone marrow suppression, aplastic anemia, idiosyncratic reaction, increased action of dicumarol and tolbutamide	Superinfection, pseudomembranous colitis, gray syndrome in neonates, staphylococcus enterocolitis
	Nausea, diarrhea, esophageal ulceration (rare)	Eosinophilia, granulocytopenia, thrombophlebitis	Superinfection, pseudomembranous colitis associated with *Clostridium difficile,* hepatic toxicity, Stevens-Johnson syndrome
	GI irritation with nausea, vomiting, diarrhea, stomatitis	Eosinophilia, thrombophlebitis	Superinfection, especially by *Candida;* cholestatic hepatitis
Neuromuscular blockade	Frequent nausea, diarrhea, colitis	Rarely neutropenia, agranulocytosis, thrombocytopenia	Superinfection including pseudomembranous colitis; hypotension with rapid IV injections
Severe muscular myopathy (rare)	GI irritation, nausea, vomiting, diarrhea	Thrombocytopenia, leukopenia, hemolytic anemia (rare)	Liver damage, organic brain syndrome

(Continued)

Table 11-11 (*Continued*)

	Hypersensitivity	Nephrotoxicity	Ototoxicity
Other Antimicrobials			
Vancomycin	Anaphylactoid reactions, chills, drug fever, skin rash, "red neck" syndrome (rare)	Nephrotoxicity with azotemia, proteinuria, hematuria	Eighth nerve damage (auditory) with blood levels greater than 60 μg/ml or continued treatment more than 10 days, in the elderly in presence of renal damage
Metronidazole (not an antibiotic)			

Penicillins in General: Adverse Effects

	Shared by all penicillins; allergic reactions, rarely anaphylactic; skin rashes, angioneurotic edema, drug fever, serum sickness	Nephropathy with serum sickness reaction, hematuria, proteinuria

Other Adverse Effects of Penicillins in Relation to Classification

	Hypersensitivity	Nephrotoxicity
Naturally occurring penicillins		
Penicillin G	As above	As above
Penicillin V	As above	As above
Phenethicillin	As above	As above

Central Nervous System Toxicity	Gastrointestinal Disturbances	Hematologic Toxicity	Other Adverse Effects
	Nausea, vomiting	Eosinophilia, neutropenia	Superinfection with gram-negative bacilli; thrombophlebitis (frequent); increased ototoxicity with other ototoxic drugs
See "Other Adverse Effects"	Nausea, vomiting, metallic taste	Neutropenia	Peripheral neuropathy (rare), seizures, encephalopathy; disulfiram-like reaction with alcohol intake
Convulsions with high doses; neuromuscular irritability; shared by all penicillins	Rarely nausea, vomiting, or diarrhea; colitis; shared by all penicillins	Hematologic changes with neutropenia or anemia shared by all penicillins	Superinfection
As above	As above	As above	Hyperkalemia, arrhythmias
As above	As above	As above	
As above	As above	As above	

(*Continued*)

Table 11-11   (*Continued*)

	Hypersensitivity	Nephrotoxicity	Ototoxicity
Other Adverse Effects of Penicillins in Relation to Classification			
Penicillinase-re- sistant semisyn- thetic penicillin			
Methicillin	As above	Interstitial nephritis and renal failure	
Oxacillin	As above	As above	
Nafcillin	As above	As above	
Cloxacillin	As above	As above	
Dicloxacillin	As above	As above	
Extended antimi- crobial spec- trum penicillins			
Ampicillin	As above	As above	
Amoxicillin			
Carbenicillin			
Ticarcillin	As above	As above	

Central Nervous System Toxicity	Gastrointestinal Disturbances	Hematologic Toxicity	Other Adverse Effects
As above	As above	Anemia, neutropenia, granulocytopenia	
As above	As above	Granulocytopenia, platelet dysfunction, thrombophlebitis	Elevated SGOT, hemorrhagic cystitis
As above	As above	As above	Elevated SGOT
As above	As above	As above	GI hemorrhage
As above	As above	As above	
As above	Diarrhea	As above	Superinfections, pseudomembranous enterocolitis, decreased effect of oral contraceptives
	Nausea, vomiting, diarrhea, glossitis, hairy tongue	Leukopenia, anemia, thrombocytopenia, agranulocytosis	Pseudomembranous colitis, elevated SGOT in infants
		Platelet dysfunction	Pseudomembranous colitis
As above		Platelet dysfunction	Hyperkalemic alkalosis, sodium overload

(Continued)

Table 11-11   (*Continued*)

	Hypersensitivity	Nephrotoxicity	Ototoxicity
Other Adverse Effects of Penicillins in Relation to Classification			
Ureidopenicillins (fourth generation) Mezlocillin Azlocillin Piperacillin	As above	As above	

(Adapted and modified from The Medical Letter on Drugs and Therapeutics, 24:21–28, 1982; and Wright AJ, Wilkowski CJ: The penicillins. Mayo Clin Proc 58:21–32, 1983)

filtration rate. In this setting, aminoglycoside antibiotics are rapidly excreted by the kidney, and the dose interval required to maintain therapeutic concentrations of the antibiotic in the blood may be as short as every 4 to 6 hours. In addition, these patients often sequester large volumes of fluid in the extravascular space and may require larger than recommended doses of antibiotic to maintain therapeutic blood concentrations. The use of pharmacokinetic dosing of aminoglycoside antibiotics has been shown to be a reliable method for maintaining therapeutic concentrations of the antibiotics and reducing their toxic complications. The use of pharmacokinetics to optimize the dosage of other antibiotics may result in improved response of patients with serious infections.

SURGICAL INTERVENTION AND ITS RELATIONSHIP TO ANTIMICROBIAL THERAPY

The use of antimicrobial agents is but one factor in the management of infection in the surgical patient. Two additional and important modalities are surgical intervention and general support. All components of therapy are interdependent, and each complements the others.

The relationship between surgical intervention and antimicrobial therapy in the management of infection depends upon the character of the clinical lesion. In some

Central Nervous System Toxicity	Gastrointestinal Disturbances	Hematologic Toxicity	Other Adverse Effects
As above	Abnormal taste, stomatitis	Leukopenia, thrombocytopenia, neutropenia, eosinophilia, prolongation of prothrombin time	Thrombophlebitis, elevated SGOT and SGPT, alkaline phosphatase, serum bilirubin, elevated serum creatinine, reduction in serum potassium

cases a surgical operation is the primary therapeutic thrust, and antibiotics assume a secondary although important position. Examples of conditions in which this approach is used are acute hemolytic streptococcal gangrene, clostridial myonecrosis, and closed-space infections. In other lesions therapeutic roles are reversed: drug use is paramount and the operation is directed at residual elements of the infection. And finally, there are other conditions in which resolution is accomplished by the use of antimicrobial agents alone.

These therapeutic interrelationships become clearer when one considers the character of the inflammatory process. If natural resolution of the initial microbial lodgment in human tissue fails, either the inflammatory reaction continues as an invasive and diffuse process or localization occurs.

In the unlocalized infection, the use of an antimicrobial drug without operative intervention is sound, provided the tissues at the site of bacterial activity are intact, well vascularized, and not threatened by pressure. Lymphangitis, cellulitis, and some serous surface infections (*e.g.*, peritonitis) in their early stages usually meet these requirements.

When the inflammatory process localizes and presents as a pyogenic abscess, tissue necrosis, or confinement within an anatomical closed space, surgical intervention is paramount. The purpose of the antimicrobial agent for localized infections such as these is to deal with residual elements of the infection and to prevent extension or dissemination to uninvolved tissue.

Surgical intervention in the management of localized infection includes one or more of the following operative procedures:

1. Incision and drainage of purulent material
2. Excision of devitalized tissue
3. Decompression of tension in an anatomical closed space
4. Relief of obstructed conduit
5. Removal of foreign body

Incision and Drainage of Purulent Material. The need to evacuate and maintain drainage of purulent collections is undisputed. Evacuation is accomplished by incision with scalpel or by aspiration using needle or trochar, under direct vision or guided by radiography or sonography. The maintenance of drainage is abetted by soft rubber tubes, or loosely inserted gauze or catheters to which gentle suction may be applied. With rare exception, antimicrobial agents administered systemically are unlikely to sterilize an abscess, but they are useful in preventing invasive infection or systemic dissemination to uninvolved tissue.

Excision of Devitalized Tissue. Surgical excision is required to assist natural separation whenever there is devitalized tissue within which infection exists or is likely to develop because of suppression of the normal vascular and cellular responses. Examples are burn wound eschar, necrotizing fasciitis, a leg that is nonviable owing to ischemia, the gangrenous vermiform appendix, and clostridial myonecrosis.

Decompression of Tension in Anatomical Closed Space. If infection is in initial stages and confined to an anatomical closed space such as tendon sheath or fascial space, antibiotics may be effective *if used early* while an intact blood supply exists, but progression of the infection, causing limitation of blood supply secondary to either pressure or vasculitis, necessitates urgent surgical intervention. In the early stages the vascular supply is intact, but rapidly developing pressure diminishes blood flow and ultimately helps to cause necrosis of tissue. The diminished blood flow also prevents access of drug that may have been effective if it had reached the area of bacterial activity. One of the aims of operation is restoration of adequate local circulation to an area that is being asphyxiated by unrelenting pressure. The surgical procedure should consist of decompression by surgical incision and should be supplemented by an appropriate preoperative and postoperative antibacterial agent.

Relief of Obstructed Conduit. Infection in various organ systems proximal or distal to a point of lumenal obstruction, due to intrinsic or extrinsic disease, is a well-known phenomenon. Examples are pyelonephritis, cholangitis, and pneumonitis secondary to obstructions of the ureter, common bile duct, and bronchial tree respectively. Under such circumstances, infection is refractory until obstruction is relieved. In most cases surgical intervention is required.

Removal of Foreign Body. Infection persists in the presence of foreign bodies such as synthetic implants, splinters of wood, kidney stones, or spicules of dead bone. The infection-potentiating effect of foreign body is widely recognized by clinicians and has been documented by anecdotal experiences; by the observations of Elek and Conen, who showed that the presence of a silk suture decreases significantly the number of staphylococci necessary to produce a subcutaneous abscess in human volunteers; and by Altemeier and Furste in their work with experimental gas gangrene.

Frequently, foreign bodies are extruded spontaneously or can be removed by relatively simple extraction, but, on occasion, surgical intervention is required.

GENERAL SUPPORTIVE MEASURES

Successful management of the patient with infection requires not only appropriately timed surgical intervention and properly selected and administered antimicrobial agents, but also measures aimed at general support. In addition to the treatment of underlying and preexisting health problems, these additional supportive measures include the following:

Rest, both general and local
Alleviation of pain
Elevation of an infected part when practical
Maintenance of normal fluid and electrolyte balance
Correction of anemia, recent blood loss, or reduced blood volume
Maintenance of adequate ventilation
Nutritional support

PREDICTION OF MOST LIKELY PATHOGEN

Valuable clues to the microorganism responsible for an infection can be gained by considering the anatomical location of the lesion, any underlying disease, a preceding operation, or the circumstances of trauma.

For instance, septicemia following urinary tract instrumentation is commonly caused by *Escherichia coli;* peritonitis following perforative appendicitis usually yields a mixture of organisms derived from the intestinal flora and includes many anaerobes; and very early cellulitis in the burn wound is often caused by streptococci. Table 11-12 elaborates this concept by listing organisms that are most likely to be associated with selected surgical infections.

Antibiotic Susceptibility Profile. Patterns of antibiotic sensitivity and resistance of certain microorganisms differ among geographic regions and even from hospital to hospital within the same region. These patterns, which change from time to time, are probably influenced by the frequency and duration with which various agents are used. Thus, it is highly desirable that each hospital laboratory maintain and distribute to its clinicians up-to-date records of the antibiotic susceptibility of frequently encountered organisms. An example of an antibiotic susceptibility profile is illustrated in Tables 11-13, 11-14, and 11-15.

(Text continues on p 221)

Table 11-12. Organisms Most Likely to be Associated with Selected Infections*

Infection
Erysipelas
Acute necrotizing fasciitis
Acute lymphangitis
Meleney's synergistic gangrene
Breast abscess
Subcutaneous abscess (not hospital-acquired)
Human bite (infected)
Abscess of hand
Abdominal wound
Gastrointestinal or genitourinary tract entered
Gastrointestinal or genitourinary tract not entered
Peritonitis following appendicitis or injury to intestine
Perirectal, appendiceal, intra-abdominal, retroperitoneal, or subphrenic abscess
Cholecystic abscess and cholangitis
Crepitant myositis
Enterocolitis following antibiotic bowel preparation
Urinary tract infection
Septicemia following burn injury
Septicemia following genitourinary instrumentation
Septicemia from contaminated intravenous solutions or associated with indwelling intravenous catheters
Septicemia from superinfections during antibiotic therapy
Primary pneumonia
Empyema
Pneumonia complicating respirator treatment or intubation
Toxic shock syndrome
Osteomyelitis
Salpingitis and tubo-ovarian abscess
Epididymitis

* Where applicable this table is to be used in conjunction with Table 11-7. (Modified from Altemeier WA, Alexander JW: Surgical infections and choice of antibiotics. In Sabiston DC Jr [ed]: Davis–Christopher Textbook of Surgery, Chap 17, pp 333–357. Philadelphia, WB Saunders, 1981)

Streptococcus
Polymicrobic, aerobes and anaerobes
Streptococcus
Microaerophilic *Streptococcus* and *Staphylococcus*
Staphylococcus, but may be polymicrobic
Staphylococcus, Streptococcus
Polymicrobic, spirochetes
Staphylococcus

Polymicrobic, *Bacteroides* important
Staphylococcus
Polymicrobic, aerobes and anaerobes

Polymicrobic, anaerobes and aerobes
Polymicrobic; *Clostridium*
Clostridium
Staphylococcus, Clostridium difficile
E. coli or other gram-negative bacilli, *Staphylococcus, Enterococcus, Candida, Chlamydia*
Polymicrobic; *Staphylococcus*, gram-negative bacilli
E. coli

Enteric bacteria, often *Pseudomonas, Serratia,* or *Mima*
Gram-negative pathogens or *Candida*
Pneumococci, *H. influenzae, Staphylococcus*
Pneumococci, *Staphylococcus*, gram-negative bacilli, *Streptococcus,* anaerobic streptococci, *Bacteroides*
Gram-negative pathogens, often *Pseudomonas*
Staphylococcus
Staphylococcus, Streptococcus, gram-negative bacilli, anaerobic *Streptococcus, Bacteroides*
Neisseria gonorrhoeae, gram-negative bacilli, anaerobic streptococci, *Bacteroides, Chlamydia*
Gram-negative bacilli, *Neisseria gonorrhoeae, Chlamydia, Mycobacterium tuberculosis*

217

Table 11-13. Antimicrobial Susceptibility Profile: Sources Other Than Urine (University of Virginia Hospital 1983)

Percent of Strains Susceptible

Organism	Number Tested	Penicillin	Nafcillin	Ampicillin	Carbenicillin	Piperacillin	Cephalothin	Cefoxitin	Cefamandole	Cefotaxime	Moxalactam	Gentamicin	Tobramycin	Amikacin	Trimethoprim/ Sulfamethoxazole	Clindamycin	Erythromycin	Vancomycin
								Penicillins			Cephalosporins			Amino-glycosides			Others	
Acinetobacter calcoaceticus	112			5	59	92	0	3	3	7	3	95	93	95	98			
Citrobacter sp.	101			5	34	78	46	46	75	89	90	88	88	98	96			
Enterobacter aerogenes	184			3	70	80	4	4	66	75	90	96	95	96	97			
Enterobacter cloacae	259			4	64	70	5	5	66	76	71	83	88	97	99			
Escherichia coli	546			67	71	76	72	98	92	99	100	98	98	99	96			
Hemophilus influenzae*	44			46														
Klebsiella oxytoca	74			11	1	96	93	100	95	100	97	100	100	95	99			
Klebsiella pneumoniae	320			8	8	84	86	97	91	100	99	91	89	99	93			
Morganella morganii	81			3	98	96	1	65	89	93	98	98	98	98	98			
Proteus mirabilis	220			91	94	94	96	95	95	98	98	100	100	100	100			
Pseudomonas aeruginosa	1383			1	55	84	1	<1	<1	9	21	79	97	89	6			
Serratia marcescens	199			5	87	100	6	68	31	99	97	100	87	93	97			
Enterococci	282	10		98													64	100
Staphylococcus aureus	1605	15	92				97									92	91	100
Staphylococci, coag. neg.	458	19	81	26			92									62	60	96

* 16 organisms = type B; 14/16 susceptible to ampicillin

Table 11-14. Antimicrobial Susceptibility Profile: Selected Isolates from Urine (University of Virginia Hospital 1983)

Percent of Strains Susceptible

Organism	Number Tested	Penicillin	Nafcillin	Ampicillin	Carbenicillin	Cephalothin	Cefoxitin	Gentamicin	Tobramycin	Amikacin	Sulfisoxazole	Trimethoprim/ Sulfamethoxazole	Nitrofurantoin	Tetracycline	Erythromycin	Vancomycin	Clindamycin
Escherichia coli	1375			75	77	73	99	99	99	99	84	95	97	80			
Klebsiella pneumoniae	273			3	2	88	96	96	96	99	67	84	66	71			
Proteus mirabilis	182			96	96	98	100	99	99	100	88	97	3	3			
Pseudomonas aeruginosa	253			0	64	0	3	78	92	96	4	3	0	2			
Serratia marcescens	32			3	59	3	44	84	59	91	50	75	6	3			
Enterococci	360	8		99									98*	26*	61*	100*	
Staphylococcus aureus	69	6	94	0		96							96	86	83	100	90
Staphylococci, coag. neg.	304	35	71	45		85							95	70	58	98	63

* Percent calculated from 196 isolates

Table 11-15. Antimicrobial Susceptibility Profiles: Selected Anaerobes (University of Virginia Hospital 1981–1983)

Organism	Number Tested	Penicillin	Carbenicillin	Cephalothin	Cefamandole	Cefoxitin	Chloramphenicol	Clindamycin	Erythromycin	Metronidazole
							Percent of Strains Susceptible			
Bacteroides fragilis	152	0	80	0	4	81	100	100	87	100
Species closely related to *B. fragilis**	71	4	87	5	12	52	99	96	81	100
Other *Bacteroides* sp.	71	61	97	66	83	92	99	100	92	99
Fusobacterium sp.	19	90	100	96	96	90	100	100	24	100
Clostridium sp., including *C. perfringens*	34	98	100	96	100	87	100	80	87	100
Anaerobic cocci	115	88	96	99	99	97	100	100	85	85

* Includes *B. distasonis* (14), *B. ovatus* (16), *B. thetaiotaomicron* (31), *B. vulgatus* (8), and *B. fragilis* groups (2)

CONTROL OF ANTIBIOTICS

Because some patients receive antibiotics without specific indications, or an agent to which the infecting organism is resistant, it is important that the hospital infection control committee and individual clinicians monitor, and in some instances restrict, antibiotic use. Such control should include reserving selected antibiotics for use in the treatment of specifically defined life-threatening infections; limiting broad-spectrum antibiotic therapy or combination therapy to patients with specific indications; voluntary restriction of certain antibiotics, based on results of in-house antibiotic sensitivity studies of selected infections; and analysis of distribution of opportunistic infections in a given hospital. Equally important is the regulation of the duration of antibiotic therapy.

SUPERINFECTION, OPPORTUNISTIC PATHOGENS, AND RESISTANCE

The equilibrium of a microbial population normally present in various parts of the body can be altered by antibiotic administration. As a result, pathogens that were present in inconsequential numbers may assume significant proportions and produce disease; this phenomenon is called superinfection. The gastrointestinal, respiratory, and urinary tracts, the skin, and the burn wound are important loci where colonization by "new" microflora may occur during or as a result of prior antibiotic therapy. Elimination of drug-susceptible organisms in a mixed microbial flora may permit the overgrowth of resistant forms, with the result of secondary infection being caused by opportunistic pathogens unresponsive to the agent being administered.

The development of this process of superinfection is influenced by the type and duration of antibiotic therapy, and it is particularly likely to occur as a sequel to prolonged therapy with broad-spectrum antibiotics or a combination of antimicrobial agents.

ANTIBIOTIC RESISTANCE TRANSFER

Antibiotic resistance may be due to inherent genes located on the bacterial chromosome or may be related to the presence of genes on ancillary genetic material, namely plasmids. Thus, bacteria may develop resistance to antibiotics by one of two mechanisms: (1) chromosomal mutations, or (2) the acquisition of antibiotic resistance genes on extrachromosomal plasmids or R-determinant plasmids.

Antibiotic resistance resulting from point mutations of chromosomal genes is a spontaneous event that occurs infrequently during the course of bacterial growth. Such mutations usually result in an alteration in components of the bacterial cell that are critical for the activity of the antibiotic. The number of resistant bacteria in a given population may thus be limited by the growth rate of the resistant strain relative to the growth rate of antibiotic-sensitive strains. Under the selective pressure of antibiotics, resistant bacteria have a growth advantage and may ultimately become the predominant organisms. Resistance acquired in this fashion is generally considered to be nontransferable between bacterial cells.

Plasmid-mediated resistance genes, in contrast, are frequently transferable between bacteria. Such transfer of resistance may be mediated either by genes on the plasmid itself or by other genetic elements such as bacterial viruses or other nonrelated plasmids. R-determinant plasmids are small, autonomously replicating cyclic DNA molecules that may carry genes encoding for resistance to multiple antibiotics. Under appropriate conditions, these plasmids can transfer between bacterial cells, conferring on the recipient bacteria resistance to multiple antibiotics. In most cases, plasmid-coded antibiotic resistance is mediated by enzymes that inactivate the antibiotic. The clinical importance of R-determinant plasmids is that they can confer resistance to all of the antibiotics to which they contain resistance genes. In addition, the formation and spread of new resistance plasmids appear to be ongoing: as newer antimicrobial agents are introduced, bacteria readily evolve mechanisms of resistance to these agents.

RECOMMENDATIONS FOR THE USE OF ANTIMICROBIAL AGENTS IN THE PREVENTION OF WOUND AND INTRACAVITARY INFECTION

The discussion to follow outlines the place of antimicrobial agents in the prevention of infection in surgical incisions, in traumatic wounds, and in bodily cavities entered by operation or by trauma. The terms *prophylaxis* and *prevention* are used synonymously and carry the meaning that the microorganism is attacked during the period of primary lodgment, prior to colonization and before either localized or invasive infection begins. In other words, the aim is to circumvent the development of clinically identifiable infection following microbial lodgment rather than to treat infection that is already established.

Surgical writings are replete with reports of laboratory studies and clinical observations aimed at assessing the value as well as the limitations of modern antimicrobial agents in preventing the development of infection in surgical patients. In 1964 Bernard and Cole at the Barnes Hospital in St. Louis reported a prospective clinical trial in 145 patients undergoing operations that are usually attended by a high incidence of postoperative wound infection. The infection rate at the operative site in a control group that received no antibiotic was 27%, whereas it was 8% in those patients who received a protective umbrella of penicillin, methicillin, and chloramphenicol, given parenterally. There had been previous prospective clinical evaluations of antimicrobial prophylaxis in surgery by others, but the protocol of this study was innovative in that antibiotics were started before operation. Moreover, administration was stopped within 4 hours after operation.

The English-language medical literature subsequent to the Bernard and Cole paper has been searched for reports of prospective, random-selection, placebo-controlled, double-blind clinical evaluations in which antibiotics were given parenterally and started before operation. A summarizing review of this survey was published in 1980 and brought up to date in 1982 (Sandusky 1980, 1982). Other reviews (Chodak, Plaut and Hirshman, Inui) and one monograph (Keighley and Burden) have addressed the subject of preventive antimicrobials in surgery. It is noteworthy that, after examining 45 articles concerned with antibiotic prophylaxis in surgery, Evans and Pollock concluded that there is room for improvement in the conduct of clinical trials.

Controlled clinical trials show that numerous antimicrobial agents, used singly or in combination and administered preoperatively, are effective in reducing the incidence of postoperative wound or intracavitary infection, or both, in an impressive list of operations, for example, in surgical procedures such as vascular reconstruction; in operations for head and neck cancer; in orthopedic procedures including fracture fixation; in gastrointestinal surgery; in colorectal operations; in biliary tract procedures; in appendectomy; and in vaginal hysterectomy. Not to be ignored are at least nine controlled clinical evaluations in which perioperative antibiotics failed to cause a statistically significant reduction in postoperation wound infection. (Bivens and associates, Brote and associates, Brown and associates, Campbell, Goodman and associates, Karl and associates, Mayer and associates, Roberts and Homesley).

Despite this lack of unanimity, it is concluded that in the clean-contaminated wound the incidence of postoperative wound infection or intracavitary sepsis, or both, can be reduced by the systemic administration of an antibiotic or a combination of antibiotics to which the offending microorganisms are sensitive, provided the drug is present before lodgment of the microorganisms.

Among the agents that have been effective in controlled clinical evaluations are penicillin, cloxacillin, nafcillin, ampicillin, piperacillin, tetracycline, gentamicin, tobramycin, rifampicin, lincomycin, cephalothin, cephaloridine, cefazolin, cefamandole, and metronidazole. It is immediately apparent that some of these agents would be inappropriate for preventive use today either because they have been superseded by more effective agents or because their use is likely to cause adverse side-effects (see Table 11-10).

Factors to be considered in selecting an antimicrobial agent for prophylaxis (prevention) include prediction of the pathogen likely to cause infection in the procedure planned, the antibiotic susceptibility profile of the community and of the respective hospital, and documented clinical experience. The potentially adverse side-effects of the drug under consideration must be weighed against the probability of benefit. When choosing a preventive agent it may be prudent, in some circumstances, to avoid one that may have to be relied upon later for treatment in the event that prophylaxis fails and infection ensues.

Effective prophylaxis requires preoperative administration of the agent timed so that tissues that will be exposed to lodgment of microorganisms during the surgical procedure will have protection against microbial colonization. Intraoperative reinforcement is necessary during long operations to ensure adequate tissue levels throughout this critical period. There is no evidence of benefit from administration beyond 24 hours. Limitation of both preoperative and postoperative use is important in reducing the probability of dose-related adverse reactions, superinfection, and the masking of signs and symptoms of developing, yet anatomically unrelated, infection. From a societal standpoint, minimal use lessens the cost as well as the possibility that resistant microbial strains will develop. The agent selected should be administered parenterally in the dosage and with the precautions usually recommended for the treatment of established infection.

Side-effects that may be adverse preclude the routine administration of antimicrobial agents to all preoperative patients. Therefore, guidelines are imperative. Broadly stated, the prophylactic use of an antimicrobial agent is indicated in those preoperative surgical patients in whom the risk of postoperative wound infection or intracavitary sepsis is great, or in whom the consequences of such infection, should it occur, would be grave. More specific selective guidelines are introduced after the following digression.

There are multiple nonmicrobial factors that influence the development of postoperative infection in a surgical patient (Chapter 9). These include local blood supply, tissue oxygenation, organic and inorganic foreign bodies, seroma, hematoma, the extremes of nutrition, and inherent or iatrogenic factors that alter the competence of host immune mechanisms. Yet microorganisms are a necessary requirement for the development of infection. Moreover, this is the only factor that can be influenced by the administration of an antimicrobial agent. The presence and density of microorganisms in tissue can be determined by the staining of a weighed and homogenized biopsy sample (see Chapter 9). Unfortunately, information based on this method is not available before operation. Therefore, if drug administration is to be started preoperatively, the decision must be made on a clinical basis.

A four-category classification of wounds is described in Chapter 3. It is based on a clinical estimation of bacterial density, contamination, and risk of subsequent infection in the wound. When used in two studies, each involving large numbers of wounds, a linear correlation between the categories in this classification and the actual incidence of infection was found (Table 11-16). Using this classification as a

Table 11-16. Incidence of Infection in Relation to Wound Classification

	Percentage of Total		Incidence of Wound Infection	
	NAS-NRC Study*	Foothills Hospital Study†	NAS-NRC Study*	Foothills Hospital Study†
Total	15,613	62,939	7.4%	4.7%
Clean	74.8%	75%	5.1%	1.5%
Clean-contaminated	16.6%	15%	10.8%	7.7%
Contaminated	4.3%	7%	16.3%	15.2%
Dirty	3.7%	3%	28%	40%
Unclassified	0.5%			

* Howard JM et al: Postoperative wound infections: The influence of ultraviolet irradiation of the operating room and of various other factors (Suppl). Ann Surg 160(2):9–192, 1964
† Cruse PJE, Foord R: The epidemiology of wound infection: a 10-year prospective study of 62,939 wounds. Surg Clin North Am 60:27–40, 1980

frame of reference, the following guidelines for the preventive use of chemotherapeutics and antibiotics in surgery were developed:

Approximately 75% of all operations are considered "clean," and in this group
the expected incidence of infection is less than 5%. If antibiotics were to be used for
all clean operations, a great number of persons would be exposed unnecessarily to
the risk of adverse drug effects. Therefore, the routine use of prophylactic antibiotics
is not recommended in all patients undergoing clean operations. Sound clinical
judgment, however, accepts their use in specific situations, such as operations
involving the insertion of permanent implants; operations that must be performed
on patients who are known to be carriers of pathogenic microorganisms (*e.g.,* nasal
carriers) or who have existing infection distant from the operative site; and operations on patients who have a history of rheumatic valvular disease or those who have
a previously implanted valve. In patients with known or suspected tuberculosis in
whom an operation is anticipated, antituberculosis therapy should be started preoperatively to prevent dissemination. Although substantive data are lacking, the use of
preventive antimicrobial agents may be beneficial in clean procedures that require
extensive dissection or that result in tissue that has diminished blood supply. The
value of such prophylaxis is unsettled in patients who require a procedure falling
into the clean category but who, because of underlying disease or therapy, have
immune incompetence.

Clean-Contaminated Operations.   Approximately one out of every six operations meets the clean-contaminated definition, and the likelihood of infection of
the wound or body cavity in an individual case is approximately 10%. The clean-
contaminated group includes some operative procedures in which the degree of
bacterial density and contamination are relatively minimal and in which the probability of infection is not great enough to justify the use of antimicrobial prophylaxis.
However, there are specific procedures covered by this definition for which the use
of these agents is recommended.

The use of prophylactic agents is recommended in the situations discussed under
the clean category and also for patients undergoing operations that require entrance
into the oropharyngeal cavity in conjunction with neck dissection; gastric resection
for carcinoma; intracavitary opening of the rectum, colon, or lower ileum or any
surgical procedure in which intestinal vascularity is compromised (*e.g.,* strangulat-
ing hernia or intussusception); entrance into the extrahepatic biliary tract in the
presence of culture-positive bile or obstruction of the tract; operations or instrumentation, including cystoscopy, that involve entering the urinary tract in the
presence of obstructive uropathy or culture-positive urine; operations on the lower
genital tract, such as vaginal hysterectomy; amputation of an extremity with
impoverished blood supply, particularly if an open ulcer is or has recently been
present; and skin grafting of open wounds.

Contaminated and Dirty Categories.   The contaminated and dirty categories combined accounted for 8% to 10% of the operations reported in the two studies
of wounds (see Table 11-16). The expected incidence of infection is high, and for

this reason the use of an antimicrobial agent is recommended for any patient whose wound is clearly identified as contaminated or dirty. Here, prophylaxis is directed not only at the wound but also at the prevention of intracavitary spread, systemic dissemination, and the development of infection in any operative incision that may be made in previously unsoiled tissue planes.

Wounds of Trauma

By definition, wounds of trauma fall into either the contaminated or the dirty and infected categories. It is here that the concept of antimicrobial prophylaxis (preventive use) may be confusing owing to apparent inconsistency in semantics. By definition, the preventive concept implies that an agent is present at the time of, or very soon after, the lodgment of microbes in a wound. In trauma, more often than not, the time lapse between injury and the possibility of administration is of sufficient length so that microbial colonization of the wound has already started. Strictly speaking, then, the use of an antimicrobial agent in such situations is more properly defined as treatment rather than prophylaxis. Even so, the routine or indiscriminate use of antimicrobial agents in a patient with a wound of trauma is to be avoided. Conversely, as in surgical wounds, prophylactic drugs may be helpful when the likelihood of infection is great. Antibiotic prophylaxis is recommended in the wound of trauma as follows:

1. *When the wound enters a joint space or when it is associated with an open fracture.* Here the problem may not be so much the probability of infection as the gravity of the consequences should infection ensue. Moreover, complete debridement may not be appropriate in every instance (see below).
2. *When there is heavy contamination.* Information on the circumstances surrounding the injury and the gross appearance of the wound itself (*e.g.,* the presence of dead or avascular tissue) are helpful in assessing the extent of the contamination. In the wound of violence, antimicrobial agents are not substitutes for careful surgical technique, namely, the excision of dead tissue, the removal of foreign material, thorough mechanical cleansing, and the reestablishment of vascular contact. Sound and careful surgery is the *sine qua non* of wound management; antimicrobials are adjunctive.
3. *When adequate debridement is not appropriate.* Adequate debridement of questionably viable tissue may not be appropriate, owing to the involvement of essential anatomical structures. This is particularly true in injuries to the tendons or fascial spaces of the hand. In such cases, even though the likelihood of infection may not be great, administration of an antimicrobial agent is desirable because the consequences of infection may be disastrous.
4. *When debridement is delayed.* Situations do occur when delay of wound care is unavoidable, owing to the need to transport the injured or for evaluation and treatment of other conditions having higher priority. In such a setting, antibiotics may make the difference between invasive infection and no infection. An intravenous antimicrobial drug should be given as soon as the patient arrives in the first emergency facility. The value of local agents prior to debridement is open to serious question in common surgical practice. It is axiomatic that locally applied drugs cannot sterilize a wound filled with blood, serum, devitalized tissue, and foreign bodies. If definitive operation must be delayed for the reasons noted above, the best means for protection against invasive infection insofar as drugs are concerned is systemic, preferably intravenous, administration.
5. *In burns.* The administration of systemic anti-infective drugs to the burn patient, with the exception of penicillin in the acute phase (the first 3 to 5 postburn days), for the

prevention of infection by Group A beta-hemolytic streptococcus and *Streptococcus pneumoniae* is ineffective and results in the early emergence of resistant strains of bacteria. Topical chemotherapeutic agents can be used to control the bacterial population of the burn wound and to prevent invasive sepsis. Systemic agents are unable to cross the interface between avascular, nonviable eschar and viable underlying tissue, thus rendering them useless in controlling the bacterial population of the burn wound. Topical chemotherapy with 10% Sulfamylon (mafenide acetate), 0.5% silver nitrate solution, or silver sulfadiazine are all effective against the common burn wound bacteria. Documentation of the effectiveness of other topical agents, such as the creams of various silver salts and gentamicin sulfate, is lacking. Moreover, the use of the latter agent has been associated with rapid emergence of organisms resistant to gentamicin.

The indications for antimicrobial prophylaxis in patients with burn-associated injuries are similar to those for any other injured patient. Concomitant disease such as tuberculosis or rheumatic fever requires appropriately modified antibiotic therapy.

6. *When the gastrointestinal tract is involved or presumed to be involved.* There is convincing evidence of the value of antimicrobial agents administered before operation when dealing with penetrating abdominal wounds provided preoperative administration is started intravenously as soon as possible (Fullen, Hunt, and Altemeier; Oreskovich and associates).

7. *In injuries prone to clostridial infection.* Certain injuries are more likely to be followed by clostridial infection than others. These include those associated with devitalized muscle, particularly in limbs with arterial insufficiency, wounds with gross contamination and retained foreign bodies, and wounds given inadequate or markedly delayed care.

Adequate surgical debridement without closure or followed by delayed closure is the keystone in the treatment of the wound likely to be infected with clostridia. In addition, penicillin G or, in the event of known allergy to this drug, another antibiotic known to be effective against the clostridia (see Table 11-1) should be administered as adjunctive therapy and should be started preoperatively. Gas gangrene antitoxin is of no value in the prevention of clinical gas gangrene. A "booster" of tetanus toxoid in those previously actively immunized or the administration of human hyperimmune antitetanus globulin in others, plus appropriate wound care, is the preferred means of tetanus prophylaxis. In certain instances of minimal contamination, a booster injection may not be necessary in patients who have received a booster within 5 years.

Preparation for Operation on Colon or Rectum

Preparation of the intestine for an elective operation that may result in fecal contamination of the operative incision or of the peritoneal cavity is aimed at reduction of intestinal content and its microbial flora. An essential part of any program of bowel preparation is thorough mechanical cleansing.

While undergoing preparation, bulk is kept low and nutritional support is maintained by the oral intake of low-residue clear liquids or with an elemental diet. In some circumstances the nutritionally depleted patient will require parenteral nutrition, including vitamins.

The meticulous use of the well-established techniques of intestinal surgery, including secondary isolation of the operative field and the use of a barrier device against soilage, are basic to the control of infection. This is true whether one uses an open anastomosis, the so-called closed method, or a stapling technique.

Employment in the early 1940s of a sulfonamide that is poorly absorbed from the gastrointestinal tract introduced a new concept in the preparation of the patient for operations on the colon or rectum. There is now agreement amongst surgeons that mechanical measures need to be supplemented by appropriately selected antimicrobial agents, but there is no unanimity of opinion on the most effective route of administration — oral, systemic, or both — or what agent to use.

Orally Administered Agents.   One method aimed at reducing the incidence of infection in colorectal surgery is the ingestion of an antimicrobial agent that is not well absorbed from the lumen of the gut and that is effective against the enteric microflora. Several commonly used single agents or combinations have been tried, but experience has shown only the following to be generally acceptable: an aminoglycoside, *e.g.,* neomycin or kanamycin (against the aerobic flora), in combination with erythromycin or metronidazole (against the anaerobic flora, particularly *Bacteroides fragilis*). Whichever combination is used, its duration should be limited to the 18- to 24-hour period immediately prior to the surgical incision in order to reduce the risk of superinfection or drug-induced colitis. Drug administration should not be started until mechanical preparation is finished.

An acceptable regimen now widely used calls for the oral administration of erythromycin base, 1 g, and neomycin, 1 g, at 19, again at 18 and again at 9 hours before the operative incision. Controlled clinical trials confirm the effectiveness of this low-dose, short-term use of these two agents in reducing significantly postoperative wound and intraperitoneal infection. (Nichols and associates; Clarke and associates). In the event that the operation must be postponed, it is advisable to stop drug preparation for several days to allow the gut to regain its normal flora and then begin anew. This is another precaution against superinfection.

Systemically Administered Agents.   Systemic agents either with or without oral agents have been effective in reducing the incidence of postoperative wound or intraperitoneal infection in operation on the colon and rectum. Numerous drugs have been used with good results, but because of potential adverse side-effects, relatively few can now be recommended for systemic use. Among those that can be recommended at this time are several agents among the broad-spectrum "second and third generation" cephalosporins and one of the "fourth generation" penicillins. These are relatively safe and of clinically proven effectiveness.

The Options.   There is no convincing evidence that one route is superior to the other or that a combination of the systemic and oral routes is more effective than either when used singly. Thus, several options are open: the systemic route alone, the oral route alone, or both.

In summary, the control of infection in colorectal operations, as is the case in surgery in general, depends upon strict attention to well-established techniques, including asepsis, the gentle handling of tissue, preoperative mechanical cleansing, and the judicious use of perioperative antimicrobial agents.

Infection-Prone Patients

Certain persons are more likely to develop infections than are others, and include those who are known carriers of pathogenic microorganisms, particularly those who carry staphylococci in the nose and throat, and those with infection at some point removed from the site of the operative procedure. When such patients require operation, even clean elective surgery, antimicrobial agents are indicated. Conversely, there are other infection-prone persons in whom systemic preventive drugs are of unproved value. These include patients at the extremes of nutrition; those who are receiving adrenocortical steroids; the aged; uncontrolled diabetics; and those whose defense mechanisms are compromised by disease or treatment, such as transplantation patients whose immune mechanism is intentionally suppressed. The administration of antibiotics places these persons at great risk of superinfection by organisms frequently unresponsive to antimicrobial therapy.

In those patients with known or suspected tuberculosis for whom an operation is anticipated, antituberculosis therapy should be started preoperatively in order to prevent dissemination of the disease. Similarly, if surgery is contemplated on a patient with known rheumatic valvular disease or with a valvular implant, prophylactic antimicrobial use is indicated.

Operations Involving the Implantation of Large Foreign Bodies

It has been shown that the presence of a foreign body results in significant reduction in the number of microorganisms necessary to produce infection in experimental animals (Altemeier and Furste) and in human volunteers (Elek and Conen). Although there are no clinical data to support their use in this setting, prophylactic antimicrobial drugs are recommended when implants are inserted into the vascular system or when a joint replacement procedure is performed.

Urinary Tract Infection

Proof is lacking that systemic antibiotics reduce the incidence of postoperative urinary tract infection in patients undergoing nonurologic operations (see Chap. 10).

Systemic preoperative antimicrobial agents are recommended when an operative incision or instrumentation (including cystoscopy) enters the urinary tract in the presence of infection or culture-positive urine (see Chap. 10), and when incision or instrumentation is required in the presence of obstructive uropathy.

Pulmonary Infection

There is no convincing evidence that antimicrobial agents administered systemically or locally reduce the incidence of postoperative pulmonary infection, or that their use will prevent colonization or invasive infection of the tracheobronchial tree in patients with a tracheostomy. Any such regimen only hastens colonization with resistant bacteria, yeasts, and fungi. The same can be said for any patient whose respiratory care includes the placement of an endotracheal tube of any variety (see Chap. 10).

Intravenous Systems Infection

There are several considerations for minimizing infection that may be introduced by means of a system used for the intravascular administration of fluids, electrolytes, blood products, or medication. These are discussed in detail in Chapter 10.

Invasive Procedures

There is no evidence that systemic or topical drug prophylaxis is indicated in any of the following invasive procedures: venipuncture, arterial puncture, arteriovenous shunt for dialysis, insertion of heparin locks, cardiac catheterization, transvenous insertion of pacemaker, aspiration biopsy, bone marrow aspiration, lumbar puncture, thoracentesis, paracentesis, joint aspiration, laparoscopy, mediastinoscopy, liver biopsy, phlebography, arteriography, lymphangiography, or cholangiography. Protection against infection in each of these procedures depends upon asepsis and antisepsis with careful nontraumatic techniques.

RABIES PROPHYLAXIS

Although antimicrobial agents are not involved specifically in measures to prevent rabies, it seems appropriate to introduce this topic at this place.

Rabies is a rare disease; nonetheless, its endemic presence in the animal life in parts of this country is reason enough for including in this manual the following guidelines on rabies prophylaxis that were prepared by the Committee on Trauma of the American College of Surgeons in August 1982.

General Considerations

Rabies occurs in many wild animals, including bats, and domestic animals, such as dogs, cats, and cattle, but rarely, if ever, in rodents. A dog or cat that remains healthy for 10 days after a bite does not have rabies, and prophylaxis for a person bitten by that animal is not indicated. A negative fluorescent antibody (FA) examination of an animal brain in an experienced laboratory is reliable evidence that the animal did not have rabies. Saliva of a rabid animal on an open wound (usually a bite) or mucous membrane constitutes exposure to rabies.

A decision to initiate postexposure prophylaxis is based upon balancing two probabilities: (1) that rabies virus was introduced into an exposed person, and (2) that a serious reaction to prophylaxis material might occur.

Principles of Postexposure Prophylaxis

Local Wound Treatment. Scrub the wound with surgical soap and water. Irrigate with saline and antiseptic solution of your choice. Debride all devitalized tissue and foreign bodies.

Indications for Immunization, Dosages, Injection Sites, and Adverse Reactions. Provide both passive and active immunization for all bite exposures, unless rabies can be excluded, and for all nonbite exposures if the animal is proven to have or is strongly suspected of having rabies.

Human Rabies Immune Globulin (RIG): Give 20 I.U./kg body weight. Infiltrate the wound with up to 50% of the material and give the remainder intramuscularly in the buttocks. RIG eliminates the hazards of sensitivity to horse serum. RIG is administered only one time, at the initiation of antirabies therapy.

Rabies Vaccine (V); Human Diploid Cell Vaccine (HDCV): Administer 1 ml intramuscularly at the same time RIG is given, but at a different site. Then give a dose of 1 ml in the arm on days 3, 7, 14, and 28 after the first dose. Check antibody titer on day 42.

The HDVC is available through state health departments or the federal Communication Disease Control Center in Atlanta, Georgia.

Nonbite exposures from escaped dogs or cats in a rabies endemic area are the only indication for using vaccine prophylaxis alone.

Adverse Reactions

RIG, or Hyperab, is the "biological of choice" for passive immunization of persons exposed to rabies. Local pain and slight febrile response may occur following the administration of RIG. Although not reported after RIG, angioneurotic edema, nephrotic syndrome, and anaphylaxis have been reported very rarely after injection of ordinary human immune serum globulin.

PREVENTIVE MEASURES OTHER THAN ANTIMICROBIAL AGENTS

The use of antimicrobial agents to prevent infection is not a measure that permits lower standards of housekeeping, antisepsis, or asepsis. Antimicrobials are not substitutes for careful surgical technique, the principal elements of which include gentleness, preservation of vascularity, hemostasis, removal of devascularized tissue and foreign particles, and anatomic closure without tension or dead space.

BIBLIOGRAPHY

ALTEMEIER WA: Infection control in the operating room and perioperative areas. In Roderick MA (ed): Infection Control in Critical Care, pp 63–71. Rockville, MD, Aspen Systems Corp, 1983

ALTEMEIER WA, FURSTE W: Studies in virulence of *Clostridium welchii.* Surgery 25:12–19, 1949

ALTEMEIER WA, HUMMEL RP, HILL EO: Staphylococcal enterocolitis following antibiotic therapy. Ann Surg 157:847–858, 1963

BARRY AL, THORNSBERRY C: Manual of Clinical Microbiology, 3rd ed, p 463. Washington, DC, American Society for Microbiology, 1980

BARZA M, LAUERMANN M: Why monitor serum levels of gentamicin? Clin Pharmacokinet 3:202–215, 1978

BERGAN T, KRODWALL EK, WIIK-LARSEN E: Mezlocillin pharmacokinetics in patients with normal and impaired renal functions. Antimicrob Agents Chemother 16:651–654, 1979

BERGER SA, NAGAR H, GORDON M: Antimicrobial prophylaxis in obstetric and gynecologic surgery: A critical review. J Reprod Med 24(5):185–190, 1980

BERNARD HR, COLE WR: The prophylaxis of surgical infection: The effect of prophylaxis antimicrobial drugs on the incidence of infection following potentially contaminated operations. Surgery 56:151–157, 1964

BIVENS MD, NEUFELD J, MCCARTY WD: The prophylactic use of Keflex and Keflin in vaginal hysterectomy. Am J Obstet Gynecol 122:169–175, 1975

BRACHMAN PS: Nosocomial infection control: An overview. Rev Infect Dis 3(4):640–648, 1981

BRÖTE L, GILQUIST J, HOJER H: Prophylactic cephalothin in gastrointestinal surgery. Acta Chir Scand 142:238–245, 1976

BROWN JW, COOPER N, RAMBO WM: Controlled prospective double-blind evaluation of a "prophylactic" antibiotic (cephaloridine) in surgery. In Hobby G (ed): Antimicrobial Agents and Chemotherapy—1969, pp 421–423. Washington, DC, American Society for Microbiology, 1970

BURKE JF: The effective period of preventive antibiotic action in experimental incisions and dermal lesions. Surgery 50:161–167, 1961

CAMPBELL PC: Large doses of penicillin in the prevention of surgical wound infection. Lancet 2:805–810, 1965

CENTERS FOR DISEASE CONTROL: Guidelines for the prevention and control of nosocomial infections. Washington, DC, U.S. Department of Health and Human Services, 1981

CHODAK GW, PLAUT ME: Use of systemic antibiotics for prophylaxis in surgery: A critical review. Arch Surg 112:326–334, 1977

THE CHOICE OF ANTIMICROBIAL DRUGS. Med Lett Drugs Ther 24:21–28, 1982

CHOW AW, PATTEN V, GUZE LB: Susceptibility of anaerobic bacteria to metronidazole: Relative resistance of non-spore-forming gram-positive bacilli. J Infect Dis 131:182–185, 1975

CLARKE AM: Prophylactic antibiotics for total hip arthroplasty—the significance of *Staphylococcus epidermidis.* J Antimicrob Chemother 5(5):493–495, 1979

CLARKE JS, CONDON RE, BARTLETT JG et al: Preoperative oral antibiotics reduce septic complications: Results of prospective, randomized, double-blind clinical study. Ann Surg 186:251–259, 1977

CRUSE PJE, FOORD R: The epidemiology of wound infection: a 10-year prospective study of 62,939 wounds. Surg Clin North Am 60:27–40, 1980

CUNHA BA, RISTUCCIA AM: Third generation cephalosporins. Med Clin North Am 66:283–291, 1982

CURRERI PW, SHUCK JM, LINDBERG RB, PRUITT BA JR: Treatment of burn wounds with 5 per cent aqueous Sulfamylon and occlusive dressings. Surg Forum 20:506–509, 1969

DAVIDSON AIG, CLARK C, SMITH G: Postoperative wound infection: A computer analysis. Br J Surg 58:333–337, 1971

EDLICH RF, SMITH QT, EDGERTON MT: Resistance of the surgical wound to antimicrobial prophylaxis and its mechanisms of development. Am J Surg 126:583–591, 1973

ELEK SD, CONEN PE: The virulence of *Staphylococcus pyogenes* for man: A study of the problems of wound infection. Br J Exp Pathol 38:573–586, 1957

EVANS M, POLLOCK AV: Trials on trial: A review of trials of antibiotic prophylaxis. Arch Surg 119:109–113, 1984

FEKETY FR, CLUFF LE, SABISTON DC et al: A study of antibiotic prophylaxis in cardiac surgery. J Thorac Cardiovasc Surg 57:757–763, 1969

FULLEN WD, HUNT J, ALTEMEIER WA: Prophylactic antibiotics in penetrating wounds of the abdomen. J Trauma 12:282–289, 1972

GAMAN W, CATES C, SNELLING CFT, LANK B, RONALD AR: Emergence of gentamicin- and carbenicillin-resistant *Pseudomonas aeruginosa* in a hospital environment. Antimicrob Agents Chemother 9:474–480, 1976

GOODMAN JS, SCHAFFNER W, COLLINS HA et al: Infection after cardiovascular surgery: Clinical study including examination of antimicrobial prophylaxis. N Engl J Med 278:117–123, 1968

GOODWIN CW JR, MCMANUS WF, PRUITT BA JR: Peritonitis and intra-abdominal infection. In Conn HF (ed): Current Diagnosis, 6th ed, pp 618–624. Philadelphia, WB Saunders, 1980

GOODWIN CW JR, MCMANUS WF, PRUITT BA JR: Burns. In Kagan BM (ed): Antimicrobial Therapy, 3rd ed, pp 397–408. Philadelphia, WB Saunders, 1980

HALASZ NA: Wound infection and topical antibiotics: A surgeon's dilemma. Arch Surg 112:1240–1244, 1977

HEIDEMANN HT, GERKENS JF, SPICKARD WA, JACKSON EK, BRANCH RA: Amphotericin B nephrotoxicity in humans decreased by salt repletion. Am J Med 75:476–481, 1983

HIRSCHMANN JW, INUI TS: Prophylaxis: A critique of recent trials. Rev Infect Dis 2:1–23, 1980

HOWARD JM et al: Postoperative wound infections: The influence of ultraviolet irradiation of the operating room and of various other factors. Ann Surg (Suppl) 160(2):9–192, 1964

HURLEY DL, HOWARD P JR, HAHN HH II: Perioperative prophylactic antibiotics in abdominal surgery: A review of recent progress. Surg Clin North Am 59(5):919–933, 1979

KARL RC, MERTZ JJ, VEITH FJ et al: Prophylactic antimicrobial drugs in surgery. N Engl J Med 275:305–308, 1966

KEIGHLEY MRB, BURDON DW: Antimicrobial Prophylaxis in Surgery. Kent, England, Pittman Medical Publishing Co Ltd, 1979

LESAR TS et al: Gentamicin dosing errors with four commonly used nomograms. JAMA 248:1190–1193, 1982

LEVINE NS, LINDBERG RB, MASON AD JR, PRUITT BA JR: The quantitative swab culture and smear: A quick, simple method for determining the number of viable aerobic bacteria on open wounds. J Trauma 16:89–94, 1976

MAYER W, GORDON M, ROTHBARD MJ: Prophylactic antibiotics: Use in hysterectomy. NY State J Med 76:2144–2147, 1976

MCMANUS WF, MASON AD, PRUITT BA JR: Subeschar antibiotic infusion in the treatment of burn wound infection. J Trauma 20:1021–1023, 1980

MILES AA, MILES EM, BURKE J: The value and duration of defense reactions of the skin to the primary lodgment of bacteria. Br J Exp Pathol 38:79–96, 1957

NEU, HC: The new beta-lactamase-stable cephalosporins. Ann Intern Med 97:408–419, 1982

ORESKOVICH MR, DELLINGER EP, LENNARD ES, WERTZ M, CARRICO CJ, MINSHAW BH: Duration of preventive antibiotic administration for penetrating abdominal trauma. Arch Surg 117:200–205, 1982

PRUITT BA JR: Infection. In Walt AJ (ed): Early Care of the Injured Patient, pp 64–83. Committee on Trauma, American College of Surgeons. Philadelphia, WB Saunders, 1982

PRUITT BA JR: Tetanus. In Conn HF (ed): Current Therapy 1982, pp 75–78. Philadelphia, WB Saunders, 1982

PRUITT BA JR, FOLEY, FD: The use of biopsies in burn patient care. Surgery 73:887–897, 1973

PRUITT BA JR, LINDBERG RB: *Pseudomonas aeruginosa* infections in burn patients. In Doggett

RG (ed): Pseudomonas aeruginosa: Clinical Manifestations of Infection and Current Therapy. New York, Academic Press, 1979

PRUITT BA JR, LINDBERG RB, McMANUS WF: Bacteriology, antibiotics and chemotherapy. In Flynn JE (ed): Hand Surgery, pp 636–676. Baltimore, Williams & Wilkins, 1981

PRUITT BA JR, O'NEILL JA JR, MONCRIEF JA, LINDBERG RB: Successful control of burn wound sepsis. JAMA 203:1054–1056, 1968

REGAMEY C, GORDON RC, KIRBY WMM: Comparative pharmacokinetics of tobramycin and gentamicin. Clin Pharmacol Ther 14:396–403, 1973

ROBERTS JM, HOMESLEY HD: Low-dose carbenicillin prophylaxis for vaginal and abdominal hysterectomy. Obstet Gynecol 52:83–87, 1978

ROSENBLATT, JE, EDSON RS: Metronidazole. Mayo Clin Proc 58:154–157, 1983

SANDUSKY WR: Use of antibiotics and chemotherapeutics in surgery. Curr Probl Surg, October 1964

SANDUSKY WR: The use of prophylactic antibiotics in surgical patients. Surg Clin North Am 60:83–92, 1980

SANDUSKY WR: Prophylactic antibiotics in surgery. Guthrie Bulletin 51:143–150, 1982

THOMPSON RL, WRIGHT AJ: Cephalosporin antibiotics. Mayo Clin Proc 58:79–87, 1983

TICARCILLIN. Medical Letter on Drugs & Therapeutics 19:17–18, 1977

TJANDRAMAGA TB, MULLIE A, VERBESSELT R, DE SCHEPPER PJ, VERBIST L: Piperacillin: Human pharmacokinetics after intravenous and intramuscular administration. Antimicrob Agents Chemother 14:829–837, 1978

WALT AJ (ed): Care of the Injured Patient, 3rd ed. Philadelphia, WB Saunders, 1982

WHELTON A, NEU HC (eds): The Aminoglycosides: Microbiology, Clinical Use, and Toxicology. New York, Marcel Dekker, 1982

WRIGHT AJ, WILKOWSKE CJ: The penicillins. Mayo Clin Proc 58:21–32, 1983

ZASKE DE et al: Gentamicin pharmacokinetics in 1,640 patients: Method for control of serum concentrations. Antimicrob Agents Chemother 21:407–411, 1982

12

The prevention and control of infection in the immunocompromised host present many complex problems. The most fundamental of these is the impaired host defenses of such patients and their consequently high risks of developing opportunistic and other types of infection. The number of such patients has progressively increased in recent years, largely because of the widespread use of various types of immunosuppressive therapy for the treatment of autoimmune diseases, the prevention and treatment of rejection associated with organ transplantation, and the management of malignant neoplastic diseases. Advances in medical and surgical care have also allowed longer survival of other groups of patients who have impaired host resistance related to trauma, existing infection, impaired nutrition, and other serious life-threatening or debilitating illnesses. The surgical intensive care unit has become a repository for such patients, and it is noteworthy that infection may be the ultimate cause of death in approximately 75% of the fatalities in patients who have been hospitalized in an intensive care unit for more than 10 days.

Although the term *immunocompromised host* is used to designate all patients with major deficiencies of host resistance that might cause an increased susceptibility to infection, it must be remembered that these deficiencies may be highly selective, broad-based in nature, and mild or severe (Table 12-1). To better understand the various types of infection that may be associated with different underlying diseases, it is often helpful to sub-divide immunocompromised hosts into two broad groupings: those with immunodepression and those with immunosuppression.

Immunodepression is most often caused by endogenous aberrations in previously healthy persons and characteristically is associated with extensive trauma, infection, or altered nutrition. Most infections in the immunodepressed host are from endogenous extracellular bacterial pathogens, although in the intensive care setting exogenous infections are frequent. Both nonspecific and specific alterations

Infection in the Immunocompromised Host

235

Table 12-1. Characteristics of Selected Immunodeficiency States

Deficiency State	Principal Effect
Humoral Defects	
Homo- or heterozygous complement deficiencies	Decrease or absence of complement component
Immunoglobulin deficiencies (IgG deficiency most common)	Decrease or absence of immunoglobulin
Tuftsin deficiency	Impaired phagocytosis
Cellular Defects	
Alteration of lymphocyte function	
B-cell dysfunction	Altered antibody production
T-cell dysfunction	Altered cellular immunity or regulatory function
Large granular lymphocytes	Decrease in natural killer (NK) cell activity (occurs with age)
Alteration of neutrophil function	
Chronic granulomatous disease (X-linked recessive in male)	No respiratory burst following phagocytosis NADH or NADPH oxidase deficiency⎫ G-6-PD deficiency (rare) ⎬ ⎭ Cytochrome b_{245} deficiency (occurs in association with oxidase defect)
Myeloperoxidase deficiency	Familial enzymatic defect in azurophilic granules
Chediak-Higashi syndrome	Defective microtubules and abnormal lysosome formation Impaired chemotaxis Partial albinism
Job's syndrome	Impaired neutrophil function in presence of increased IgE
Undefined Acquired Defect	
Adult immunodeficiency syndrome	Decrease in T helper – T suppressor ratio Lymphopenia Anergy

Hemolytic complement analysis
Antigen-specific immunoelectrophoresis
or immunodiffusion

Quantitative γ globulin assay

Tuftsin assay

Quantitative γ globulin assay
Response to specific antigens

Skin testing
Mitogen response
Flow cytometry with monoclonal
antibodies

Flow cytometry with monoclonal
antibodies

NBT reduction test
Chemiluminescence assay
Radioisotope assay of glucose metabolic
pathways
Analysis of spectrum of oxidation-
reduction difference of cytochrome b_{245}

Peroxidase stain of blood smear
Quantitative peroxidase assay

Abnormal azurophilic granules in
neutrophils on blood smear
Abnormal platelet morphology and
function
Chemotactic assay

Chemotactic and bacterial killing assays
IgE assay
Eosinophil count

Assay of β_2 microglobulin ($\uparrow$)
Thymosin α_1 assay ($\uparrow$)
Lymphocyte count ($\downarrow$)
Flow cytometry with monoclonal
antibodies
Skin testing

in host defense are numerous, but the primary alterations predisposing to infection are abnormalities of phagocytic function, particularly of neutrophils. In most patients with abnormal phagocytic function, protein nutritional support is insufficient or endogenous mediators that suppress host resistance are present. Many of the endogenous host-altering substances are associated with activation of the complement sequence, such as may occur with severe multisystem trauma, thermal injury, or infections.

In contrast, *immunosuppression* is associated with the administration of drugs or irradiation that alters immune function. When cytotoxic drugs are given, leukopenia is the most important predisposing factor to infection, and the majority of infections are endogenous in origin, especially involving aerobic enteric bacteria. Abnormal lymphocyte function is a cardinal feature of chronic immunosuppression, and a substantially larger number of infections are caused by intracellular pathogens such as viruses and fungi.

Meakins and MacLean have recently advocated skin testing as a nonspecific indicator of host defense mechanisms in patients who are at risk for development of postoperative infection and mortality. While delayed hypersensitivity to intradermal injection of recall antigens (*e.g., Candida,* mumps virus, purified protein derivative, *Trichophyton,* and streptokinase-streptodornase) mainly reflects a compromise in cell-mediated immunity, it also correlates well with impairment of mediators of host defense mechanisms for humoral and phagocytic functions. Sequential testing can be used as an indicator of outcome or response to treatment, because correction of underlying predisposing factors, malnutrition, trauma, shock, or infection can in many instances restore normal reactivity.

TYPES OF INFECTION: THEIR INCIDENCE AND IMPORTANCE

The Immunodepressed Host

Extracellular bacterial pathogens cause the most common types of infections occurring in the immunodepressed host. As an example, most patients with burn areas greater than 50% of the body surface develop burn wound infections and bacteremic events. The major pathogen following burn injury in the United States at the present time is *Staphylococcus aureus,* although the gram-negative enteric bacteria are also important etiologic agents. *Pseudomonas aeruginosa,* once the predominant pathogen following burn injury, now occurs as a major pathogen in only approximately 10% of serious burn-related infections.

Infections caused by fungi, *Pneumocystis carinii,* and herpesvirus occur in the immunodepressed host, usually after marked suppression of endogenous flora by antimicrobial therapy. Infections in postoperative patients in the intensive care unit are more likely to be caused by gram-negative enteric bacteria, but *Staphylococcus aureus* is also a significant pathogen there. The intracellular pathogens, although still infrequent, are more common in the intensive care unit than following burn injury or trauma, and also usually appear following intensive antibiotic therapy for extracellular bacterial pathogens.

The Immunosuppressed Host

There has been extensive experience with infections in patients receiving immuno-suppressive therapy for renal transplantation. Only a decade ago, approximately 30% of patients receiving a cadaveric renal allograft died within the first year following transplantation, and half of these deaths were related to infections. In spite of other advances in this field, infection has remained a serious problem. Most transplant patients develop cytomegalovirus infection, and many have infections caused by other pathogens in the herpesvirus group, including herpes zoster, herpes simplex types I or II, or Epstein-Barr virus infection. *Pneumocystic carinii* infection, once a serious and usually lethal pathogen, has almost disappeared as a cause of post-transplant infection, but legionellosis has appeared as a successor. Most of the infections in transplant patients are felt to be related to macrophage abnormalities caused by intensive chronic immunosuppression, particularly in association with steroids. In patients who have depression of cell-mediated immune function, typi-fied by those treated with antilymphocyte globulin, intracellular pathogens become of paramount importance. The most important of these are *Listeria monocytogenes, Mycobacteria, Nocardia,* and *Salmonella. Cryptococcus neoformans* and *Candida* are the most important yeast pathogens; *Pneumocystis carinii* and *Toxoplasma gondii* are the most common protozoan pathogens; and *Strongyloides stercoralis* is the most common helminth pathogen. Both primary and reactivation types of infection may occur.

Patients receiving cytotoxic drugs for the treatment of cancer develop infections primarily related to neutropenia. The frequency of infection rises directly as the neutrophil count drops below 500/ml, and infections are especially common when the count is below 100/ml. Gram-negative bacteremias are the most common type of infection, the organisms that colonize the lower alimentary tract being the ones most frequently causing infection. It is surprising that *Bacteroides fragilis* is an infrequent pathogen.

DIAGNOSTIC CONSIDERATIONS

When infection is suspected in the immunocompromised host, early collection of specimens or body fluids for diagnostic study is essential since there is a close relationship between survival of the patient and the rapidity of diagnosis and treatment. The antimicrobial agent chosen should provide the narrowest spectrum possible to decrease the chance that resistant flora and other opportunistic microor-ganisms will emerge, while still providing broad enough coverage to protect against the large majority of potential life-threatening pathogens. With accurate diagnosis, antimicrobial therapy can usually be directed toward a single organism.

Pulmonary Infection

Although all infectious complications constitute major threats to the immunocom-promised patient, involvement of the lung is the most common form of infection, and it is associated with a high mortality. Interpretation of sputum cultures in patients with pulmonary infections can be difficult and misleading, because the organisms isolated may represent only saprophytic colonization unless large numbers of a single microorganism (usually pneumococcus) are seen in association with large numbers of neutrophils in gram-stained smears. In order to obviate this problem, a number of invasive techniques should be considered. The particular procedure chosen depends upon the appearance of the pulmonary infiltrate and the general condition of the patient.

Transtracheal Aspiration.   Usually, transtracheal aspiration is the approach of first choice because it reveals the diagnosis in 90% of bacterial, 50% of nocardial, 20% of *Aspergillus,* and 20% of *Pneumocystis* infections. Although contraindicated in the uncooperative or hypoxemic patient, it can be performed very safely in others, even in the thrombocytopenic patient, as long as the patient's platelet count is greater than 50,000/ml.

The procedure can be performed at the bedside under local anesthesia. A catheter-sheathed 16- to 20-gauge needle is introduced through the cricothyroid membrane into the trachea. The needle should be angulated, with the tip directed caudad so that the catheter will be passed into the lower trachea and not into the oropharynx. After removal of the needle, specimens can be obtained through the catheter. If a sample cannot be aspirated, 5 ml of normal saline (without a bacteriostatic agent) can be instilled through the catheter and aspirated. Specimens should be gram stained immediately, and processed using methenamine silver staining for *Pneumocystis* and fluorescent antibody for *Legionella pneumophila.* Cultures should be obtained for viral, bacterial, and fungal organisms. Complications such as hematoma, cellulitis, and subcutaneous emphysema are rare but have occurred in approximately 10% of cases in reported series. Usually, the risk of any particular technique should be weighed against the risk of failure in establishing a definite diagnosis.

Percutaneous Needle Biopsy.   Percutaneous needle biopsy of the lung has proven to be of value in the diagnosis of infection since it allows for direct sample of the area of concern. It is performed with a thin-walled 18-gauge or smaller special needle through which material can be aspirated. If no sample is obtained, up to 5 ml of sterile saline may be injected and immediately aspirated for appropriate sampling. This technique can be used to sample lesions as small as 2 cm or less in diameter with a positive diagnostic yield of 76%. The patient must be sufficiently alert and cooperative to be able to suspend respirations for periods of 5 seconds or longer while the needle is intermittently and progressively advanced into the lesion. Complications of this procedure include pneumothorax in 26% of cases, 10% to 15% of which require tube drainage. Although this technique has been most useful in diagnosing peripheral nodular pulmonary lesions, it has been also used in diffuse lung disease.

Bronchoscopy and Open Lung Biopsy.   Before proceeding to an open biopsy, consideration should be given to flexible fiberoptic bronchoscopy with bronchial washings and transbronchial biopsy. This procedure can reduce the need for thoracotomy, particularly in those patients with diffuse lung disease suspected of being cytomegalovirus or *Pneumocystis* infection, who are not critically ill at the time of examination. Because of oropharyngeal contamination, this technique is frequently unreliable for the diagnosis of bacterial infections. Performed under fluoroscopy, bronchial washings and brushing can be obtained and submitted for appropriate culture.

Open lung biopsy provides adequate tissue for both histological and bacteriological examinations. Performed through a limited anterior thoracotomy, it can be done under general or local anesthesia with a specific diagnostic yield of between 60% and 80%. Reported nonspecific diagnoses including interstitial pneumonitis and fibrosis reflect the effects of earlier treatments, radiation therapy, or drug toxicity.

Diagnosis of Legionnaires' Disease. The diagnosis of legionnaires' disease, which is commonly manifested as a rapidly progressive lobar pneumonia, can be difficult, because the gram stain does not readily stain the bacterium in pulmonary secretions, and also because the organism has fastidious growth requirements. *Legionella pneumophila* grows optimally at 35°C under 2% CO_2 in Mueller-Hinton agar containing 1% hemoglobin and 1% Isovitale X or F-G agar containing L-cysteine hydrochloride and soluble ferric pyrophosphate. The best specimens for culture growth are lung pleural fluid and transtracheal aspirates, since sputum and bronchial washings can be contaminated with other bacteria that will interfere with the slow-growing *Legionella pneumophila*. Rapid diagnosis can be made by direct immunofluorescent antibody (DFA) staining of the sputum, transtracheal aspirates, pleural fluid, or bronchial washings. Serologic diagnosis is suggested either by a single high titer > 1:256 or by a fourfold rise late in the course of the disease.

Atypical Mycobacterial Disease. Lately an increasing number of nontuberculous or atypical mycobacterial infections have been reported in the compromised host. Whereas *Mycobacterium tuberculosis* spreads by personal contact, atypical mycobacteria are found in the environment from which they spread to man. The diagnosis of these infections in the immunocompromised patient cannot be made solely upon the isolation of a particular organism; rather, it must be correlated with clinical features suggestive of an atypical mycobacterial infection. The organisms responsible for these atypical infections have different sensitivities to the antimicrobial agents to which *M. tuberculosis* is sensitive. In the laboratory, strains of these microorganisms can be differentiated from *M. tuberculosis* because they are niacin negative. Also, they can be differentiated further into four subgroups by the variations in their pigmentation and growth characteristics.

Abdominal Infections

In patients who are on immunosuppressive drugs such as steroids, the classical signs of tenderness and inflammation may be completely lacking. Thus the possible presence of an intra-abdominal infectious process should be considered in patients with occult fever even in the absence of usual clinical features.

Radiological Studies.   Radiological studies to be considered in patients with suspected intra-abdominal abscesses include a plain radiograph of the abdomen, water-contrast radiopaque studies of the gastrointestinal tract when alimentary leakage is suspected, and the newer noninvasive imaging modalities now available. Other conventional radiological studies such as plain abdominal films, barium contrast studies, and angiographic studies are often inconclusive and difficult to perform in critically ill patients. The latter offer diagnostic advantages for precise localization and planning for proper surgical treatment of intra-abdominal abscesses.

Ultrasound.   Imaging of abscesses with ultrasound may be helpful in their diagnosis and localization. Since it is not possible to distinguish an abscess from a cyst, lymphocele, hematoma, or loculation of ascitic fluid by this technique, it is important to correlate the obtained information with that from other diagnostic methods as well as with clinical data. Needle aspiration under ultrasound guidance with bacteriological and cytological studies may permit differentiation between an abscess and other fluid-filled cavities. The advantages of ultrasound imaging are that it allows a rapid, simple, inexpensive, noninvasive evaluation of the critically ill individual and permits localization of abscesses of the subdiaphragmatic, intrahepatic, subhepatic, pelvic, and retroperitoneal areas in a high percentage of cases. However, a negative test should not be taken as an indication of the absence of intra-abdominal abscess, particularly in an immunocompromised patient.

Computed Tomography.   Computed tomography (CT) is another diagnostic technique using ionizing radiation to provide useful information in the diagnosis of intra-abdominal abscesses in the immunocompromised patient. An outstanding feature is its capability of detecting the presence of a focal lesion and ascertaining its size, shape, position, density, and relationship to other regional anatomical structures.

The presence of gas or air fluid levels on roentgenograms may also be helpful, but their differentiation from tumors, hematomas, lymphoceles, or necrotic tissue in these patients may be difficult; thus, CT findings must be correlated with the symptoms and physical signs of sepsis and the results of needle aspiration or other drainage.

The general advantages of computed tomography in immunocompromised patients include its noninvasiveness, its wide applicability, patient acceptance, and diagnostic sensitivity. Unlike sonographic evaluations, which are operator dependent, CT provides reproducible contrast images and permits visualization of the costophrenic angles, diaphragm, lesser sac, and retroperitoneal space. CT scans of the upper abdomen also demonstrate the presence of intrahepatic lesions such as abscesses, cysts, tumors, or dilated biliary ducts.

Percutaneous Aspiration and Drainage.   As an important adjunct to ultrasound and computed tomography, percutaneous aspiration and drainage may be used, both as a diagnostic maneuver and as a means of inserting catheters for surgical guidance and, in some instances, definitive percutaneous drainage. Lesions amenable to this type of drainage are usually unilocular abscesses that can be reached safely through a percutaneous route.

This method is contraindicated in patients in whom abscess cavities cannot be reached safely percutaneously without involvement of other adjacent structures. Since control of sepsis is especially important in the immunocompromised patient, open local or transperitoneal surgical drainage should not be delayed if resolution of the infection is incomplete after percutaneous drainage.

Radionucleotide Scanning. Radionucleotide scanning may also be helpful in identifying and localizing obscure septic processes not demonstrated on routine or other studies. Radiopharmaceutical agents such as ^{67}Ga (gallium 67) and ^{111}In (indium 111) have been used as scanning agents. Gallium will accumulate in parts of the body where neutrophils infiltrate. Thus, gallium scanning does not distinguish between an inflammatory phlegmon and an isolated loculation of purulent material or abscess. False positive results have been reported following accumulation of gallium in the gastrointestinal tract in certain tumors, and in other inflammatory conditions such as Crohn's disease and pseudomembranous colitis.

A newer technique of localization of obscure abscesses using autologous leukocytes labeled with ^{111}In has been introduced. Experimental animal studies have demonstrated better accumulation in abscesses of the ^{111}In-labeled leukocytes than with ^{67}Ga, with the added advantage of a shorter period of study. Also, abscess to liver, spleen, and kidney ratios were severalfold higher with ^{111}In-labeled leukocytes. Several preliminary clinical trials have confirmed the usefulness of ^{111}In-labeled leukocytes in identifying abscesses. Pitfalls of this technique have included accumulation of labeled leukocytes in infarcts, accessory spleens, and early postoperative wounds. ^{111}In may give slightly better results than ^{67}Ga, but neither is accurate enough or fast enough to be very useful in immunocompromised patients for whom an early accurate diagnosis is mandatory and may be lifesaving.

Nuclear Magnetic Resonance. Nuclear magnetic resonance (NMR) is a new technique under current evaluation because of its potential for providing soft-tissue imaging more safely than other modalities. Whereas NMR images are in some ways similar to CT scans, the physical principles underlying the NMR phenomenon are entirely different from those related to x-rays. Essentially, when atomic nuclei are placed in a magnetic field and stimulated by radiowaves of a particular frequency, they will re-emit some of the absorbed energy in the form of radio signals. NMR images can be constructed to receive data from a single point, a plane, or a three-dimensional volume in the sample at the same time. Other advantages of NMR over CT imaging are that vascular structures are readily distinguishable, and there is better contrast resolution of soft-tissue images. This promising technique needs critical study.

Bone Marrow Biopsy. Bone marrow biopsy can be helpful in evaluating disseminated granulomatous infections in some patients. In two recent series of disseminated histoplasmosis, the diagnosis was established in half of the patients by careful histological examination of the bone marrow, and in the recent experience at the University of Cincinnati Hospital, recipients having febrile syndromes were diagnosed as having histoplasmosis by this means.

Diagnosis of Viral Infections.   Different techniques are available for the laboratory diagnosis of viral infections. Meaurement of antibodies by antibody tests are more readily and cheaply performed than virus isolations; however, they require adequately spaced serum samples. Thus, diagnosis often is not confirmed until convalescence. Serial samples of serum need to be tested; the first sample should be collected as soon as possible after the onset of the illness, the second one 2 to 3 weeks after. A fourfold rise in serum antibody is considered diagnostic of a recent infection. Viral humoral immune responses are useful not only as an indicator of the patient's immune status, but also as a determinant of the need for immunization.

Procedures for quantifying antibodies in virus diseases are based on classic antigen – antibody reactions. Commonly used procedures include complement fixation, neutralizing antibodies, immunofluorescence, hemagglutination inhibition, precipitin testing, and radioimmunoassay.

Virus isolation is usually required when new epidemics occur or when treatment of the disease is indicated. It is also used to confirm a presumptive diagnosis made by microscopic observation or when a given clinical picture may be caused by other agents. Since some viruses are known to persist in humans tested for long periods of time, the isolation of a given virus like herpesvirus, poliomyelitis virus, echovirus, or coxsackieviruses from a patient does not always prove that agent is the cause of the current disease. A clinical and epidemiological pattern must be consistent with the infection for that particular virus.

It is important to remember that many viruses may be demonstrated only in the first few days of the illness. Thus, collection of material for virus identification studies should be done early in the course of the disease. The choice of specimens includes throat swabs, vesicle fluid, spinal fluid, urine, biopsy tissue, stools, nasal washings, and blood specimens.

Viruses multiply only inside living cells; thus, cell culture techniques are most widely used for isolating viruses from clinical specimens. When cells that have been specifically attacked by a virus show changes reflecting injury, it is designated as a cytopathic effect. Different cell lines can be used for isolation of viruses; these include cynomolgus monkey kidney cells for myxoviruses and enteroviruses, human epithelial cells for respiratory syncytial and adenoviruses, and human foreskin cells for the growth of human cytomegaloviruses.

The ability to grow in certain cell lines plus a cytopathic effect are characteristic for a particular virus. Inhibition of viral growth by using specific antisera can also be used to confirm the identity of a particular agent. Certain viruses that do not produce a characteristic cytopathic effect will produce hemagglutination. In periodic testing, a positive test result is presumptive evidence of the presence of certain viruses, for example, orthoviruses and paramyxoviruses (such as those causing influenza A and B, parainfluenza types I, II, and III, and mumps).

Inoculation of a susceptible animal is used to isolate neurotropic viruses causing encephalitis. Infant mice are inoculated intracerebrally. Viruses isolated after death from the animal brain are subsequently inoculated in another infant mouse. Inoculation of a mouse with specific antisera that prevents its death helps in identifying the involved virus.

Histological examination by compound light microscopy will allow easy visualization of inclusion bodies, which can be typical for certain viruses, for example, Negri bodies for rabies virus, Guarnieri's bodies for vaccinia and variola viruses, and "owls eye" inclusions for cyclomegalic viruses in enlarged cells. These inclusion bodies, representing either viral particles or remnants of earlier virus replications, can be found either in the cytoplasm of the parasitized cells where these viruses usually replicate, as in the case of RNA viruses, or in the nuclei, as in cytomegalovirus.

The *electron microscope* can be used to visualize typical herpesvirus particles in tissues such as brain specimens, in Pap smears, or in serum taken from superficial vesicles; reovirus-like agents in stool specimens; or hepatitis B virus in urine specimens. Viral antigens can also be detected in biopsy and autopsy specimens by the use of fluorescein-labeled (or peroxidase-labeled) antibody and enzyme-linked immunoabsorbent assay (ELISA).

SPECIAL PREVENTIVE CONSIDERATIONS

Prophylactic Antibiotics

Prophylactic antibiotics have been found to be useful for the prevention of wound infections in immunocompromised hosts when given for a very short period of time during the perioperative and intraoperative periods. The indications for their use are, in fact, almost identical to those recommended for normal hosts (see Chap. 11). However, prevention of systemic or local infections not related to the surgical wound by the use of prophylactic antibiotics in immunocompromised hosts is usually not effective because the period of increased risk is much longer, and the antimicrobial agents must be given for a prolonged period of time. With prolonged use, changes in the resident microbial flora of the intestinal tract and epithelial surfaces occur regularly, with the result that resistant pathogens and sometimes disastrous infections may emerge spontaneously. Nevertheless, there are highly specific situations in which prolonged administration of prophylactic antibiotics may be beneficial. Selective decontamination of the gastrointestinal tract using prophylactic trimethoprim-sulfamethoxazole with or without polymyxin or amphotericin B has been found to selectively diminish the Enterobacteriaceae and other aerobic organisms without significantly suppressing enteric anaerobes, which apparently rarely cause infections in leukopenic patients. Thus, for patients undergoing intensive chemotherapy, selective decontamination of the gastrointestinal tract during brief periods of granulocytopenia appears to be of value. The use of broad spectrum, nonabsorbable antibiotics and the use of prophylactic systemic antibiotics in themselves are generally ineffective in the immunocompromised host. Long-term daily prophylactic penicillin therapy has been advocated by some authorities to prevent pneumococcal infections in splenectomized patients. However, restricting penicillin therapy to periods of upper respiratory infections and vaccinating splenectomized patients with pneumococcal vaccine appears to be a more rational and highly effective approach.

Immunization

Numerous vaccines and immunization procedures have been tried for the prevention of infections in the immunocompromised host. A pneumococcal vaccine that contains 14 polysaccharide antigens is one of the few vaccines, however, that has been shown to be effective. This vaccine will substantially reduce the rate of infection in patients who are asplenic, who are immunosuppressed for renal allografts, or who have the nephrotic syndrome. However, effectiveness of the vaccine is greatly diminished in patients being treated for active Hodgkin's disease or multiple myeloma because of the impaired antibody responses of such patients. It is also more effective when given prior to splenectomy rather than after.

Pseudomonas vaccines have been evaluated experimentally and clinically for the prevention of serious *Pseudomonas* infections in burned patients. Multivalent vaccines against *Pseudomonas* in some trials have resulted in approximtely an 80% reduction in the incidence of death from burn wound sepsis or septicemia caused by this organism. However, the overall incidence of serious infection has not been reduced in modern burn units.

Influenza vaccines consisting of killed virus antigens are generally considered to be safe. However, although they produce satisfactory antibody responses in renal transplant recipients, there is no proof that they actually reduce active disease or its complications. The efficacy of hepatitis B vaccine has been established recently in a healthy patient population; it is also expected that patients with renal failure may benefit from such vaccines despite attenuated antibody response (see Chapter 10). Trials of an attenuated live cytomegalovirus (CMV) vaccine in transplant patients indicate that humoral responses can be induced, but clinical protection is not conferred following transplantation since cell-mediated responses are compromised by the associated immunosuppression. The protective value of any of these vaccines in patients with an acquired immune deficiency syndrome has not been established.

Laminar Air Flow

In the highly immunosuppressed and leukopenic patient in total reverse isolation, laminar air flow apparently can reduce the acquisition of potential pathogens, and infections are reported to be decreased by about 50% as compared with control groups in prospective studies. The use of laminar air flow combined with reverse isolation plus oral nonabsorbable antibiotics also appears to reduce the number of infections, as compared with conventional treatment of patients with neither reverse isolation nor oral nonabsorbable antibiotics. On the other hand, the final outcome in patients with malignant disease does not seem to be changed.

Prophylactic Granulocyte Transfusions

Prophylactic granulocyte transfusions from HLA-identical siblings has resulted in a reduced incidence of septicemia in the severely granulocytopenic patient. When granulocyte transfusions are received from non-HLA-identical donors, however, there has been a high incidence of transfusion reaction and allosensitization, rendering this technique relatively ineffective.

Reduction of Cross-Contamination

Reduction in acquisition of new organisms is an important aspect of care of the immunosuppressed patient. Perhaps the most important method for reducing cross-contamination is hand-washing by physicians, nurses, attendants, and others before and after their contact with each patient. Other methods include strict attention to detail in housekeeping procedures as outlined in Chapter 15: proper decontamination of fomites, the exclusion of fresh flowers or plants from the patient's room, and a low-microbe diet. Standard reverse isolation techniques have been found to be of little value in the immunosuppressed patient.

Nutritional Support

Nutritional support for the prevention of infection is beyond the scope of this discussion. However, it seems to be clear that altered nutrition may have a profound influence on resistance to infection. Protein malnutrition is found frequently in hospitalized patients, particularly those who are hypermetabolic as a consequence of trauma or infection. In severely burned patients, not only is it necessary to increase the total caloric intake, but apparently a greater percentge of that intake should be in the form of high-quality proteins. Dietary regimens have been found to be helpful for the support of host resistance in the already infected patient and in patients undergoing chemotherapy. It has also become clear that a protein-restricted diet may have adverse effects on host defense and resistance to infection in the uremic patient.

Immunomodulating Drugs

Immunomodulating drug usage for the prevention of infection in the immunocompromised host has been explored only recently. Several agents have been tested in burned animals and found to increase resistance to bacterial infections of the burn wound; these include *Corynebacterium parvum* vaccine (Burroughs Wellcome Company), TP-5 (the active pentapeptide of thymopoietin; Ortho Pharmaceutical Corporation), and CP-46,665 (Pfizer Laboratories). Other agents that may increase host resistance to infection in normal animals and sometimes in malnourished animals include muramyl dipeptide, levamisole, CP 20, 961, and lithium carbonate. Lithium carbonate can also reduce the incidence of leukopenia in patients undergoing chemotherapy. At least two of these agents, *Corynebacterium parvum* vaccine and TP-5, are undergoing clinical trials for the prevention of infection in burn patients. The role of these agents in the immunocompromised patient, while promising, has yet to be established.

SPECIAL THERAPEUTIC CONSIDERATIONS

Granulocyte Transfusions

Granulocyte transfusions have been available for clinical use for 15 years, but considerable controversy still remains about their proper utilization as a result of the complex biologic and clinical situations for which granulocytes are transfused. This form of therapy has been applied most effectively in patients with profound neutropenia from iatrogenic marrow aplasia due to cytotoxic or chemotherapeutic agents.

Leukocytes can be harvested from donors by continuous flow centrifugation techniques or by filtration leukophoresis. The filtration technique has given better yields, but the continuous flow technique has been associated with better *in vitro* function of the collected cells. Better results have been obtained when cells were harvested from ABO-compatible, HLA-identical donors, or from relatives, in an effort to decrease the incidence of alloimmunization and transfusion reactions. It is important to emphasize that leukocyte transfusions, when indicated, are second in priority to the prompt and appropriate use of antibiotics in the septic immunocompromised person.

The transfusion of granulocytes is usually recommended for patients in whom recovery of the bone marrow is anticipated when their peripheral blood count contains less than 1000 granulocytes per cubic millimeter during infection. A daily transfusion of more than 10^{10} granulocytes is required, and this will increase the number of granulocytes in the patient only by several hundred per cubic millimeter. Granulocyte transfusions have no proven benefit in patients with normal granulocyte counts but with abnormal granulocyte function associated with bone marrow suppression caused by sepsis.

Passive Immunization

Passive immunization may be considered for management of the immune deficiency patients. While both antibody and nonspecific opsonins of the complement system are absolutely essential for normal resistance to infection by most bacterial pathogens, a considerable *in vivo* reserve exists. Patients with predominantly B-cell defects (hypogammaglobulinemia) and abnormal antibody responses have been treated successfully with gamma globulin injections for prevention of infection. In contrast, patients with cellular immune deficiency do not benefit from treatment with gamma globulin. In a recent study, it was demonstrated that low levels of serum opsonins (IgG, C3, properdin, factor B) were not associated with bacteremic episodes unless abnormal phagocytic function was also present. In another controlled study of patients with large burns, the routine administration of plasma resulted in no difference in levels of opsonic proteins and no clinical benefit in the late burn course. The administration of plasma should therefore be of value in patients who are expected to be markedly deficient in blood opsonins, such as severely malnourished or hypermetabolic patients having sepsis who respond poorly to conventional therapy.

Investigation of the opsonophagocytic requirements for *Pseudomonas aeruginosa* have shown that nearly all of the isolates have an absolute requirement for specific antibody, and also that active infection of burn wounds with *P. aeruginosa* can cause selective consumption of the specific protective antibody in the patient's serum. For these reasons, pooled gamma globulin might confer benefit, but only in highly selected patients. Hyperimmune anti-*Pseudomonas* gamma globulin has been shown to have therapeutic benefit both experimentally and clinically, but it is not commercially available.

Impairment of the function of the reticuloendothelial and macrophage systems, which may appear during severe sepsis, has been attributed to depletion of opsonic fibronectin. Cryoprecipitate infusion in septic patients with organ failure has been reported to result in rapid reversal of this opsonic deficiency with improvement of pulmonary, renal, and peripheral vascular function. There is no firm evidence that opsonic protein is a regulator of bacterial phagocytosis, and improvement has been attributed to clearing of blood-borne particulate products of sepsis and stabilization of endothelial surfaces by plasma fibronectin. The clinical value of fibronectin therapy has yet to be established.

Another interesting approach has been the development of antisera against key antigenic bacterial cross-reacting determinants. Human antiserum is raised against the *Escherichia coli* J5 mutant; this antigen is considered to be similar to the core antigen of most gram-negative bacteria. In a recent clinical trial in patients with gram-negative bacteremia, J5 antiserum, added to surgical and antimicrobial treatment, showed a beneficial effect in reducing deaths when compared with controls.

Surgical Excision

The importance of surgical excision must be emphasized. In the treatment of surgical infections, antibiotic agents and other supportive measures frequently serve only as adjuncts to surgical drainage of collections of pus, or excision or debridement of necrotic infected tissues that may serve as a pabulum for toxin production and further infection.

Changes in color of the burn wound associated with an unexplained toxic state often indicate the presence of invasive fungal infection. Such a lesion usually has a necrotic center surrounded by a rapidly expanding area of inflammation that presents as purplish discoloration. Prompt biopsy of the involved area will help to demonstrate hyphae invading viable tissue. This finding confirms the diagnosis. Organisms associated with this infection include *Aspergillus, Mucor, Candida,* and *Geotrichum* species, and others. Such infections have been seen with increasing incidence in other disorders associated with decreasing host resistance, particularly in patients with malignancies of the lymphoid and reticuloendothelial systems, and in those with diabetes mellitus and acidosis.

Both *Aspergillus* and *Mucor* can invade the paranasal sinuses and extend to the orbit and brain. In this desperate situation, extensive and early radical debridement along with amphotericin B therapy is essential for the patient's survival.

Necrotizing fasciitis is another rapidly progressive infection that may affect the subcutaneous tissue and fascia in the immunosuppressed patient. It may be accompanied by severe systemic toxicity. The factors that predispose a patient to a rapidly progressive clinical course are unknown, but diabetes, anemia, and renal failure are often found in association. Synergistic bacterial surgical infections are frequent and may include both aerobic and anaerobic gram-positive and gram-negative microorganisms. Early diagnosis and prompt radical surgical incision and debridement are essential for successful treatment, along with appropriate antimicrobial therapy.

TREATMENT OF SPECIFIC INFECTIONS IN THE IMMUNOCOMPROMISED HOST

In the critically ill immunocompromised host, it is imperative to initiate treatment without undue delay. The knowledge of bacterial sensitivity patterns associated with a presumptive diagnosis of the offending organism will frequently lead to selection of proper antibiotics until sensitivities are available. So-called shotgun therapy is to be discouraged except in severe established infections when death of the patient appears probable before sensitivity tests would be available.

Precise identification of the microorganisms involved is necessary both for treatment and for suggestions of potential sources. Direct examination of gram-stained smears of pus or secretions will often reveal the nature of the infecting organism. When there is an immediate need for information about antibiotic sensitivity of the organism, direct sensitivity tests may be done by plating exudate directly on blood agar and simultaneously testing with sensitivity disks. Definitive information can thus usually be obtained within 12 hours.

Bacterial Infections

Although unusual pathogens are important in this clinical setting, the common bacteria such as *Staphylococcus aureus, Escherichia coli, Klebsiella, Proteus,* and *Enterobacter* are the most frequent causes of serious infections, most of them arising from the patient's endogenous flora. It is important to remember that a patient who develops an infection in the hospital or while receiving antibiotics may have an altered aerobic flora with antibiotic-resistant organisms. Specific antibiotic therapy of these organisms is discussed in Chapter 11 and is similar for the immunocompromised host. In leukopenic patients, however, bactericidal antibiotics may be preferable to bacteriostatic ones.

Listeriosis. *Listeria monocytogenes* is a small gram-positive aerobic or microaerophilic coccobacillary organism that can produce a bacteremia in patients with impaired cell-mediated immunity without any apparent primary source. In the immunosuppressed person with listeriosis, meningitis may present with acute, subacute, or complete absence of meningeal signs except for persistent headache and fever, although focal brain infection with localizing neurological sepsis is rare. Clinical suspicion along with these findings should suggest the need for a lumbar puncture for diagnosis. The organism is susceptible to most of the common antibiotics including ampicillin, penicillin, erythromycin, tetracycline, and gentamycin. Ampicillin (12 – 14 g per day IV) or penicillin G (2,000,000 units IV every 2 hours) with or without aminoglycosides is the preferred treatment. In patients with neurological involvement, therapy should be continued for 2 weeks after defervescence.

Legionnaire's Disease. Legionnaire's disease is caused by the *Legionella* species of bacteria. Clinically, it presents with fever, leukocytosis, pulmonary infiltrate, and a toxemic state with mental confusion (Fig. 12-1). Treatment for Legionnaire's disease or suspected infection is erythromycin in dosage of 2 to 6 g/day intravenously. Higher doses are needed for more severe infections. After clinical response,

Fig. 12-1. A left upper lobe infiltrate in a 55-year-old white man, which occurred after his second cadaver kidney transplant. Diagnosis of legionellosis was made by fluorescent antibody technique. Despite treatment with erythromycin, the patient died of progressive lobar pneumonia.

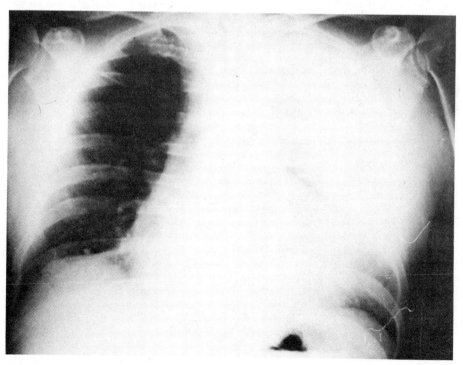

oral administration may be started. Erythromycin is given for a minimum of 3 weeks.

Nocardiosis. Nocardial infections may occur in immunosuppressed patients, usually as a pneumonitis, either lobular or lobar. The *Nocardia* species were misclassified as fungi because of their filamentous appearance, but they are clearly bacteria, staining gram-positive as well as acid-fast. The primary route of pulmonary infection is the inhalation of spores. It may progress to tissue necrosis with abscess formation and cavitation. The appearance on the chest roentgenogram may be acute lobar consolidation, cavitary abscess, empyema, hilar adenopathy, or solitary nodules (Fig. 12-2). An open lung biopsy may be required for definitive diagnosis. Clinical findings include cough, fever, chills, and copious purulent or bloody sputum. Metastatic brain involvement through hematogenous spread should be ruled out if possible in any patient with nocardiosis.

Nocardia infection in the immunocompromised patient requires at least 4 to 6 months of therapy with high doses of sulfonamide or trimethoprim with sulfa-

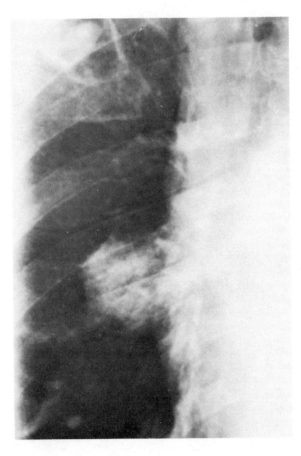

Fig. 12-2. An infiltrate in the right lower lobe due to aspergillosis, and also a "fungus ball" due to *Nocardia* in a 58-year-old white man, a post-renal transplant patient. Diagnosis proven by autopsy.

methoxazole. Sulfonamides including sulfisoxazole are given in divided doses every 6 hours for a total daily dose of 6 to 10 g. Combination therapy with ampicillin and erythromycin may be needed in the patient that cannot tolerate sulfonamides.

Mycobacterial Infections.   Since tuberculosis in the immunosuppressed patient is unusual, its prevention or treatment is indicated only in the patient with a grossly abnormal chest x-ray, a recent tuberculin test conversion, or a history of past untreated infection.

For prophylaxis, isoniazid (INH) is the only drug recommended, although it may cause hepatotoxicity. The usual dosage is 5 mg/kg body weight per day for 1 year. For patients with active tuberculosis, two-drug therapy is indicated: INH and ethambutol. The dosage is 25 mg/kg body weight per day for 6 to 8 weeks, followed by 15 mg/kg/day. In patients with advanced cavitary pulmonary disease, miliary tuberculosis, or pericarditis, INH, ethambutol, and streptomycin are required. Streptomycin must be given parenterally; the average dosage is 1 g daily for the first 2 to 8 weeks of therapy followed by 1 gm twice a week. The excretion of streptomycin is by way of the kidneys, and dosage should be adjusted in patients with renal failure. Rifampin, a fat-soluble molecule excreted by the liver, rivals INH in its efficacy; dosage is given as 600 mg/day in a single dose. Because of its potential for hepatotoxicity, it should be used with caution in the immunosuppressed patient.

Viral Infections

Viral infections in the immunocompromised host can occur as acute, chronic, or recurrent diseases. Protection against most of these is under the control of cell-mediated mechanisms rather than humoral immunity. Persistent infections may occur with all the human herpes groups of viruses: herpes simplex virus, varicella zoster virus, Epstein-Barr virus, and cytomegalovirus.

Herpes Simplex Virus Infection.   Infection with herpes simplex virus (HSV) is related to either of two serotypes: HSV-1 is primarily transmitted by infected saliva and is a major cause of herpes labialis, gingivostomatitis, and encephalitic and corneal infections. HSV-2 is a sexually transmitted disease that causes herpes genitalis and neonatal infections. Widespread systemic involvement with HSV-2 can also cause pneumonitis, hepatitis, and encephalitis (Fig. 12-3). Diagnosis can be made by finding characteristic multinucleated giant cells using cytological and histological techniques. Also, the virus grows readily on a variety of cell cultures, and diagnosis by characteristic cytopathic changes can be made within 24 to 48 hours. Topical agents like idoxuridine (IDU), vidarabine, and trifluridine (trifluorothymidine), which provide high local concentration, have proven useful in the treatment of superficial herpes keratitis. Except for the treatment of ocular infections, however, use of these agents has not been of much value. Parenteral adenine arabinoside (ara-A) has been found to reduce both morbidity and mortality of HSV encephalitis and neonatal herpes in the immunologically intact patient. Acyclovir (acycloguanosine) is a nucleoside derivative with great therapeutic promise since it

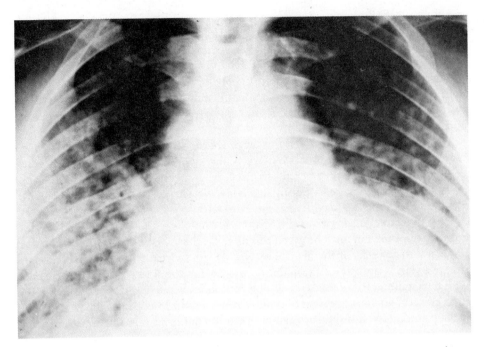

Fig. 12-3. Bilateral lung infiltrate consistent with herpesvirus pneumonia that occurred in a 25-year-old white male patient after he received a living donor transplant. The patient improved without treatment.

has been found effective against herpes simplex. Prophylactic and therapeutic intravenous acyclovir has been proven to reduce virus shedding and lesions in transplant recipients. This observation suggests that such therapy, although successful in preventing active HSV replication, was not able to eradicate the virus. Since most antiviral agents are only effective against the replicating virus, the possibility of combining them with interferon to achieve this goal is being investigated and studies are in progress. Interferon apparently has the capability of rendering these cells resistant to subsequent virus infection by inducing the production of cellular enzymes that block viral production. The major therapeutic efforts in the compromised host should be directed toward reducing the level of immunosuppression and preventing superinfection.

Varicella-Zoster Virus Infection.   Varicella-zoster virus (VZV) infection is presumably acquired through the respiratory tract or skin, or is disseminated by way of the blood to skin and visceral organs. The lung has usually been the major target organ. This virus is thought to persist within the sensory ganglia following infection. When host defense is impaired, it travels down the sensory nerve to the skin to produce zoster vesicles. Humoral antibody may have a protective role against infection as evidenced by the beneficial effect of prophylactic zoster immune globulin or plasma in immunosuppressed children at risk for infection. Prophylaxis by a live VZV vaccine is also being evaluated. Treatment for established infection consists of ara-A in doses of 10 mg/kg/day. This treatment started early in the course of the disease has been successful in healing vesicles and preventing the formation of new vesicles. Human leukocyte interferon in large doses $(1.7-5.1 \times 10^5$ units/kg/day) may significantly decrease cutaneous dissemination when compared with placebo treatment.

Epstein-Barr Virus Infection. Epstein-Barr virus (EBV) is the causal agent of infectious mononucleosis, and it is also associated with Burkitt's lymphoma and nasopharyngeal carcinoma. It is of importance in the immunosuppressed patient because it may be transmitted through blood transfusions and because reactivation of EBV infection is common, especially in the transplant patient. Primary EBV infection may occur as a pneumonia or a disseminated lymphoproliferative disorder. Although there is no treatment available for EBV infection, therapy does not appear necessary in most situations. In patients with severe clinical manifestations, however, reduction of the level of immunosuppression or its discontinuation may be indicated.

Cytomegalovirus Infection. Cytomegalovirus (CMV) is the most common pathogen causing morbidity and mortality in transplantation patients. In those patients with disordered cell-mediated immunity, it can cause a variety of clinical diseases including pancreatitis, hepatitis, pneumonia, retinitis, and gastrointestinal ulcerations (Fig. 12-4). Multiple blood transfusions have been associated with primary CMV infection in both normal and immunosuppressed patients. Transfusion of stored blood, blood from seronegative donors, and blood products that are poor in leukocytes should lower risk of CMV transmission. The risk appears to be greater for primary CMV infection when seronegative live recipients receive grafts from seropositive donors. However, reactivation of the virus is also responsible for a substantial number of infections. A major concern in patient management is the reduction in the level of immunosuppression in order to prevent serious bacterial or fungal infection. Live attenuated CMV vaccines have been developed for administration to seronegative recipients of allografts from seropositive donors. In preliminary testing, these vaccines have failed to produce protection following transplantation, since cell-mediated responses are attenuated by associated immunosuppression. Antiviral agents like ara-A have not been effective in transplant recipients.

Viral Hepatitis. Viral hepatitis presents a severe clinical problem in the immunocompromised host, and these patients also represent significant hazards for transmission of hepatitis to other patients and medical personnel. Although several lines of evidence suggest that cellular immunity may be important in defense, absence of humoral antibody can lead to quite severe infections. Two types of virus, A and B, have been demonstrated to be etiological agents in this infection. There is increasing evidence that one or more additional viruses exist, commonly referred to as non-A, non-B agents, and that these are responsible for most of the infections.

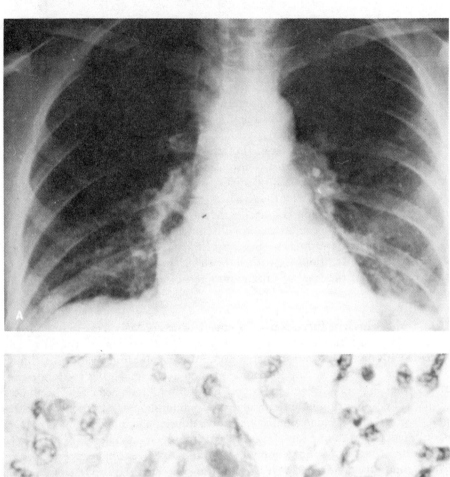

Fig. 12-4. (A) A left lobe infiltrate in a 24-year-old white man 8 weeks after receiving a living related transplant. Open lung biopsy provided the diagnosis of cytomegalovirus. Improvement occurred without treatment. (B) Photomicrograph of lung biopsy from same patient showing cytomegalovirus.

Prevention of hepatitis depends primarily on limiting contact with individuals who have hepatitis infections. Since there is no treatment for the established infection, prophylaxis becomes extremely important when exposure has occurred. In hepatitis A exposure, 0.01 ml of immune serum globulin (ISG) per pound of weight given IM early in the incubation period will prevent symptoms and jaundice in exposed contacts. Hepatitis B immune globulin (HBIG) is recommended only for individuals who have high risk exposure such as accidental oral, percutaneous, or mucosal contact with blood or body fluids infected with hepatitis B. It is given in two doses of 0.04 ml/kg body weight, 1 month apart. Patients whose blood is anti-HBs positive do not require immunoprophylaxis. HBIG and conventional gamma globulin have not been shown to be effective against non-A, non-B hepatitis. Renal allograft recipients who are HBs Ag carriers or infected with non-A, non-B hepatitis have been shown to have a low probability of graft rejection and these patients have a late excessive rate of late nonhepatic infection. Thus, the conservative use of immunosuppressive drugs is warranted under these circumstances. The efficacy of two different hepatitis B vaccines has recently been established in healthy patient populations, and it is expected that patients with renal failure may benefit from such vaccines despite the evidence of attenuated response of some patients with uremia to hepatitis B vaccines (Chap. 10).

Fungal Infections

Opportunistic infections by fungi are commonly associated with high mortality rates in the immunocompromised patient. They may occur either as a reactivation of a latent infection or as a new opportunistic infection. In the first category are included disseminated histoplasmosis, coccidioidomycosis, and blastomycosis. New opportunistic infections are more often caused by *Cryptococcus neoformans, Aspergillus fumigatus,* and *Candida albicans.* Not only are these infections difficult to diagnose, but treatment by most antifungal agents may exert toxic effects.

Amphotericin B, a polyene macrolide antibiotic obtained from *Streptomyces nodosus,* is the most reliable and effective antifungal agent. Its antifungal effect resides in its ability to combine with cytoplasmatic membrane sterols in fungi. Associated toxic side-effects include nephrotoxicity, fever, cardiovascular collapse, and potassium wasting; these side-effects represent serious limitations of the drug. Therapy usually begins with a 1-mg dose test to determine if the patient will develop a fever. This dose is then increased by 5-mg increments daily up to the full therapeutic dose. A common goal is 60 mg per day with a total dose of 1 to 3 g. Depending on the mycosis being treated, the duration of therapy is usually 6 to 12 weeks. If the creatinine rises above 3 mg/ml, the dose is lowered by 10 to 20 mg, or the interval between the doses can be increased (up to 3 days). Since cerebrospinal fluid levels may be inadequate, intrathecal or intracisternal injections are occasionally given in patients with fungal meningitis. Hydrocortisone, diphenhydramine, and salicylates may be used to limit side-effects. Amphotericin B has been used with other antifungal agents in an effort to reduce its toxicity and increase the therapeutic effect. Since it combines with cell membranes and increases permeability, other agents can gain entrance into the fungal cell in larger quantities.

Aspergillosis. In immunocompromised patients, *Aspergillus fumigatus* and *Aspergillus flavus* are the most common isolated pathogens causing aspergillosis. Factors predisposing to infection are impairment in neutrophil and T-lymphocyte function.

The organism tends to invade blood vessels, causing clotting and infarction of tissue with hematogenous spread to distal organs, brain abscesses being common and usually leading to a fatal outcome. It can also occur in the lung as a diffuse interstitial infiltrate, lobar consolidation, or focal cavitary lesions with a fungus ball or aspergilloma (Fig. 12-5). Multiple infections are common, and aspergillosis may complicate cytomegalovirus infection and bacterial pneumonia, or develop along with nocardiosis or tuberculosis. The agent of choice for treatment is amphotericin B.

Cryptococcosis. Cryptococcosis is another fungal infection that may be associated with defects in cell-mediated immunity. The major clinical infections are in the lungs and central nervous system (Fig. 12-6). Although the typical finding in the lung is a mass or segmental consolidation, occasionally with some cavitation, it can occur with nodular lesions that resemble bronchogenic carcinoma. Miliary disease may develop in patients with the most profound defects in host resistance. Mixed

Fig. 12-5. Photomicrograph of lung at autopsy in a 28-year-old white woman who developed fever and a diffuse lung infiltrate after a kidney transplant. She was treated for rejection and died after a massive gastrointestinal hemorrhage. Autopsy showed aspergillosis.

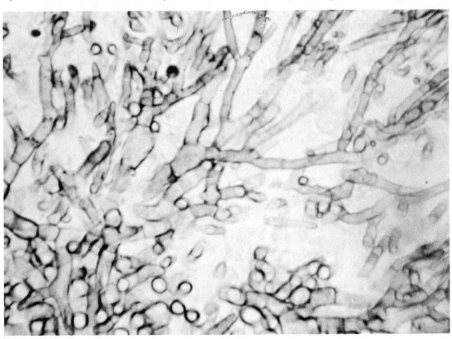

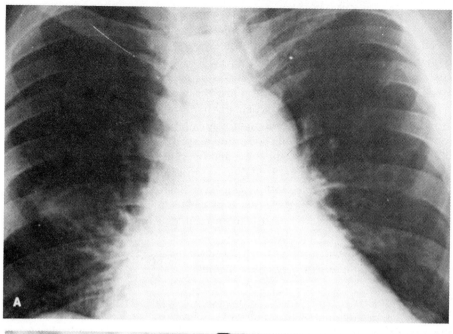

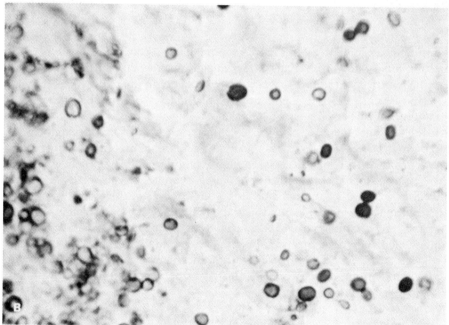

Fig. 12-6. (*A*) Cryptococcal lung infection in a 47-year-old black man, a cadaver kidney recipient, 3 years after transplantation. He underwent a right lobectomy for right lower lobe nodule and was treated with amphotericin B for 40 days (total of 1347 mg). He recovered. (*B*) Photomicrograph of lung depicting the *Cryptococcus* pneumonitis.

infections with nocardiosis, tuberculosis, or aspergillosis may also occur. Lung biopsy is the preferred method of diagnosis. Histopathological material shows a yeast form with an unstained capsular halo using hematoxylin-eosin or silver stains. In the immunosuppressed patient, pulmonary cryptococcus infection should lead to a search for disseminated disease, particularly in the meninges, and spinal tap should be performed. The diagnosis depends on the isolation of the organism or demonstration of cryptococcal antigen in the body fluid. Cryptococcal meningitis may present with fever and persistent headache only, and fully developed meningismus is rare.

Appropriate treatment is combined therapy with amphotericin B, 0.3 to 0.5 mg/kg/day, and 5-fluorocytosine, 150 mg/kg/day. Since 5-fluorocytosine, a cytosine antimetabolite, is absorbed by the gastrointestinal tract and excreted undamaged by glomerular filtration, the dose must be reduced in patients with renal failure. The few toxic side-effects include bone marrow depression. Since cerebrospinal fluid levels can be inadequate, intrathecal injections are indicated for patients who are not responding to amphotericin B systemic therapy.

Histoplasmosis.   Histoplasmosis may occur as a primary infection in the lung where spores are engulfed by macrophages and replicate intracellularly in the yeast phase. Local inflammation produces areas of interstitial pneumonitis. Draining lymph nodes are involved, and hematogenous spread of the organism follows. The appearance of the chest x-rays may vary from a few areas of alveolitis to an extensive diffuse nodular infiltrate (Fig. 12-7). Symptomatic recovery from the primary infection usually follows, leaving a few calcifications visable on the chest x-ray. Chronic infection can lead to cavitary lesions, mainly in the upper lobe, that may mimic tuberculosis. Also it can present as solitary nodules that must be differentiated from bronchogenic carcinoma.

In the immunosuppressed patient, disseminated disease may occur as endogenous reactivation. The clinical picture is usually variable and nonspecific with persistent fever with or without pulmonary symptoms. Physical examination is not diagnostic and usually consists of nonspecific lung findings with lymphadenopathy and hepatosplenomegaly. Early diagnosis is made by means of histopathological specimens, obtained from bone marrow aspiration or biopsies that reveal macrophages crowded with small yeasts. Cultures may take several weeks to become positive. Complement fixing serologic reactions against yeast antigens with high or rising titers are found in convalescent specimens and are also diagnostic. Amphotericin B is the indicated treatment for chronic cavitary or disseminated histoplasmosis. A dose from 500 mg to 2 g total has been recommended.

Blastomycosis.   *Blastomycosis,* caused by *Blastomyces dermatitidis,* has also been noted in immunocompromised hosts. The infected spores are inhaled into the lungs where an early inflammatory response occurs with invasion by macrophages. Cell-mediated immunity develops later. Acute pulmonary blastomycosis presents with symptoms like acute pneumonia. The radiological appearance is quite varied, and a diffuse infiltrative pattern with bilateral involvement of both lower lobes may be observed. Most clinical cases present as chronic pulmonary disease with chronic

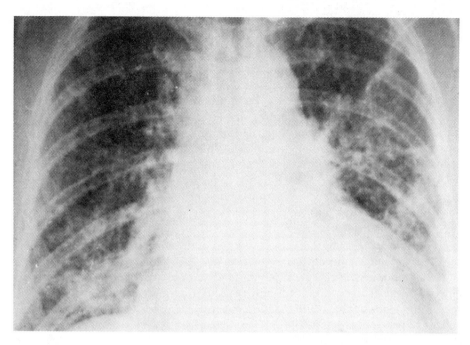

Fig. 12-7. Pulmonary histoplasmosis diagnosed by open lung biopsy in a 55-year-old white woman who was a living donor renal transplant recipient. She recovered after treatment with amphotericin B (total of 1600 mg).

cough and low-grade fever. Hematogenous spread may produce a picture of miliary disease in the lung, and may spread throughout the body with involvement of skin, bone, or genitourinary tract. Nodular lesions can be mistaken for carcinoma. Unilateral disease may mimic tuberculosis. Diagnosis depends upon identification of the yeast in the sputum or histopathologic examination of biopsy specimens. In the severely ill patient, treatment consists of the administration of amphotericin B.

Coccidioidomycosis. Coccidioidomycosis caused by the fungus *Coccidioides immitis,* is another infection that may occur in the immunosuppressed patient. The disease is endemic in the southwestern United States. Infection occurs by inhalation of the infective arthrospores, which elicits an inflammatory reaction in the alveoli of the lung with exudation predominantly of polymorphonuclear cells. A specific T-cell-mediated immunity against the maturing spherules follows. Disseminated disease can result following a primary infection or reactivation of chronic infection. It begins with persistent or recurrent fever, and can progress rapidly with development of meningitis and involvement of the spleen, lymph nodes, and verrucous cutaneous lesions. Single nodular masses seen in x-rays of the chest can mimic carcinoma. Diagnosis of meningitis can be facilitated by spinal tap with demonstration of the complement-fixing antibody in the spinal fluid.

Amphotericin B remains the treatment of choice, but is less effective against *C. immitis* than against other fungi. The usual dose is 500 mg to 2 g, intravenously, but in disseminated disease, a prolonged course of 4 to 5 g is indicated. Intrathecal injections may be needed for meningeal involvement, and are given until complement-fixing antibodies in cerebrospinal fluid remain negative.

Miconazole or ketoconazole may be of value in patients who do not respond to amphotericin B therapy. Their exact role in treatment of this infection is yet to be defined, but it is important to note the lack of significant renal, hepatic, or bone marrow toxicity. Miconazole, a synthetic antifungal compound, acts by its ability to damage the fungal plasma membrane by its interference with ergosterol synthesis. Dosages are 0.6 to 1 g IV every 8 hours. Ketoconazole, another imidazole derivative, has similar action but better oral absorption. Dosages of 200 to 400 mg by mouth in single daily doses are recommended.

Candidiasis.   Candidal organisms are part of the normal bowel flora of man and also constant inhabitants of the mouth, pharynx, and upper airways. Different types of cellular immune defects predisposing to *Candida* infection vary with the type of infection. Mucocutaneous infections may occur in patients with altered T-lymphocyte – mononuclear phagocyte function, whereas invasive candidiasis is more often related to neutrophil defects in function. One of the most common factors predisposing patients to invasive *Candida* infections is the direct access to the circulatory system by way of an intravenous catheter, particularly a hyperalimentation line. Long-term treatment with broad-spectrum antibiotics that suppress normal flora and allow the number of *Candida* organisms to increase is another important determinant.

For the prevention of candidiasis and fungemia in immunocompromised persons, oral nystatin in high doses appears to be useful in reducing the numbers of *Candida* in the intestine. Also, oral ketoconazole may prove to be helpful in preventing colonization by *Candida.*

Oral candidiasis may produce esophagitis by direct extension. Patients usually complain of dysphagia, and the diagnosis is confirmed by barium swallow or esophagoscopy. Oral and esophageal candidiasis can be treated with oral nystatin in large doses of 10 million units four times a day. Nystatin suppositories or lozenges may be used orally; they should be allowed to melt, and then be swallowed. If there is no response to this therapy in 24 to 48 hours, amphotericin B should be administered intravenously in dosages of 0.25 to 0.5 mg/kg/day for 2 weeks.

Although primary *Candida* pneumonia is rare in the immunosuppressed patient, *Candida* organisms are frequently part of polymicrobial superinfections. Diagnosis of this infection can only be proven by lung biopsy. Treatment consists of intravenous amphotericin B in doses of 1 mg/kg, with or without added 5-fluorocytosine.

Overgrowth of local candida organisms in the bowel or mucosal surfaces can penetrate into the tissues and produce intermittent seeding into the bloodstream, producing disseminated candidiasis. The demonstration of candidemia indicates the presence of disseminated candidiasis and the need for systemic anticandidal therapy. Perhaps the major site of metastatic seeding is to the kidney, and the presence of candiduria may indicate disseminated candidiasis. Candidal endophthalmitis is a frequent complication of sustained candidemia and is easily diagnosed by examination of the eye. Another site of metastatic infection that may be of diagnostic help is the skin, since such lesions can be biopsied. Invasive candidiasis should be treated with the combination of intravenous amphotericin B and 5-fluorocytosine along with correction of any disposing factors, such as removal of intravenous and urinary catheters, discontinuing broad-spectrum antibiotics, control of diabetes, and decreasing immunosuppressive therapy, if possible. In candidal endocarditis, surgical removal of the infected valve may become necessary. Patients with the septicemic form of candidiasis may have brain involvement, with multiple cerebral microabscesses and neurological signs. Treatment requires systemic or intrathecal amphotericin B with or without 5-fluorocytosine.

For treatment of bladder colonization or local invasion, removal of the catheter should be enough; if not, the bladder may be irrigated with amphotericin B, 50 mg in a liter of sterile saline through a Foley catheter twice a day.

Parasitic Infections

Pneumocystis Pneumonia. *Pneumocystis carinii* is an intracellular parasite with both cystic and trophozoite stages. The cyst contains up to eight oval bodies, termed sporozoites, which are best seen in silver-stained smears of infected fresh lung preparations. Rapid diagnosis can be made by Giemsa-stained imprints, but the Gomori–methenamine–silver nitrate stain is the most reliable (although time consuming) procedure for identification of cysts.

P. carinii is acquired by airborne human transmission or by reactivation of a latent asymptomatic infection. Cytomegalovirus infection can predispose to or coexist with *P. carinii*. Clinically, *P. carinii* infection occurs with fever, nonproductive cough, and progressive dyspnea with hypoxia, as determined by blood gas readings. These changes may precede x-ray findings. The typical radiological appearance is a diffuse bilateral interstitial alveolar infiltrate. Since transtracheal aspiration will demonstrate the organism only in 15% to 20% of cases, a lung biopsy is usually necessary for definitive diagnosis.

Trimethoprim–sulfamethoxazole has been successfully used to treat most cases of pneumocystis infection. It is administered over 14 days at dosages of 20 mg of trimethoprim and 100 mg of sulfamethoxazole/kg/day by mouth in three or four doses. A parenteral form is available, the dose being approximately 50% of the recommended oral dose. For prophylaxis, 5 mg of trimethoprim and 20 mg of sulfamethoxazole/kg/day in two divided doses may be effective. If during a 72- to 96-hour period of observation, the condition of the patient treated with trimethoprim–sulfamethoxazole has worsened, pentamidine should be added to the therapeutic regimen.

Toxoplasmosis. Although fewer cases of toxoplasmosis than *Pneumocystis carinii* infection have been reported in the recent literature, toxoplasmosis may occur in the very same patients who are susceptible to pneumocystosis. *Toxoplasma gondii,* an obligate intracellular parasite, causes toxoplasmosis, which is endemic worldwide (Fig. 12-8). Patients with Hodgkin's disease and those receiving immunosuppressive therapy are most commonly affected. Infection can result from reactivation of or primary acquisition of the organism. The clinical disease occurs with fever, malaise, diffuse lymphadenopathy, hepatosplenomegaly, and maculopapular rash. Neurological manifestations with focal signs and seizures can predominate, along with diffuse encephalopathy and meningoencephalitis. Diagnosis is based upon demonstration of trophozoite forms in the body fluids and tissues, and the finding of toxoplasma antibodies of specific type and titer.

Pyrimethamine (a diaminopyrimidine) and a sulfonamide are active against the trophozoite forms and interactive synergistically when used in combination. Pyrimethamine is given in a loading dose of 100 to 200 mg followed by maintenance to a total dose of 1 mg/kg/day. Sulfadiazine, or a triple sulfa mixture, are the most active sulfonamides against *T. gondii*. Sulfadiazine is given to adults in dosages of 100 mg/kg/day divided into four hourly doses after a loading dose of 50 mg/kg. Such combined therapy may be necessary for a month or longer, with careful monitoring of renal, hepatic, and hematologic functions.

Fig. 12-8. Photomicrograph showing diffuse pulmonary infiltrate caused by toxoplasmosis in a 21-year-old white man who had received his second cadaveric transplant 3 weeks after his first transplant. He died of progressive pulmonary insufficiency, and autopsy confirmed the diagnosis of toxoplasmosis.

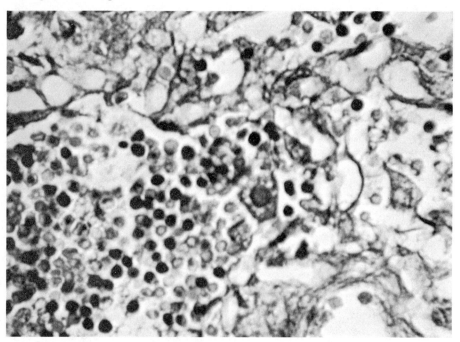

Strongyloidiasis. Strongyloidiasis is an infection caused by *Strongyloides stercoralis,* an intestinal nematode, which can cause disseminated disease involving the heart, liver, skeletal muscle, adrenals, pancreas, kidneys, and central nervous system in the immunocompromised patient. Patients present with a combination of pulmonary and gastrointestinal symptoms associated with eosinophilia. Pulmonary involvement causes hemorrhagic infiltrates. In the gastrointestinal tract, severe ulcerating hemorrhagic enterocolitis may serve as a portal of entry for bacterial and fungal superinfections. Diagnosis is made by examining aspirated duodenal contents for the presence of larvae, which may also be found in transtracheal aspirates. Examination of the stool is negative in 70% of the cases. For treatment, the agent of choice is thiabendazole in doses of 25 mg/kg twice daily for 15 days. Alternative treatment is mebendazole in doses of 100 mg twice a day for 15 days.

ACQUIRED IMMUNE DEFICIENCY SYNDROME (AIDS)

Since June 1981, when the Acquired Immune Deficiency Syndrome (AIDS) was first described, over 1000 cases of life-threatening opportunistic infections with or without Kaposi sarcoma have been reported.

These illnesses appeared suddenly with a remarkable geographic distribution that favors concentration in major urban centers. Although most of the patients have been homosexual men and intravenous drug abusers, the disease has also been reported in heterosexual Haitian patients living in Florida, male patients with hemophilia, and prison inmates.

Major clinical manifestations of the syndrome are Kaposi sarcoma and/or infections with a variety of opportunistic pathogens including *Pneumocystis carinii, Toxoplasma gandii, Candida, Cryptococcus,* and various *Mycobacterium* species. Infections are usually overwhelming, with high mortality.

Prodrome includes onset of leukopenia several months before diagnosis consistent with a prolonged incubation period, which is followed by anorexia, fever, weight loss, and lymphadenopathy.

Although humoral immunity is unchanged, there is impairment of cellular immunity, cutaneous anergy, and diminished lymphocyte proliferation response to various mitogens and antigens; also, there is a decreased number of T helper/inducer cells and inversion of the normal helper/inducer cell to T suppressor/cytotoxic ratio. The similarity in epidemiologic patterns of the syndrome and hepatitis B is so striking that the possibility of an infection or chemical agent transmissable by blood or blood products must be considered.

Although it is not known why some patients develop immune deficiency associated with viral infections, whereas others with similar viral exposures do not, possible explanations include the following:

Repeated viral infection before resolution of previous infection
Genetic factors modifying the host's ability to respond to infections (frequency of HLA-DR 5 is increased among homosexual men with Kaposi sarcoma)

Heavy narcotic use or nitrate exposure
Antigen stimulation from repeated transfusions or inoculations, which may blunt immune
response and contribute to the susceptibility to infection

Increasing reports of AIDS in different groups of patients underscores the public
health hazard and concerns brought by this new outbreak.

BIBLIOGRAPHY

Alexander JW, Good RA: Fundamentals of Clinical Immunology. Philadelphia, WB
Saunders, 1977

Allen RC, Pruitt BA Jr: Humoral phagocyte axis of immune defense in burn patients. Arch
Surg 117:113–140, 1982

Altemeier WA, Alexander JW: Surgical infections and choice of antibiotics. In Sabiston
DC Jr (ed): Christopher's Textbook of Surgery, 12th ed, pp 333–357. Philadelphia, WB
Saunders, 1981

Bose B: Letter to the editor: *Pseudomonas* immunoglobulin and vaccine in burn patients.
Lancet 1:435, 1981

Castellino RA: Etiologic diagnosis of focal pulmonary infection in immunocompromised
patients by fluoroscopically guided percutaneous needle aspiration. Radiology 132:563–
567, 1979

Coleman ER, Black RE, Welch DM, Maxwell JG: Indium-111 labeled leukocytes in the
evaluation of suspected abdominal abscesses. Am J Surg 139:99–104, 1980

Davidson M, Tempest B, Palmer D: Bacteriologic diagnosis of acute pneumonia: Comparison of sputum, transtracheal aspirates, and lung aspirates. JAMA 235:158–163, 1976

Dick G (ed): Immunological Aspects of Infectious Disease. Baltimore, University Park Press,
1979

Ellis MJ: Transbronchial lung biopsy via the fiberoptic bronchoscope: Experience with 107
consecutive cases and comparison with bronchial brushing. Chest 68:524–532, 1975

Garner JS, Simmons BP: Guideline for Isolation Precautions in Hospitals. Atlanta, U.S.
Department of Health and Human Services, Infection Control of CDC, 1983

Gerzof SG, Robbins AH, Birkett DH, Johnson WC, Pugatek RD, Vincent ME:
Percutaneous catheter drainage of abdominal abscesses guided by ultrasound and computed tomography. Am J Radiol 133:1–8, 1979

Greenman RL, Goodall PT, King D: Lung biopsy in the immunocompromised hosts. Am J
Med 59:488–496, 1975

Haaga JR, Craig G, Weinstein AJ, Cooperman AM: New interventional techniques in the
diagnosis and management of inflammatory disease within the abdomen. Radiol Clin
North Am 17:485–513, 1979

Howard RJ, Balfour HH, Simmons RL: The surgical significance of viruses. Cur Probl
Surg 16:3, 1977

Johnson WC, Gerzof SG, Robbins AH, Nabseth DC: Treatment of abdominal abscesses:
Comparative evaluation of operative drainage versus percutaneous catheter drainage
guided by computed tomography or ultrasound. Ann Surg 194:510–519, 1981

Jones RJ, Roe EA: Controlled trial of *Pseudomonas* immunoglobulin and vaccine in burn
patients. Lancet 2:1263–1265, 1980

McNeil B, Sanders R, Alderson PO, Hessel SJ, Frieberg H, Siegelman SS, Adams DF,
Abrams HL: A prospective study of computed tomography, ultrasound and gallium
imaging in patients with fever. Radiology 139:647–653, 1981

Meakins JL, Christou NV, Shizgal HM, MacLean LD: Therapeutic approaches to anergy
in surgical patients. Ann Surg 190:286–295, 1979

Munda R, Alexander JW, First MR, Gartside PS, Fidler JP: Pulmonary infections in
renal transplant recipients. Ann Surg 187:126–133, 1978

MUNSTER AM, HOAGLAND HC, PRUITT BA JR: The effect of thermal injury on serum immunoglobulins. Ann Surg 172:965–969, 1970

PENNINGTON JE, FELDMAN MT: Pulmonary infiltrates and fever in patients with hematological malignancy assessment of transbronchial biopsy. Am J Med 62:581–587, 1977

RUBIN RH, YOUNG LS (eds): Clinical approach to Infection in the Compromised Host. New York, Plenum Publishing Corporation, 1981

SANFORD JP: Legionnaire's disease the first thousand days. N Engl J Med 300:654–656, 1979

SARAL R, BURNS WH, LASKIN OL, SANTOS GW, LIEBMAN PS: Acyclovir prophylaxis of herpes simplex virus infections. N Engl J Med 305:63–66, 1981

SCHIFFER CA: Principles of granulocyte transfusion therapy. Med Clin North Am 61:1119–1131, 1977

SIMMONS RL, HOWARD RJ (eds): Surgical Infectious Diseases. New York, Appleton-Century-Crofts, 1982

SZMNNESS W, STEVENS CE, HARLEY EJ et al: Hepatitis B vaccine: Documentation of efficacy in a controlled clinical trial in a high-risk population in the United States. N Engl J Med 303:833–841, 1980

THAKUR ML, COLEMAN RE, WELCH MJ: Indium-111-labelled leukocytes for the localization of abscesses: Preparation, analysis, tissue distribution, and comparison with gallium-67 citrate in dogs. J Lab Clin Med 89:217–228, 1977

VERHOEF J, PETERSON PK, QUIE PG (eds): Infection and the Compromised Host: Pathogenesis, Prevention and Therapy. Netherlands, Elsevier/North Holland Biomedical Press, 1980

WALTZER WC, STERIOFF S, ZINCKE H, BERNATZ PE, BREWER MJ: Open-lung biopsy in the renal transplant recipient. Surgery 80:601–610, 1980

WARDEN GD, MASON AD, PRUITT BA JR: Evaluation of leukocyte chemotaxis in vitro in thermally injured patients. J Clin Invest 54:1001–1004, 1974

WARDEN GD, MASON AD JR, PRUITT BA JR: Suppression of leukocyte chemotaxis in vitro by chemotherapeutic agents used in the management of thermal injuries. Ann Surg 181:363–369, 1975

ZIEGLER EJ, McCUTCHAN JA, FIERER J, GLAUSEN MP, SADOFF JC, DOUGLAS M, BRANDE A: Treatment of gram-negative bacteremia and shock with human antiserum to a mutant Escherichia coli. N Engl J Med 307:1225–1250, 1982

13

Architectural design is important to the overall efficiency of a surgical suite. It affects not only utilization patterns and materials handling, but also traffic and commerce in and around the suite. To a certain extent architectural design also affects the effectiveness of the air handling system, equipment, and personnel, thereby affecting the quality of surgical care and the incidence of wound infection. However, attempts to demonstrate a direct effect of architecture upon the incidence of surgical infection have met with frustration, largely because of the multitude of factors involved. Perhaps for this reason more than any other, we have had to base our architectural decisions upon indirect evidence, past experience, deductive reasoning, and related information.

The surgical environment generally is organized into a series of four functional systems:

1. Surgical support systems (the environment)
2. Traffic and commerce (the activities)
3. Communication and information (the record)
4. Administration (the management)

SURGICAL SUITE DESIGN

The design of a surgical suite is dictated largely by available space, performance requirements, and the prevailing art form of the day. Virtually any operating room is usable, although certain limitations may be imposed by its design. In general, operating rooms are now made without windows for better control of insects, temperature, and humidity. Although windows in the operating rooms are to be avoided, visual access to the outside world somewhere in the suite is recommended by Beck for the sake of employee morale.

Efforts or attempts at providing a safer operating room environment have centered around the following:

1. Modification of building codes, architectural and engineering principles, and guidelines to meet the needs of surgeons and nurses, and of anesthesia, x-ray, and other diagnostic equipment

Hospital Design Requirements for Safe Surgery

2. Improvement in electrical and mechanical function, including emergency power supply
3. Elimination of explosion hazards
4. Control of the presence and activities of unskilled personnel
5. Control of infection

The margin of permissible error in operating room design is great, and equally good operations may be performed in many different types of suites. Furthermore, there is no firm evidence that one surgical suite design holds any demonstrable advantage over any other in the control of infection. In general, four basic designs for infection control in surgical suites have emerged, each with variations:

1. The central corridor or hotel plan
2. The double corridor or clean-core plan
3. The peripheral corridor or racetrack plan
4. The grouping or cluster plan

Most operations can be comfortably performed in operating rooms approximately 20 × 20 feet. For open heart surgery, operating rooms of 24 × 24 to 28 × 30 have been recommended. While special facilities and equipment are important for specialty practice, it is desirable, when possible, to construct all operating rooms approximately the same size within a surgical suite for multi-purpose and more economical use. "Prep" and induction rooms adjacent to the operating rooms offer possible time-saving and other advantages in anesthesia and other preoperative preparations as required for the individual case.

At present, hospital planners seem to prefer an architectural form that provides a peripheral corridor around the surgical suite (racetrack plan). The ostensible purpose of this corridor is to offer a "semi-clean" thoroughfare within the suite. This floor plan is predicated on the premise that a patient and his surgical team are "cleaner" before the operation than they are afterward; therefore, they should enter the operating room from a clean core and leave by way of a less clean peripheral corridor. Elaborate traffic patterns have been drawn up in an attempt to enforce this concept, but in practice these patterns are only imperfectly followed. Moreover, the valuable space assigned to peripheral corridors is too often used for open storage of large pieces of equipment because of insufficient storage space in operating suites.

Laufman has recommended that "rather than designing for an unrealistic division of one type of clean traffic from another type of clean traffic, it would be more practical simply to make sure that: (a) people in scrub clothes do not mingle with people in street clothes; (b) all used instruments and disposable materials are containerized as they leave the operating room on their way to being processed or disposed of; (c) used surgical gowns, gloves, and drapes are left inside the operating room and not worn in movement; (d) distribution inside the surgical suite is accomplished with economy of movement and least congestion by means of appropriate location and size of clean storage areas; and (e) interior janitorial closets and other cleaning facilities such as wet vacuum outlets, cleaning equipment storage space, and so on are properly heated and adequate."

For open heart surgery, a room in the clean area may be designated as a "pump room" in which extracorporeal pump-oxygenators and all other essential equipment are stored, conditioned, and maintained. The room serves as a combination storage area and workroom in which the pump is maintained and prepared for use. An alternative plan is to use the pump room primarily for setup of the pump, and to store most of the supplies in a central sterile supply department, requisitioning them as needed. Variations of these plans depend upon available space and the method preferred by the open heart cardiac surgery team.

In large surgical suites, the grouping of operating rooms into clusters of four has proven to be an efficient configuration, especially for materials handling. A supply port at the center of each cluster, with convenient access to each operating room, is more efficient than the central corridor design in which some operating rooms are close to the supply source and others are far from it.

The interface between the operating room and public corridors of the hospital should be designed with a double set of doors separating the corridors of the surgical suite from other areas. Such a design can help control airborne contamination by providing an area for dilution of air from the corridors with the more highly filtered air in the operating suite, and by serving as a convenient place to transfer patients from hospital carts to operating room carts. Door control is important both at the entrance to the suite and in the individual operating room.

A series of tests have shown that a doormat with a tacky surface placed at the entrance to the operating room exerts no demonstrable effect on the bacterial population of cart wheels or shoes that traverse this mat. In other cases in which the mat had been traversed previously, the second set of wheels or shoes were shown to have picked up bacteria deposited during the preceding trip. Similarly, sponge rubber or sponge plastic mats or patches of carpeting that were soaked with a strong antiseptic solution may have been self-sterilizing, though this did not affect the bacterial content of cart wheels or shoe soles that traversed them. The antiseptic solutions require a contact time of at least 30 seconds; taking a few steps over such a soaked mat, therefore, will do little for bacterial control but could cause a person to slip on the wet floor.

It has been demonstrated that circulating particulate matter in the air tends to settle on horizontal surfaces, the largest being the floor. Dried, previously settled particles on the floor may be recirculated by the activity of occupants and by air systems that are not provided with adequate exhaust vents. These particles are constantly being generated from the skin and hair of personnel within the room despite the addition of highly filtered air coming into the room. Frequent wet cleaning using appropriate techniques appears to be one means of minimizing this problem (see Chap. 8). Another is to cover more adequately the hair and skin of all personnel in the operating room with barrier apparel.

Surface Materials

Because hard, smooth, nonporous surfaces do not permit the adherence of bacterial particles as readily as rough surfaces, and because such surfaces are easier to clean, it is reasonable to propose that all surface materials in an operating room be as hard and smooth as possible. Ideally, these surfaces should be as free as possible of seams, joints, and crevices. For many years ceramic tile was considered to be the most practical material for lining operating room walls, but if the grouting between the tiles was rough, it was shown to harbor bacteria. A smooth, hard grouting material is now available. Seamless walls using polyester coating or "liquid tile" have been advocated by some. Hard-finish epoxy paints over plaster board are *not* recommended; Hinshaw has reported the frequency of their damage. Laminated walls of polyethylene over brown plaster, covered by an epoxy paint or vinyl (possibly with a photomural), will stand up best.

A variety of conductive seamless floorings may be provided, including stone terrazzo, plastic terrazzo, and hard vinyl, all of which should be able to withstand flooding and wet-vacuuming. The wall–floor junction should be curved or coved to permit adequate cleansing.

Ceiling material varies greatly but should be able to withstand repeated washings with germicidal detergent cleaners. Polyester film or metal-faced ceiling tiles with a porous core for absorbing sound have been recommended.

Scrub Area

Scrub sinks should be used strictly for hand-washing and not as depositories for specimens or for rinsing infected instruments. A newly designed scrub sink operates without handles or pedals of any kind; the stream of water is activated either by a photoelectric beam or by the proximity of the person using it, and is shut off automatically a few seconds after the user walks away.

Air Handling

Wound infections in modern surgery are preponderantly the result of contact contamination, either with an endogenous (patient-generated) source or by permeation of the surgical team through ineffective barrier materials (Chap. 10). It is important to emphasize again that there are two sources of airborne organisms that may be significant in an occupied operating room: the air that is delivered to the room by the ventilating system, and the personnel. The latter are more likely to be a source of contamination and more difficult to control, but both sources must be dealt with. The ability of a ventilation system to remove generated aerosols can be mathematically expressed by the equation used by Bourdillon and Colebrook. The rate of biological decay of a substance at any moment is proportional to the concentration present at that moment and to the rate of removal. With increasing concern over postoperative infection, generated in part by increasing medicolegal and economic considerations, considerable research on air handling systems has been undertaken. Such research has been concentrated on either ultraviolet irradiation or forced-air filtration systems. Figure 13-1 demonstrates the variation of bacterial and particle counts related to operating room proceedings during an operation.

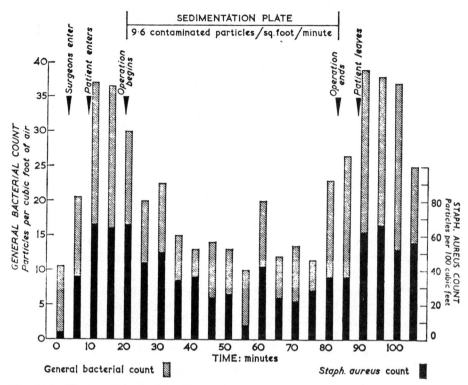

Fig. 13-1. Results of air sampling during an operation. The general bacterial counts indicate the number of contaminated particles in each cubic foot of air. The black areas indicate, on a different scale, the number of particles contaminated with *Staphylococcus aureus.* Clearly shown are the increased counts caused by the arrival and departure of the patient and by activity of the nursing staff during the operation, this being especially marked towards the end of the operation. (Williams RE: Hospital Infection: Causes and Prevention. Chicago, Year Book Medical Publishers, 1966)

As indicated in the standards of the Joint Commission on Accreditation of Hospitals (JCAH), the ventilation system should provide an effective controlled, filtered air supply in designated critical areas, including the operating room, recovery room, and surgical intensive care unit.

Airborne microorganisms and their influence on surgical infection have been studied particularly by orthopedic surgeons. This opportunity is available to them because they perform large numbers of identical operations with the same teams and in identical environments, with the ventilating system as the only variable.

The Committee on the Operating Room Environment (CORE) of the American College of Surgeons has published comments on the use of special air systems for operating rooms, which states, ". . . there is no conclusive evidence at this time that laminar clean airflow, in itself, has a favorable influence on the incidence of surgical infections." This statement has not been altered by the committee over the last decade.

Today, good practice dictates that filtered air be introduced at the ceiling and exhausted near (within 3 inches of) the floor. Although the "Minimum Requirements of Construction" of the Public Health Services presently require 25 air changes, including 5 units of outside air, it is suggested in the proposed 1983 guideline that this be reduced to 20 changes with 4 units of outside air. Air from areas of contamination or odor problems should be exhausted to the outside.

Organ transplant, burn, and foreign body implant units may require additional provisions for air quality control. Much obviously can be achieved, even in these operations, by meticulous observance of aseptic methods, limitation of traffic, interdiction of talking, and keeping all doors closed.

In the studies of Hart and Nicks, ultraviolet irradiation destroyed 75% to 95% of viable bacteria settling on shielded culture plates in the operating room. In the Five University Study, however, ultraviolet irradiation did not reduce the incidence of infection in any type of wound except in a refined clean case, in which a 25% decrease was noted. Irritation of and damage to the skin and eyes of surgical personnel must be guarded against. The effect of ultraviolet irradiation on airborne bacteria is discussed in Chapter 8.

More recently, several air handling systems have been studied. Efforts have been concentrated on the manufacture of laminar, or unidirectional, flow systems with high efficiency particulate air filters (HEPA filters) and passive exhausts to maintain positive pressure in the operating room relative to the corridor and adjoining rooms. These systems may use either fresh or recirculated air, or both. Fresh air systems require costly cooling, heating, humidifying, and dehumidifying equipment but eliminate the hazards of accumulation of anesthetic gases that are not degraded. The subject of exhaustion of anesthetic gases from the operating room environment has assumed increasing importance since the publication of the first edition of this manual. This problem will affect the architectural design of the operating room areas, but probably will not affect their design in relation to infection control functions. Recently, gas-scavenging devices have made it possible to recirculate up to 80% of the air without fear of accumulation of gases.

Some engineers have shown that laminar flow systems cannot deliver unidirectional airflow in an operating room in which personnel or patients are moving, or in which there are movable overhead lights, suction apparatuses, heat sources (i.e., people, including the patient), electrocoagulation units, and lights. Any of these may produce turbulence. With the use of unidirectional flow, air samplers placed inches from the surgical incision produced bacterial counts at or near zero levels — a 10- to 18-fold reduction compared to control levels without mass airflow. An objection raised to horizontal laminar flow is that placement of all activity must be downstream from the operative site to prevent possible contamination. In addition, the opening and closing of operating room doors allow corridor air to enter despite pressurized operating rooms. In spite of these objections, so-called laminar flow systems of either vertical or horizontal design with HEPA filters are now in use and have been able to exchange 15 to 100 cubic feet of air per minute. These systems deliver vertically sterile air into an empty operating room. Where there were no sterile precautions and with normal activity in a room, particle counts of up to one billion/cubic foot of air have been found. With laminar flow units, or with a good vertical mass flow air system with well-placed, active exhaust filters low on the walls, particle counts below one per cubic foot may be achieved.

More conventional turbulent flow systems with 5-μ filters have been shown to produce dramatic reduction in particle counts in functioning operating rooms. Colony counts of bacteria on culture plates in operating rooms near to and remote from the operative site have been significantly reduced by such air handling systems. The literature is replete with evidence of the ability of the laminar or turbulent systems with various filtration devices to produce substantial reductions in particle counts and bacterial colony counts.

The microbiological profiles of operating room air have varied widely, depending on many factors including type of ventilation and surgery, number of people, degree of activity, and environmental controls. A hospital built many years ago may yield an average of approximately 10 colony-forming units (CFU) of bacteria/cubic foot of air during surgery. Higher levels are generally detected before and after surgery, and during preparation and clean-up. Somewhat lower levels of 5 to 6 CFU/cubic foot of air may be detected in newer operating rooms in community hospitals in which shorter surgical procedures are performed and fewer people are present in the operating room. The definition of microbiologically clean air was created by a committee representing surgeons, engineers, and microbiologists, creating the three classes listed in Table 13-1. It was approved by CORE and may be helpful in setting standards for a good operating room environment.

A number of studies have been performed on infection rates in laminar flow operating rooms, including the incidence of wound sepsis after total hip prosthesis, with conflicting and confusing results. Infection rates in one study were reduced from 8.9% to 1.3% over a 6-year period (Charnley). Because a number of innovations, including the double-glove technique, unidirectional airflow, and helmeted surgical masks, were developed during this period, it is difficult to determine the relative importance of any one of them (Laufman). In another large study, the infection rates in a vertical laminar flow operating room and two conventionally ventilated operating rooms were investigated over a 4½-year period. The infection rates in the two control rooms were 1.14% and 0.93% during a total of 8253 procedures, whereas the infection rate in the laminar airflow room was 0.79%

Table 13-1. Classification of Microbiological Clean Air Approved by the Committee on Operating Room Environment (CORE)

Maximum number of bacterial particles per cubic foot	Maximum number of bacterial particles per cubic meter	Maximum number of particles in total sample test of ( ) feet
1	35	(30) 30
5	175	(30) 150
20	700	(10) 200

during 3408 surgical procedures (Whitcomb). The difference between control and study groups was not statistically significant.

It has been established that certain surgical procedures are more likely to result in infection than others (Chap. 2). Such procedures include those in which implants are placed and in which strong suction is used. In most surgical procedures, the suction effluent is discarded. However, in coronary bypass procedures there are additional suction lines to aspirate from the wound blood that is returned to the heart–lung machine for recirculation to the patient. When this line is not aspirating blood, it is drawing room air at the rate of 1.5 to 2 cubic feet each minute, which is mixed with blood that is eventually recirculated to the patient. One hour on coronary bypass will expose the patient to a minimum of 900 CFU (10 CFU/cubic foot/minute × 60 minutes). This observation does not consider the fact that most airborne bacterial particles probably exist as clumps of two or more organisms. Infections in patients undergoing these procedures have been shown to be caused by the same strain of organism as that isolated from the operating room air and the heart–lung machine during surgery.

Some orthopedic procedures have been associated with relatively higher infection rates, since smaller infective doses are required because of poor blood supply to the involved tissues and the large size of foreign materials placed in them. "Late" infections have also been a problem of such orthopedic procedures.

In a multicenter study from England, Scotland, and Sweden, 8000 records of total hip or knee replacement operations were studied for the incidence of sepsis (Lidwell and associates). In the patients whose prostheses were inserted in an operating room ventilated by an ultraclean-air system, the incidence of joint sepsis confirmed at reoperation within the next 1 to 4 years was about half that of patients who had had the operation in a conventionally ventilated room at the same hospital. When whole-body exhaust suits had been worn by the operating team in an operating room ventilated by an ultraclean-air system, the incidence of sepsis was about a quarter of that found after operations performed with so-called conventional ventilation. When all groups in the trial were considered together, the analysis showed an incidence of 1.5% deep infections after operations in the control group, and 0.6% in the ultraclean-air groups. The design of the study did not include a strictly controlled test of the effect of prophylactic antibiotics, but their use was associated with a lower incidence of sepsis than in patients who had received no antibiotic prophylaxis, 0.6% vs. 2.3%.

This study, the largest and best controlled of the studies published on the subject, demonstrates that ultraclean air is preferable to so-called conventional air. The problem in transferring these results to American experiences is the difference in what is called "conventional" air supply in the United States compared with that in England, Scotland, and Sweden. A code-accepted, properly installed and maintained conventional air system in American operating rooms is basically a vertical flow, unidirectional air system, delivering a minimum of 25 changes per hour of HEPA filtered air into an operating room. The air is exhausted low on the walls with an active exhaust system, which helps to maintain directional air flow. Joint-replacement operations done in such conventional operating rooms and with good barrier containment of the surgical team carry infection rates equally as low as those found in the British study. Although the British study was well-designed, it provides no information on matching the types of airborne bacteria with those found in the infected wounds. Also, only imprecise information is presented on the possibilities of contact contamination in the infected cases. The fact that the coverall exhaust-ventilated suit worn by the surgical team further lowered the incidence of infection a full 50% from that resulting from operations performed in ultraclean-air rooms with so-called conventional clothing makes one wonder what the incidence of infection would be if the surgeons wore coverall exhaust-ventilated suits in a conventional air operating room. In other words, the study did not isolate the effect of barrier containment alone. It is obvious that wound infection control is a multiple-discipline pursuit, and every effort should be made to control all environmental factors as well as those related to surgical technique and hygienic measures. The lack of proven effectiveness was chief among the reasons for the decision of CORE not to recommend laminar airflow for general use in operating rooms.

Halls, Corridors, Closets, and Cabinets

Surgical suites in hosptials that were built many years ago often have improperly ventilated corridors. Many of these corridors have no independent ventilation of their own but rely upon air escaping from operating rooms. The heavier traffic in the corridors generates a high airborne particle count. As a result, the frequent opening and closing of doors, and leaving doors ajar during operations, may constitute hazards related to airborne contamination. Several studies have confirmed the fact that airborne particles may be swept into the operating rooms by the motion of the doors and the movement of people and objects through the doorways.

In newer surgical suites, more attention has been paid to clean air circulation in the corridors of the operating room suite. Under these circumstances, the temperature differential between operating room and corridor is lessened, and other environmental factors such as humidity, pressure, and air changes approach those of the operating rooms. The only difference between the air in the operating room and that in the corridors is one of pressure. National Fire Protection Association (NFPA) Code 56 requires a 10% pressurization of the operating room air over that in the corridors.

Similarly, it is suggested that closets, offices, storage space, and all other areas within the surgical suite be ventilated in a similar manner as the operating room. The principle underlying this method of ventilation is to minimize the collection and egress of settled dust particles from such areas into the air of the surgical suite. Another suggestion that has been considered to be of possible use in minimizing accumulation of dust particles on horizontal surfaces is the use of wire or perforated shelving throughout the surgical suite (Laufman). It has been shown that such shelving accumulates fewer dust particles and bacteria than solid surfaces.

Consideration is also being given to the use of perforated or wire shelving in cabinets and of a multivented surface in the ceiling of cabinets, through which clean air is brought through the clean air duct system (Laufman). Under these circumstances, the cabinetry constitutes one of the cleanest parts of the operating room rather than a place where dust particles accumulate and are wafted into the room every time the cabinet doors are opened.

The need for infection control impinges on the practice of and construction for ambulatory surgery. It seems reasonable to provide an operating room for ambulatory surgery with the same design, equipment, and practices for infection control as used for inpatient surgery. The same would be true for preoperative preparation and immediate postoperative care.

Another important matter of planning concerns intercommunication in the operating suite. Frequent messages (related to housecleaning, orderlies, attendants, and nursing personnel) may interrupt the concentration of the surgeon and influence his judgment and technical skills. Such systems should be properly installed to permit efficiency of operation without disturbing other than the individual for whom a message is intended.

RECOVERY ROOMS, INTENSIVE CARE UNITS, AND OTHER SURGICAL SPECIAL CARE AREAS

Bacteriological testing has shown that recovery rooms and intensive care units as they exist in most hospitals are conducive to cross-infection. In these units, beds are often as close as 0.60 meter (2 feet) from each other, sometimes separated by cloth curtains, sometimes not. The air is poorly circulated and, in some instances, stagnant and odoriferous. Attendants and nurses often go from patient to patient, treating them without washing their own hands, often because there are no facilities for washing. If this is the case, hand-washing substitutes can be of some assistance. Because of personnel shortage or budgetary considerations, many recovery rooms are closed in late afternoon, making it necessary for any patient requiring an emergency operation or others operated on in the afternoon or evening to go directly to an intensive care unit. This unit usually is located some distance from the operating room and, like its recovery room counterpart, designed with virtually no isolation between patients. Thus, the high-risk postoperative patient may be exposed to patients with established or potential infections. Many intensive care units have one or two isolation rooms, but such rooms, when available, are usually in a distant, almost inaccessible part of the intensive care unit.

Many recovery rooms have rules under which a patient with an infection, or one at whose operation pus was encountered, is deprived of recovery room care and is sent directly to a nursing floor, often with no special attention to isolation precautions. For these reasons and others related to the quality of patient care, some recovery rooms are now being designed as an important component of the clean surgical suite. Adequate square footage should be allocated to permit the enclosure of every bed with glass and metal walls and a foldaway front for every cubicle. A small hand-wash sink should be built into every cubicle near the doorway. A minimum of 10.8 square meters (120 square feet) should be provided for every cubicle. It is recommended that an appropriately designed recovery room suite offer excellent vision of every patient and permit necessary monitoring and access to every bed of all the usual lifesaving facilities and equipment. The air-handling characteristics, including ventilation, should be comparable to those for the operating rooms. All contaminated, soiled, and waste materials in the intensive care unit and recovery room as well as the operating room should be collected and sealed in plastic bags at the site of origin with minimum handling by personnel wearing rubber gloves. Wastes, secretions, excretions, and blood-stained material, particularly from patients in isolation, should be sealed in impervious plastic containers for prompt handling and transport within the hospital.

The cubicle design of special care areas, including recovery rooms and surgical intensive care units, should provide for forward or backward isolation precautions to be carried out on any patient requiring them. If clinical judgment dictates that a patient be kept in the intensive care unit for longer than a day, the design and construction of such units should make it possible to do so without fear of the patient's tracheostomy becoming contaminated from a source in the ICU and without fear that his draining wound will endanger other patients. To those who would defend the open ward on the grounds that it provides more ready access to patients in case of emergency, one can point out that the glass and metal cubicle provides better surveillance than opaque curtains. If the cubicle is built so that the entire front folds away, access in case of emergency is virtually unlimited for any number of people and any kind of equipment, and with much less disturbance to other patients in the unit. Directional airflow can be used as an additional curtain for the protection of the patient and the disposal of shed bacteria-bearing particles that are airborne.

BIBLIOGRAPHY

ALLEN P, REYNOLDS DA: Clean air operating environments. Br J Hosp Med 20:591–598, 1978

ALTEMEIER WA: Infection control in operating rooms and perioperative areas. In Roderick MA (ed): Infection Control in Critical Care. Rockville, Maryland, Aspen Systems Corporation, 1983

BECK WC: Handwashing substitute for degerming. Am J Surg 135:728, 1978

BECK WC, FRANK F: The open door in the operating room. Am J Surg 125:592, 1973

BECK WC, MEYER RH: Health care environment: The user's viewpoint, p 128. Boca Raton, FL, CRC Press, 1982

BERNARD H: Personal communication. January, 1983

BOTZENHART K: Hygienic significance of constructional and instrumental arrangements within the hospital. Hefte Unfallheilkd 132:110–121, 1978

BOURDILLON RB, COLEBROOK L: Air hygiene in dressing rooms for burns or major wounds. Lancet 1:601, 1946

CDC GUIDELINES ON INFECTION CONTROL. Infect Control 3:52–72, 1982

CHARNLEY J: Postoperative infection after total hip replacement with special reference to air contamination in the operating room (Internal Publication No. 38). Wrightington Hip Centre, 1978

CORIELL LL, BLAKEMORE WS, McGARRITY GJ: Medical applications of dust-free rooms. JAMA 203:1038, 1968

DEFINITION OF SURGICAL MICROBIOLOGIC CLEAN-AIR COMMITTEE ON OPERATING ROOM ENVIRONMENT. Bulletin of the American College of Surgeons, 61(1):19–21, 1976

FLOURNOY DJ, MUCHMORE HG, FRANCIS EB: Nosocomial infection linked to handwashing. Hospitals 53(15):105–107, 1979

HARGISS CO: The patient's environment: Haven or hazard? Nurs Clin North Am 15(4):671–688, 1980

HART D: Bactericidal ultraviolet radiation in the operating room. JAMA 172:1019, 1960

HART D, NICKS J: Ultraviolet radiation in the operating room: Intensities used and bactericidal effect. Arch Surg 82:449, 1961

HINSHAW JR: Hospital Special Care Facilities, p 83. New York, Academic Press, 1981

HINSHAW JR: Unbacked dry wall construction: A problem in the operating room. Bulletin of the American College of Surgeons 67:6, 1982

HINSHAW JR: Minimum requirements of construction and equipment for hospital and medical facilities. Washington, DC, U.S. Department of Health and Human Services, Health Resources and Services Administration, 1982

LAUFMAN H: Philosophical and Architectural Program for a Surgical Center in a General Hospital (private publication). New York, Montefiore Hospital and Medical Center, 1969

LAUFMAN H: Operating room systems as seen by a surgeon. Hospitals 44:56, 1970

LAUFMAN H: What's wrong with our operating rooms? Am J Surg 122:332–343, 1971

LAUFMAN H: Surgical hazard control: Effect of architecture and engineering. Arch Surg 107:552, 1973

LAUFMAN H: Current status of special air-handling systems in operating rooms. Med Instrum 7:7, 1973

LAUFMAN H: Architectural and engineering aspects of the operating room environment. Bull Soc Int Chir 33:1, 1974

LAUFMAN H: Editorial: The infection hazard of intensive care. Surg Gynecol Obstet 139:413–414, 1974

LAUFMAN H: Design, devices, and discipline in operating room infection control. Med Instrum 12(3):158–160, 1978

LAUFMAN H: Airflow effects in surgery. Perspective of an era. Arch Surg 114:826–830, 1979

LIDWELL OM, LOWBURY EJL, WHYTE W, BLOWERS R, STANLEY SJ, LOWE D: Effect of ultraclean air in operating rooms on deep sepsis in the joint after total hip or knee replacement: A randomized study. Br Med J 285:10–14, 1982

MALE CG: Theatre ventilation: A comparison of design and observed values. Br J Anaesth 50(12):1257–1263, 1980

MILLAR KJ: The impact of a new operating theatre suite on surgical wound infections. Aust NZ J Surg 49(4):437–440, 1979

NELSON JP: Asepsis and perioperative infection prevention. Infection in Surgery 2:39, 1983

PROPOSED RECOMMENDED PRACTICES FOR TRAFFIC PATTERNS IN THE SURGICAL SUITE. AORN J 32(6):1040–1048, 1980

PUTSEP E: Modern Hospital: International Planning Practices, pp 168–194. London, Lloyd–Luke Ltd, 1979

SARUBBI FA JR, KOPF HB, WILSON MB, MCGINNIS MR, RUTALA WA: Increased recovery of *Aspergillus flavus* from respiratory specimens during hospital construction. Am Rev Respir Dis 125(1):33–38, 1982

SCANNELL JH, BROWN GE, ELLISON RG, GROVES LK, LAUFMAN H, SABISTON DC JR, SLOAN HE, WHEAT MW: Optimal resources for cardiac surgery: Surgery Study Group of Inter-Society Commission for Heart Disease Resources. Circulation 44:221–236, 1971

SELL JC: Mechanical needs in the operating and delivery suites. Hospitals 48:79–84, 1974

WALTER CW: Prevention and control of airborne infection in hospitals. Ann NY Acad Sci 352:312–330, 1980

WALTER CW, KUNDSIN RB: Floor as a reservoir of hospital infections. Surg Gynecol Obstet 111:412, 1960

WALTER CW, KUNDSIN RB, BRUBAKER MM: The incidence of airborne infection during operation. JAMA 186:908, 1963

14

A major part of control against the spread of infection is the maintenance of a clean hospital environment. Although it is impossible to maintain a sterile environment short of a "life island" or isolation system of some sort, the density of bacteria, particularly pathogenic bacteria, can be minimized by adequate housekeeping techniques. The hospital patient is constantly exposed to the circulating air and dust, to objects with which he has contact, and to the personnel who provide his care. Whereas it is difficult to define a precise level of contamination necessary to increase the infection rate, it is generally agreed that the number of bacteria in the environment should be minimized and controlled. It is oversimplification to say that with a sterile environment and microbe-free patients there would be no infection. Obviously we cannot reach the perfect situation, but it is important that we strive toward the goal.

All persons in many types of environment are in daily contact with millions of bacteria, and the opportunities for contamination are legion. The average person has a number of defense systems at work to prevent contact or contamination from becoming overt infection. In the hospital patient, on the other hand, these defenses may be interfered with either by his injury or disease, or by the treatment being given (Chaps. 5, 9, 10, and 12). It is particularly important, therefore, that his environment be kept as free of pathogenic organisms as possible. No one questions the need for a sterile environment in the operating room, and high standards are demanded there. It is also reasonable to expect similar, although less rigid, standards to be provided in other patient areas.

This chapter has been designed to provide a set of plans for maintaining cleanliness in the surgical patient care areas and in the surgical intensive care unit. A similar plan should apply to ambulances, their patient care equipment, and their personnel. For those special housekeeping procedures designed for the operating rooms and suite, see Chapter 8.

No attempt has been made to evaluate all of the methods, schedules, cleansing agents, and so forth,

Housekeeping Techniques for the Prevention and Control of Infections

but it is hoped that the following guidelines will provide some idea of what is involved and how to develop or correct a given system should the need arise. A method of control is recommended to periodically evaluate the effectiveness of the cleaning procedures and to document the same.

The overall housekeeping plan has been subdivided into the following categories so that quick reference to a specific situation can be made:

1. Personal cleanliness and safety
2. Housekeeping of patient floors
3. Housekeeping after the discharge of a patient
4. Cleaning of isolation rooms
5. Light (maid) housekeeping of intensive care units
6. Heavy (porter) housekeeping of intensive care units
7. Housekeeping of the operating room suite

Each of these categories is discussed and recommendations are made according to composite plans in operation at several large general hospitals. Routine environmental bacteriological sampling is not recommended, but the Center for Disease Control recommends it if there is a local problem.

PERSONAL CLEANLINESS AND SAFETY

An effective way of helping to prevent illness and injuries is to practice good personal cleanliness and safety habits.

Good Grooming Habits

Housekeeping employees are in constant contact with refuse that harbors microorganisms. It is important, therefore, that good personal habits be developed and followed. The following recommendations apply to all employees of the housekeeping department:

1. Keep hair clean and neat.
2. *Men:* Shave every day or, if bearded, maintain a well-groomed and clean beard.
3. Wash hands as often as needed during the day. Clean and trim fingernails for appearance and safety.
4. Keep uniforms clean and neat.
5. Keep shoes clean. Wear rubber heels to prevent noise in walking and for safety.

Safety Habits

Since accidents may mean time lost for key and supporting personnel skilled in isolation and infection control techniques, they should, if possible, be avoided. Constant alertness and prompt reporting of possible safety hazards helps in this regard. Some of the most common accidents that involve housekeeping personnel are

1. Falls due to
   a. Objects on stairs or in corridors

b. Mop handles and brooms in passageways
c. Soap film, detergents, or water on floors
d. Improper cleaning of floors
e. Water and snow tracks on floor
f. Unsteady ladders
g. Caution signs not placed as required
2. Cuts due to glass, needles, or razor blades in waste receptacles
3. Skin irritation due to improper use of cleaning solutions and failure to wear rubber gloves
4. Strains and bruises due to swinging doors and lifting of heavy objects
5. Smoking in corridors and patient areas, particularly near oxygen tanks or equipment

Working Habits and Decorum

Since each worker represents the housekeeping department and the entire institution, his manner should be quiet, courteous, and reserved. He should speak quietly and never shout to fellow workers. Working as quietly as possible and reporting noisy equipment is recommended.

Always knock on a patient's door before entering, being courteous at all times. Avoid indulging in long conversations with patients or discussing their illnesses. If patients want to talk about their health, they should be advised politely to talk with their doctor. Refer all patient requests, such as raising the bed, getting cigarettes, water, food, or anything pertaining to patient care, to the nurse in charge.

Maids, attendants, or porters should always leave the room when a doctor or nurse enters for a professional call to ensure privacy and confidentiality.

HOUSEKEEPING OF PATIENT FLOORS
Light Housekeeping

The light housekeeper is responsible for cleaning all rooms, corridors, and hub areas on the patient floors.

Equipment

Light-housekeeping cart
Double mopping unit with wringer
  on cart
Mop handle and heads
Treated sweeping tool
Treated sweeping cloths
Counter and radiator brush
Dustpan
Squeegee for window
  washing
Putty knife
Metal polish

Bowl cleaner kit
Two-section plastic pail
Gloves
Razor blade envelopes
Notebook and pencil
Furniture polish
Screwdriver
Phenolic-detergent-disinfectant
  solution with dispenser
Bags for trash and clean and
  soiled cloths
Plastic bags

Procedure.   Report to assigned patient floor with light-housekeeping cart, equipment, and supplies. Plastic liners, paper towels and cups, toilet tissue, and hand soap, if not furnished by nursing service, are available on each patient floor and should be included on the cart.

Prepare solutions at light-housekeeper's closet for treating cleaning cloths and washing floors as follows:

1. Add appropriate amount of water to a suitable detergent-disinfectant and lint-suppressing agent in one section of the plastic pail. In the other section, add 1 quart of water. Use this solution for treating cleaning cloths.
2. Add water and manufacturer's recommended amount of a suitable detergent-disinfectant in one of the mop pails and 2 gallons of water to the other mop pail. Use this solution to wash floors.

From the utility room on the patient floor, pick up paper towels and cups, toilet tissue, and hand soap, and place on maid's cart.

Check with head nurse on the patient floor for any special instructions, such as precautions to be taken for certain rooms, rooms to be washed, discharges, and so forth.

Patient rooms should be cleaned as follows:

1. Place light-housekeeping cart near the wall and the door of the room to be cleaned. Make sure that your equipment does not rub against the wall or block the corridor or door.
2. Knock on the door of the room and explain to the patient that you are the housekeeping maid and will clean the room. Take care not to disturb the patient. Do not visit or carry on a conversation with the patient.
3. Empty and clean all wastebaskets and ashtrays. Make sure that there are no smoldering cigarettes or ashes in the ashtray. At least daily, replace plastic liners as required.
4. Damp-dust all furniture including bureau, chairs, cushions, tables, footstool, and floor lamp, including the base and globe. Wash and polish mirrors. If bed is vacant, damp-dust bed rails, legs, headboards, and footboards. Damp-dust window sash and ledge, and top and base of radiator. Check and replace light bulbs in the floor lamp as needed.
5. Wash the sink including the underside and pipes. Use porcelain cleaner if sink is spotted and stained. Wash shelf over sink. Wash and polish mirror over sink. Damp-dust paper towel and cup holders and refill if necessary. Damp-dust light bulb over sink; check light bulb and replace as needed.
6. Wash bathtub and tile around tub, and damp-dust shower curtain rod.
7. Using bowl cleaner kit, wash inside of the toilet bowl. Using cleaning cloths, wash both sides of toilet seat, and underside and back of toilet bowl. Wash water tank including underside and pipes. Refill toilet tissue holder as necessary. Leave an extra roll of toilet tissue in room.
8. Spot-wash walls around sink, toilet, light switch, call button, and doors.
9. Check drapes and cubicle curtains. If soiled, change.

10. After all furniture and equipment has been cleaned, wet-mop the floor as follows:
    a. Place the clean mop in the pail with the phenolic detergent-disinfectant solution, wring out the mop, and wash a section of the floor. Start at the back of the room and work toward the door. Make sure to move chairs and so forth.
    b. After washing the first section of the floor, place the mop in the pail, wring it out, and wash another section of the floor. Repeat this procedure until the entire floor, including that in the bathroom, has been washed.

Damp-sweep and wash each patient room floor daily. Change solutions as required. Change dusting cloths and cleaning cloths for each room. Place soiled cloths in the designated bag on maid's cart and bring to housekeeping at the end of the workday.

In addition to the above, in two patient rooms daily

1. Wash windows, damp-dust window shades/venetian blinds, hinges, and door closer and jamb, and wash both sides of door.
2. Polish all chrome, doorknobs, and plates on door; damp-dust and polish cubicle curtain rods.
3. Wash wastebaskets. Clean vents. Dust tops of high cabinets and lockers.

In patient bathroom, toilets, and public toilets

1. Clean sinks, toilets, and bathtubs daily as above.
2. Wash sitz baths with detergent-disinfectant solution. Be sure to wash the outside of the tub and to spot-wash wall around it.
3. Wash shower stalls daily with detergent-disinfectant solution. Wash floors in showers daily and scrub once a week.
4. Keep sanitary disposal units in public toilets empty. Clean unit and place a clean bag in it daily.
5. Damp-dust window ledges, sash, and top and bases of radiators daily. Damp-dust and spot-wash window shades/venetian blinds, doorjambs, closers, hinges, and doors once a week. Wash windows once a week.
6. Polish all chrome, doorknobs, and plates once a week.

Dust corridors with treated dustcloths and wash daily. At times, it may be necessary for the maid to dust the corridor floor. Corridor windows should be washed once a week. Damp-dust window shades, ledges, and sash, and top and base of radiator daily.

In nurses' stations, utility rooms, flower room, conference rooms, treatment rooms, laboratory rooms, linen closets, and maid's closet

1. Wash outside of wastecans in "soiled" utility room.
2. Damp-dust all furniture daily.
3. Dust and wash floors daily.
4. Wash and damp-dust sinks, toilets, mirrors, and paper towel and cup holders daily and refill as needed.

5. Wash bedpan flushers daily. Use bowl cleaner in flusher and phenolic detergent-disinfectant solution for outside and underside.
6. Once weekly, wash windows; damp-dust window shades, venetian blinds, and doors including hinges, closer, and jamb; polish all chrome door-knobs and plates; and damp-dust vents and tops of cabinets.

In contaminated rooms the following procedures are to be carried out by the light housekeeper:

1. Wear a *gown and mask* in all instances when cleaning a contaminated room.
2. Dust and wash the floor daily.
3. Damp-dust and wash all furniture, toilets, sinks and bathrooms as for a regular room. Wastebaskets are to be emptied by nursing personnel.
4. All cloths used in a contaminated room should be considered contaminated. Change solutions for each contaminated room and use clean cloths in each room.

Rooms of discharged patients on each floor are normally cleaned and prepared for new admissions by the "discharge-cleaning" team. At times, because of the work load, it may be necessary for the light housekeeper to wash the furniture of a discharge unit and clean as follows:

1. Vacuum rugs as necessary.
2. Operate wet-dry vacuum as necessary.
3. Pick up and dispose of trash as required.
4. Move small items of furniture and equipment.
5. Report to supervisor items needing repair or in excess, and light bulbs needing to be replaced.

Housekeeping After Patient Discharge

The discharge-cleaning team on duty is responsible upon notification for the cleaning and preparing of patient rooms for new admissions. All rooms from which a patient has been discharged are to be cleaned and prepared for new admissions by the discharge-cleaning team(s). At times, because of the number of discharges, it will be necessary to have the floor maid help by cleaning the furniture.

During periods when the discharge rate is low, the team may perform such other work as assigned by the supervisor.

Equipment

Maid's cart
Double mopping unit with wringer
  on cart
Mop handles and heads
Treated sweeping tool
Treated sweeping cloths
Counter and radiator brushes
Dustpan
Small squeegee for window washing
Putty knife

Clean dustcloths
Two-section plastic pail
Gloves
Razor blade envelopes
Notebook and pencil
Furniture polish
Screwdriver
Phenolic-detergent-disinfectant
  solution with dispenser
Plastic bags

Metal polish   Discharge packs for bed making
Bowl cleaner kit   Toilet seat bands
Oilcan

Cleaning Solutions. *For cleaning the floor,* prepare 1% phenolic detergent-disinfectant solution as follows:

Place 3 gallons of water in one of the mop pails. Add the manufacturer's recommended amount of phenolic detergent-disinfectant solution. In the other pail, place 2 gallons of clean water. Add the amount of phenolic detergent-disinfectant solution recommended on the label. Use the two-pail mopping system without exception when washing a floor.

For treating dustcloths and cleaning cloths, prepare 1% phenolic detergent-disinfectant solution as follows:

Place 2 quarts of water in one section of the double pail (plastic). Add the recommended amount of phenolic detergent-disinfectant solution. In the other section of the pail, place 2 quarts of water. Add the phenolic detergent-disinfectant at the dilution recommended by the manufacturer.

Use clean floor-sweeping cloths, dustcloths, and cleaning cloths for each room. Place soiled cloths in the appropriate bag on the cart.

Procedures.
Unoccupied Rooms

1. Proceed to the room to be cleaned. Place equipment against the wall near the door. Be sure the corridor and door are not blocked.
2. Obtain a clean laundry bag from the linen room on the floor and place it over the back of a chair in the room.
3. Strip the bed as follows:
   a. Remove pillow case and place in the middle of the bed. Place the pillow on the chair.
   b. Remove bedspread, top sheet, blanket, and cloth drawsheet from under mattress; starting at the head of the bed, fold these toward the foot of the bed and away from your body. Place in laundry bag.
   c. Remove bottom sheet as above and place in laundry bag.
   d. Close laundry bag and place it down laundry chute.
4. Remove nursing utensils to utility room.
5. Empty and clean wastebaskets.
6. Clean the bed as follows:
   a. Raise the head and foot of the bed. If manual or electric hi-lo bed, raise to highest position.
   b. Using clean cloths treated in 1% phenolic detergent-disinfectant solution, wash the bed rails, legs, spring, head- and footboards, and castors. If bed is electric, wipe off electric cord and outside of motor. Make sure to disconnect the electric cord before moving the bed.
   c. Wash plastic mattress cover and pillow covers.

    d. Spray or wipe the mattress with commercially available disinfectant.

7. After the bed has been cleaned, make it up as follows:

    a. Obtain a discharge pack and place on chair.

    b. Make sure the mattress has a clean cover.

    c. Place bottom sheet with wide hem at head of bed and right side up. Fold sheet under the mattress 10 inches at the top; bottom edge should be flush with bottom edge of the mattress. Make mitered corners at head and tuck rest of the sheet under mattress to foot of bed.

    d. Place draw sheet 10 inches from head of bed and tuck under mattress.

    e. Place top sheet with wide hem at head of bed and right side down. Fold sheet under mattress 10 inches at bottom. Make mitered corners and tuck in 10 inches along side.

    f. In cold weather and in air-conditioned rooms, place blanket on bed.

    g. Place spread on bed 18 inches from top of mattress. Fold under at foot of mattress and miter corners.

    h. Fold top sheet over top edge of spread and blanket.

    i. Place pillowcase on pillow and place pillow on bed with open end facing away from door.

    j. If only one person is making the bed, do one side at a time, repeating the procedure on the other side.

8. After the bed has been made, clean remainder of discharge unit.

    a. Wash both sides of chair and stool cushions, inside and outside of bedside table, overbed table and bureau, and floor lamp, including washing inside of globes and base, and wiping off electric cord. Clean and wipe castors on all furniture.

    b. Wash the sink, including underside and pipes, medicine cabinet and mirror, paper towel and cup holders, towel rack, and light globe. Polish chrome.

    c. Wash bathtub or shower, including tile and shower curtain rod. Polish chrome.

    d. Wash inside of toilet with bowl cleaner. Wash both sides of toilet seat, toilet tank, and underside of toilet with cloth treated with phenolic detergent-disinfectant solution.

    e. Place razor blade envelope on shelf over sink and place seat band on toilet seat.

    f. Wash inside of window. Damp-dust shade or venetian blind, window sash, and inside and outside of ledge.

    g. Damp-dust top and base of radiator(s).

    h. Wash inside and outside of wall lockers, including door.

    i. Spot-wash door and frame, and damp-dust door closer and hinges.

    j. Using the treated floor-sweeping cloth and tool, dust floors including bathroom. Start at the back of the room and work toward the door. Pick up trash with the counter brush and dustpan at the door.

    k. Using double mopping unit and floor cleaning solution, place mop in the prepared solution. Wring out and wash a section of the floor, starting at the back of the room.

        After washing one section of the floor, place the mop in clear water and wring out. Place the mop in the prepared solution, wring out, and wash another section of the floor. Repeat as above to wash remainder of floor. Damp-dust baseboards.

Occupied Rooms. The procedure for cleaning an occupied room is the same as for an unoccupied room. In cleaning and preparing occupied rooms, take care not to disturb the patient remaining in the room.

Isolation Rooms. If the discharge-cleaning team is to clean an isolation room, the procedure for cleaning the furniture and the floor is the same as for unoccupied rooms, except tht *the nursing service is responsible for stripping the room.*

CLEANING ISOLATION ROOMS

Equipment for maid or discharge-cleaning team
   Maid cart with equipment and supplies
Equipment for porter

Wall washing ladder and equipment	Mop head and handle
Sponge mop	Double pail mopping unit
Cleaning cloths	Dustpan and broom
Floor sweeping tool and treated cloths	Gloves
Phenolic detergent-disinfectant solution	Isolation gown and masks

Procedure. The isolation rooms may be cleaned by the discharge-cleaning team or by a porter and the maid on the floor on which the room is located.

1. Assemble equipment, prepare solutions, and report to the room to be cleaned.
2. *Nursing personnel are responsible for stripping the room.* If the room is not stripped, notify the supervisor who will check with the nursing service.
3. Prepare the following solutions:
   a. Washing ceilings and walls: Add 3 gallons of water and the manufacturer's recommended amount of phenolic detergent-disinfectant solution in one pail. Add 2 gallons of water to the other pail.
   b. Damp-dusting and washing furniture: Add 2 quarts of water and the manufacturer's recommended amount of phenolic detergent-disinfectant solution in one section of the double pail. In the other section, add 1 quart of water.
4. Prepare the dust cloths and cleaning cloths by placing them in the phenolic detergent-disinfectant solution and wringing out by hand.
5. Put on a gown and mask.
6. Take supplies, including double pail and cleaning cloths, into the room.
   a. Wash furniture, starting with the bed, as described previously. Make sure to leave furniture in the room.
   b. After all furniture has been washed, place it outside of room in the corridor. One person must remain in the room to push furniture to the door; a second person must place it in the corridor. The person leaving the room must

remove gown and mask before doing so. Make sure to place the furniture near the room and close to the wall, so that the corridor is not blocked.

   c. Take into the room the equipment needed to wash walls, ceilings, sinks, toilets, and so forth. Be sure to don gown and mask on entering room.

   d. Using the sponge mop, wash ceilings, walls, toilets, as follows:

     (1) Place the sponge mop in pail containing the phenolic detergent-disinfectant solution, wring it, and wash a section of the ceiling. After washing one section of the ceiling, place the sponge mop in the pail with water only, wring it, place it in the pail with the phenolic detergent-disinfectant solution, wring it again, and wash another section of the ceiling. Repeat this procedure until all of the ceiling has been washed.

     (2) After the ceiling has been washed, wash the walls using same procedure as above.

     (3) Damp-dust cubicle and drapery rods, light globes, window shades, venetian blinds, outlet boxes, inside and outside of wall locker, and all pipes in the room.

     (4) Wash windows, including sashes and ledges, and top and base of radiators.

     (5) Wash sink, medicine cabinet, glass shelf over sink, light globe over sink, paper cup and towel holders. Make sure to wash underside of sink and pipes.

     (6) Wash the bathtub and tile around the tub. Damp-dust the shower curtain rod.

     (7) Using the bowl cleaner, wash inside the toilet bowl. Using the cleaning cloths, wash the toilet seat on both sides, underside of toilet, toilet tank, and pipes.

   e. After all the equipment, walls, ceilings, and so forth have been washed, damp-mop the floor. Start at the back of the room and work toward the door. Pick up trash with dustbroom and dustpan; place it in a paper bag, staple it, and place a red tag on it; put it in the utility room with other refuse bags.

   f. After damp-sweeping the floor, wash the floor as described previously. Make sure to use fresh detergent-disinfectant solution. Damp-dust baseboards.

7. When the room is clean, remove your gown and mask, place them in a laundry bag, close and tag with a red tag, and place it down the laundry chute.

8. Obtain cubicle and window drapes and hang as required.

9. Place furniture back in its proper place in the room. Notify housekeeping office that the room is ready and the bed can be made.

10. Important points to remember in cleaning the isolation room are

   a. Wear cap, gown, and mask while in the isolation room. *Never leave the room without removing gown and mask.*

   b. Always wear disposable plastic or clean, heavy work gloves when cleaning.

   c. Consider equipment and cloths used in the room as contaminated. Wash and clean them with 1% phenolic detergent-disinfectant solution before removing them from the room.

   d. Change solutions for each room. Use clean cloths for each room.

   e. *Wash hands often, and particularly after removing gloves following handling of contaminated material.*

HOUSEKEEPING OF THE INTENSIVE CARE UNIT
Light Housekeeping

Equipment

Maid's cart
Double mopping unit with wringer
  on cart.
Mop handle and heads
Treated sweeping tool
Treated sweeping cloths
Counter and radiator brushes
Broom and dustpan
Dusting and cleaning cloths
Canvas kit with tools
Metal polish
Squeegee for window washing

Spray bottles for washing windows
  and spot washing
Toilet bowl cleaner with kit
Two-section plastic pail
Rubber gloves
Razor blade envelopes
Notebook and pencil
Furniture polish
Phenolic detergent-disinfectant
  solution with dispenser
Plastic bags as needed

Procedure.   Report to assigned area and prepare cleaning solutions as follows:

1. *Floors.* Place 2 gallons of water in each pail. In one pail put manufacturer's recommended amount of phenolic detergent-disinfectant solution.
2. *Washing and dusting furniture.* Place one-half gallon of water in each side of double pail. Put the manufacturer's recommended amount of phenolic detergent-disinfectant solution in one side of the pail.

After preparing solutions, clean rooms as follows:

1. *Bathroom.* Wash and polish sink, mirror, shelf over sink, and pipes under sink, paying particular attention to underside and side of sink. Clean inside of toilet with toilet bowl cleaner. Wash outside of toilet, including back and base, using detergent-disinfectant solution. Replace paper supplies and hand soap as needed. Empty and clean wastebaskets and sanitary pad holder. Spot-wash as necessary. If porter is not available, dust and wash floor. Polish chrome as needed.
2. *Hospitality Room.* Dust and polish all furniture. Empty and clean wastebaskets and ashtrays. Wash top of stove and front of refrigerator. Clean sink and work area. Polish chrome as needed. Spot-wash as needed. Remove soiled dishes. Replace paper supplies. Dust window ledge, and tops and bases of radiators. If porter is not available, dust and wash floor.
3. *Office-Conference Rooms.* Dust and polish all furniture, telephone, files, and shelves. Polish as needed. Dust windowsills and wash windows as needed. Empty and clean all wastebaskets and ashtrays. If porter is not available, dust and wash floor.
4. *Utility Rooms and Toilet.* Wash and clean all sinks, toilets, and bedpan flusher. Dust shelving as needed. Wash windows in cabinets as needed. If porter is not

available, dust and wash floors. Polish all chrome as needed. Replace paper supplies.

5. *Kitchen.* Wash and clean sink, top of stove, refrigerator, and shelves. Wash windows in cabinets as needed. If porter is not available, dust and wash floor. Polish all chrome as needed. Replace paper supplies.

6. *Patient Areas.* Daily, empty and clean all wastebaskets and replace plastic liners. Dust all furniture and polish as needed. Wash sinks, making sure to clean underside and pipes. Dust windowsills and shelving, including cabinets. Wash blinds as needed. Wash windows as needed. Spot-wash walls as needed. If porter is not available, dust and wash floor. Replace paper supplies.

7. *Discharge.* Strip bed and remove soiled linen to basket in linen room. If utensils are soiled, clean them. Wash all furniture in room including bed. Spot-wash as needed. Empty and clean all wastebaskets. Dust and wash floor if porter is not available. Remake bed, and obtain clean utensils and place in bedside cabinet. Change cubicle curtains as needed. Replace paper supplies. Polish all chrome, dust blinds, and wash inside of windows.

Heavy Housekeeping

Equipment

Cart
Double mopping unit with wringer on cart
Mop handle and heads
Treated sweeping tool and cloths
Rubber gloves
Dustpan and broom

Phenolic detergent-disinfectant solution with dispenser
Supplies for washing windows, spot-washing, wall-washing, and polishing chrome
Canvas kit with tools

Procedure. Report to assigned area and prepare cleaning solution for floor, as follows:

Place 3 gallons of water in one pail with the manufacturer's recommended amount of phenolic detergent-disinfectant solution. In the other pail, place 1 gallon of water only. Place wringer on pails so that mop wrings into the pail with the 1 gallon of water.

Clean rooms as follows:

1. *Hospitality Room.* Dust and wash floor.
2. *Nurses' Station and Head Nurse's Office.* Wash corridor window inside and out, making sure to clean window track slides. Dust and wash floor.
3. *All Other Rooms and Corridors.* Dust and wash floors. If nursing personnel are around bed when cleaning it, ask them politely to move. On discharge or transfer of patient, assist maid in cleaning all furniture, remaking bed, and cleaning soiled utensils and replacing with clean utensils. Dust and wash floor.
4. *Washing Windows.* Wash all windows in ICU on rotation basis or as required, including windows between patient units, outside windows, and windows in cabinets.

5. *Cubicle Curtains.* Change cubicle curtains as required and at least once a month on a rotation basis.
6. *Doors.* Wash on rotation basis or as required.
7. *Soiled Linen.* Collect all soiled linens in a covered basket and place down chute. Check soiled utility room for soiled linens when first reporting for work, after lunch, and just prior to finishing the workday.
8. *Refinishing Floors.* As required and in coordination with head nurse, strip, scrub, and refinish floors.
9. *Doctors' Lounge, Locker, and Shower Rooms; Nurses' Lounge, Locker and Shower Rooms; Offices; and Storage Rooms in OR Suite and Intensive Care Unit (ICU).* Empty and clean all wastebaskets and reline with plastic bags; empty and clean all ashtrays and urns; clean sinks, toilets and urinals. Replace paper supplies as needed. Wash mirrors, and paper towel and cup dispensers. Dust and wash floors. Check lights and replace bulbs as needed.
10. *Trash.* Place trash in wastecans and take either to incinerator room for burning or can room for discard, as required. Pick up trash in ICU daily on a scheduled basis. Take trash from ICU except for empty cartons and from wastebaskets, *etc.,* (which should be left at can room) to incinerator room.
11. *Venetian Blinds.* Clean on rotation basis.
12. *Wall Washing.* Walls should be washed as required and scheduled. When a unit closes for a period of time, it should be housecleaned, with the walls washed and floors refinished as needed.

HOUSEKEEPING OF THE OPERATING ROOM SUITE

Directions for cleaning the operating room suite are given in Chapter 8.

GENERAL SUMMARY

Although phenolic detergent-disinfectant solutions are generally recommended, excessive hardness of the local water supply may cause formation of metallic plaque with use of such agents. This plaque may harbor microorganisms and make adequate cleaning impossible until it is removed from the surface concerned. In such a situation, use of a nonphenolic detergent-disinfectant solution, such as a quaternary ammonium compound, may be preferable.

In general, dusting and sweeping are avoided or minimized, and all surfaces are either wet-mopped, wet-vacuumed, or wiped with a damp cloth to avoid creating microbe-laden aerosols. Special attention must be given to air ducts and grills to remove any adherent dust or other particulate matter that could form an aerosol. Each week all floors must be thoroughly cleaned with a floor-scrubbing machine, followed by wet-vacuuming. Carpets should be vacuumed daily, with focal areas cleaned as necessitated by soilage. Carpets also should be shampooed monthly, or more often if soilage is evident.

All debris and trash should be enclosed in impermeable bags for disposal, to prevent contamination of other areas or people by contact.

This chapter has attempted to define the need for good housekeeping and to describe recommended techniques in order to provide the patient the best possible protection against the development of an infection from his immediate room and corridor environment. Several detailed methods have been outlined as an approach to specific problems. It should be possible to modify these methods to fit any local situations. Additional information is available in the form of various pamphlets published by the American Hospital Association, Chicago, Illinois, or the Center for Disease Control, Atlanta, Georgia.

BIBLIOGRAPHY

ANDERSON K: *Pseudomonas pyocyanes* disseminated from an air-cooling apparatus. Med J Aust 1:529, 1959

AYLIFFE GAJ, BABB JR, COLLINS BJ, LOWBURY EJL: Transfer areas and clean zones in operating suites. J Hyg (Camb) 67:417, 1969

AYLIFFE GAJ, COLLINS BJ, LOWBURY EJL: Cleaning and disinfection of hospital floors. Br Med J 2:442, 1966

AYLIFFE GAJ, COLLINS BJ, LOWBURY EJL: Ward floors and other surfaces as reservoirs of hospital infection. J Hyg (Camb) 65:515, 1967

BANASZAK EF, THIEDE WH, FINK JN: Hypersensitivity pneumonitis due to contamination of an air conditioner. N Eng J Med 283:271, 1970

BOTZENHART K: Hygienic significance of constructional and instrumental arrangements within the hospital. Hefte Unfallheilkd 132:110–121, 1978

CABRERA HA: An outbreak of *Serratia marcescens* and its control. Arch Intern Med 123:650, 1969

CENTER FOR DISEASE CONTROL: PHS Publication No. 71-8043. Public Health Service, Department of Health, Education, and Welfare, 1970

CENTER FOR DISEASE CONTROL: Disinfectant Fogging, an Ineffective Measure. National Nosocomial Infection Study Report 1971, 3rd quar. (DHEW Publication No. [CDC] 72-8149). Washington, DC, U.S. Government Printing Office, 1972

CLEANING HOSPITAL FLOORS. Hospitals 44:86, 1970

CROSS DF, BENCHIMOL A, DIMOND EG: The faucet aerator—a source of *Pseudomonas* infection. N Engl J Med 274:1430, 1966

DETAILED PROCEDURES FOR AREA CLEANING. Exec Housekeeper 26(11):26, 28–31, 1979

FINK NJ, BANASZAK EF, THIEDE WH, BARBORIAK JJ: Interstitial pneumonitis due to hypersensitivity to an organism contaminating a heating system. Ann Intern Med 74:80, 1971

FITZWATER JL: Scrub sinks harbor potential danger. AORN J 1:36, 1963

FOSTER WD: Environmental staphylococcal contamination: A study by a new method. Lancet 1:670, 1960

GABLE TS: Bactericidal effectiveness of floor cleaning methods in a hospital environment. Hospitals 40:107, 1966

GUIDELINES FOR HOSPITAL ENVIRONMENTAL CONTROL. U.S. Department of Health and Human Services, Public Health Service, Center for Disease Control, 1981

HERMAN GL, HIMMELSBACH CK: Detection and control of hospital sources of flavobacteria. Hospitals 39:72, 1965

JOHNSON HK: True and false economy in housekeeping supplies. Hospitals 37:110, 1963

JONES FA: Letter to the editor: Cleaning hospital wards. Br Med J 280(6210), 1980

KAHN G: Depigmentation caused by phenolic deterent germicides. Arch Derm 102:177, 1970

KELSEY JC, MAURER IM: The choice of disinfectants for hospital use. Monthly Bulletin, Ministry of Health & Public Health Laboratory Service 26:110, 1967

KINGSTON D, NOBLE WC: Tests on self-disinfecting surfaces. J Hyg 62:519, 1967

KRESKY B: Cross-infection on a pediatric contagion unit: A program for control. Clin Pediatr 4:699, 1965

KUIPERS JS: Investigation and treatment of floors of patients' rooms: A study with an agar cylinder. J Hyg 66:625, 1968

LaFAVE E, PRYOR AK, McDUFF CR: A new method for decontaminating mops. Hospitals 41:83, 1967

LITSKY BY: Use of sterile mops reduces contamination. Hosp Manag 100:46, 1965

LITSKY BY, LITSKY W: Investigations on decontamination of hospital surfaces by the use of disinfectant-detergents. Am J Public Health 58:534, 1968

LOWBURY EJL, AYLIFFE GAJ, GODDES AM, WILLIAMS JD: Control of Hospital Infection, 2nd ed, pp 63–104. Philadelphia, JB Lippincott, 1981

McDADE JJ, FAVERO MS, MICHAELSEN GS, VESLEY D: Spacecraft sterilization technology (1965). NASA-SP 108:51, 1966

PHILMON G SR: Scrupulous housekeeping is crucial to infection control, says consultant. Laund News 6(8):110–121, 1978

SYKES G: The sporicidal properties of chemical disinfectants. J Appl Bact 33:147–156, 1970

WALTER G, FORIS S: Pitfalls in disinfectant evaluation. Soap and Chemical Specialties 43:45, 1967

WALTER CW, KUNDSIN RB: The floor as a reservoir of hospital infections. Surg Gynecol Obstet 111:412, 1960

WELLS WF, RILEY EC: An investigation of the bacterial contamination of the air of textile mills with special reference to the influence of artificial humidification. J Ind Hyg Toxicol 19:513, 1937

WILLIAMS D: Role of housekeeping is essential to health-care infection control. Laund News 7(4):15, 1981

WILSON MG, NELSON RC, PHILLIPS LH, BOAK RA: New source of *Pseudomonas aeruginosa* in a nursery. JAMA 175:1146, 1961

WYPKEMA W, ALDER VG: Hospital cross infection and dirty walls. Lancet 2:1066, 1962

15

MICROBIOLOGY

High-quality laboratory support is an essential component of good patient care. This is particularly true of the function of the microbiology laboratory in the prevention and control of infections, although dependable and skilled support in clinical chemistry, serological techniques, hematology, and other technical areas is also very important. A technically competent, well-trained microbiology staff is essential, and a close-working liaison must exist between the surgeon, microbiologist, and infection control committee. The modern general hospital microbiology laboratory requires someone with an advanced degree or training who can direct work in the areas of microbiology, mycology, parasitology, virology, serology, and immunology. The laboratory staff should be regarded as participating members of the surgical team and their assistance should be sought in developing policies and plans of treatment. An integral part of any epidemiologic investigation should include sampling and culture of the environment or personnel to determine environmental or personnel reservoirs. Clinicians using the laboratory should become familiar with its work, since specimens are selected and taken more intelligently when it is known what the laboratory can do, how it is done, and how the results can be interpreted.

The role of the laboratory in the control of surgical infections can be considered to be largely in three general areas: diagnostic bacteriology, epidemiological investigations, and environmental control programs within the operating rooms and in the surgical services. The effective management of patients with surgical infections necessitates constant surveillance of hospital practices and regular assessment of antibiotic sensitivity of causative organisms in order to employ intelligent therapy in urgent situations. In this regard, the monthly publication and distribution to the clinical staff of an antibiotic profile table for the more prevalent microorganisms isolated by the laboratory from infected patients in that hospital or area is recommended (see Chap. 11).

Surveillance and monitoring should also include identification of clusters of infection, epidemiological surveys to identify environmental or personnel sources of infection, and environmental sampling to assess the effectiveness of housekeeping procedures, if such are in doubt. This surveillance, including microbiological sampling and culture, should be under the supervision of the hospital infection control committee or its epidemiologist and should be coordinated with the respective chief of the clinical service and the microbiologist (see Chap. 4). Routine sampling and culture of materials commercially purchased as sterile need not be done unless contamination is suspected. If evidence of contamination is noted, the Center for Disease Control and the U.S. Food & Drug Administration should be notified.

Principles of Microbiological Diagnosis

Laboratory support begins, and may fail, with the culture techniques employed by the clinician or technician. It is the responsibility of the physician to recognize the need for culture and to use the proper method and timing for the collection of the culture material in cooperation with the appropriate laboratory personnel. If in doubt, the physician should consult the microbiologist or pathologist.

To ensure adequate microbiological diagnosis, the following rules are recommended:

1. Carefully obtain the representative and appropriate specimen for the type of disease and organism anticipated (*i.e.,* cultures of pus from the walls of abscesses rather than their centers only; samples of the interfacing tissues between normal and infected tissue; and, in epidemiological surveys, culture of the throat for streptococci and of the nose and throat for staphylococci). Contact plates are recommended for use in culturing burn wounds, but swab cultures are usually employed for culturing other surgical wounds.
2. Collect specimens (prior to the initiation of antimicrobial therapy when possible) by means of aseptic techniques, and transport material in a sterile container, using transport media appropriate for the specimen concerned. Only personnel familiar with specimen collection requirements should obtain the cultures. A greater yield will be obtained from blood cultures if they are taken during the acute phase of infection and, specifically, before or early in the beginning of a temperature rise. If blood cultures suspected of being positive are reported negative, obtain three cultures within a 12- to 24-hour period. Anaerobes should be suspected and carefully sought.
3. Properly identify and label each specimen and record the specific tests desired. It is also important to provide the microbiologist with a presumptive diagnosis and information on antibiotic therapy if it is being employed.
4. Ensure appropriate transport and timely delivery to the laboratory of each specimen. Transportation requirements vary with the organism involved (*e.g.,* suspected meningococcal infections require bedside inoculation of the culture media, but urine cultures may be stored in a refrigerated state until media inoculation is undertaken). Blood cultures must be incubated immediately and maintained at 35° to 37°C. Any swab culture requires either immediate inoculation or storage in holding or transport media. For cultures of suspected anaerobic infections, obtain the material in an anaerobic condition, and use an anaerobic transport device immediately after obtaining the culture and prior to laboratory processing. Regardless of storage or transport considerations, optimal han-

dling of any culture specimen necessitates timely delivery of the specimen to the laboratory by a responsible person.

At the time of culture, submitting additional specimen material for direct gram-stained smears may permit a presumptive diagnosis, thus enabling the initiation of appropriate therapy at the earliest possible moment. Alternatively, by coordination with the microbiologist, this examination can be obtained in the laboratory.

Laboratory Processing of Specimens

Upon receipt of a specimen in the laboratory, the processing to be done includes plating of the material on primary, selective, and enrichment media, and, if required, animal inoculation.

Media selected for broad spectrum isolation of organisms are blood agar (sheep, rabbit, or human blood, in that order of preference), nutrient agar (TSA is widely used), and enrichment cultures in brain–heart infusion broth. Gram-negative bacteria are sought on blood agar and selective substrates including EMB, MacConkey's, and SS agar, especially for Enterobacteriaceae including enteric pathogens. *Pseudomonas aeruginosa* is selectively grown on cetrimide agar. Gram-positive cocci are sought on blood agar and phenylethyl alcohol blood agar. Other media are becoming increasingly important in diagnosing more obscure and complex infections. Thioglycolate broth and chopped meat broth are used in enrichment media for anaerobes. Bacteroides species and other nonclostridial anaerobes are sought on sheep or rabbit blood agar with menadione added. If mycoplasmas are potentially present, the specimen should be planted on special hypertonic media. The increasing incidence of fungi associated with the use of catheters and as saprophytic infections in gravely ill patients indicates that Sabouraud's dextrose agar may be a desirable substrate to be included in the culture battery. The problem of viruses is always to be considered, and suitable specimens should be available if extracts are to be inoculated into living cells or live animals.

Another consideration relevant to culturing is the fact that we frequently use disinfectants in hospital practice, including chlorine, formaldehyde, gluteraldehyde, iodine, mercurials, phenolics, and the quaternary ammonium compounds. A very helpful medium that neutralizes these disinfectants is thioglycolate, to which has been added sodium thiosulfate, sodium bisulfate, polysorbate 80 or Tween 80, and lecithin. Direct microscopic examination can be carried out on specimens from the area of infection if coordinated with the microbiology staff. Following growth in the culture media, colony morphology, gram staining, biochemical tests, pigment production, motility, serology, phage typing, and a number of other tests will assist in speciation and grouping of the organisms. Antibiotic sensitivities, always necessary for organisms isolated from blood cultures and usually necessary for other material obtained from other serious infections, are carried out following confirmation of bacterial growth. Prompt reporting of results is necessary and may be lifesaving.

Prerequisites for a Microbiology Laboratory

The microbiology laboratory must be capable of performing the following for the support of a surgical service:

1. Established aerobic and anaerobic culture techniques for isolation and identification of all bacteria in specimens, including swabs, exudates, transudates, tissue biopsies, blood, urine, sputum, and any other samples submitted
2. Quantification of the bacterial density in urine and sputum, as well as biopsy and autopsy tissue samples
3. Isolation and presumptive identification of fungi and yeast, including saprophytic species
4. Antibiotic sensitivity testing, including at least diffusion methods and preferably tube and agar plate dilution techniques (All sensitivity testing techniques have limitations that influence their interpretation. The physician should familiarize himself with these techniques and be aware of their limitations.)

    Much attention has been focused recently on variables influencing bacterial antibiotic sensitivity testing. By refined techniques it is possible to demonstrate a small but significant influence of a number of variables that superficially might not appear to be important, such as the effects of a difference in incubation temperature between 35° and 37°C. Similar effects have also been noted for many other variables. The Center for Disease Control study has been reassuring, since it indicates that the ultimate results of sensitivity testing (*i.e.,* labeling an organism sensitive, resistant, or intermediate) can be carried out with a high degree of reproducibility among community hospital laboratories despite the presence of these uncontrolled variables (Bennett). This finding is of considerable practical importance.
5. Assaying of antibiotic levels in blood, body fluids, and tissues
6. Acid-fast bacillus microscopy and culture
7. Environmental sampling, including surface sampling with swab and contact plates (usually Rodac), and air sampling (impinging techniques, such as that using the Anderson Air Sampler, are optimal, but settling plate studies may be used)
8. Monitoring of patients to establish the bacterial flora characteristic of infections in the particular hospital
9. Surveying of ward personnel when needed to assess the presence of "carriers," as in staphylococcal and streptococcal local "epidemics"
10. Maintenance of liaison with reference laboratories such as the Center for Disease Control (CDC) and public health department laboratories to facilitate specific typing of pertinent pathogens uncovered by the above studies. (The laboratory should be able to quick-freeze samples for shipment to such laboratories.)

In addition, periodic review of culture data is necessary to detect variations in resident flora. It is also advisable that periodic reports of culture results and the sensitivities of organisms causing infections be published and distributed to all professional staff members (see Chap. 11). Such reports are helpful in identifying infection rates and clusters of infection, and in permitting rational selection of initial antimicrobial therapy in life-threatening infections before culture results are available. These reports also aid in eliminating indiscriminate use of antibiotics (Tables 15-1 and 15-2).

Table 15-1. *Staphylococcus aureus* Antibiotic Sensitivity Data, Burn Unit: Monthly Summary, Dec. 1, 1983, to Jan. 1, 1984

Antibiotic	Resistant		Intermediate		Sensitive		Total Number
	%	No.	%	No.	No.	%	
Amikacin	0.00%	0	1.14%	1	87	98.86%	88
Gentamicin	18.39%	16	2.30%	2	69	79.31%	87
Tobramycin	9.09%	8	10.23%	9	71	80.68%	88
Ticarcillin	12.50%	11	5.68%	5	72	81.82%	88
Mezlocillin	16.09%	14	4.60%	4	69	79.31%	87
Piperacillin	15.48%	13	20.24%	17	54	64.29%	84
Moxalactam	2.74%	2	76.71%	56	15	20.55%	73
Cefotaxime	2.74%	2	0.00%	0	71	97.26%	73
Cefoperazone	7.41%	6	7.41%	6	69	85.19%	81
Cefsulodin	3.41%	3	1.14%	1	84	95.45%	88
Sulfadiazine	2.86%	2	15.71%	11	57	81.43%	70
Methicillin	0.00%	0	0.00%	0	70	100.00%	70
Cephalothin	2.27%	2	3.41%	3	83	94.32%	88
Vancomycin	0.00%	0	0.00%	0	88	100.00%	88
Kanamycin	0.00%	0	0.00%	0	67	100.00%	67
Chloramphenicol	1.39%	1	4.17%	3	68	94.44%	72
Tetracycline	1.41%	1	0.00%	0	70	98.59%	71
Ampicillin	1.39%	1	2.78%	2	69	95.83%	72
MK0787	3.49%	3	2.33%	2	81	94.19%	86
Clindamycin	0.00%	0	0.00%	0	71	100.00%	71
Penicillin	76.06%	54	9.86%	7	10	14.08%	71
Erythromycin	0.00%	0	0.00%	0	71	100.00%	71
Streptomycin	0.00%	0	0.00%	0	71	100.00%	71

Table 15-2. Quarterly Blood Culture Review, Burn Unit: Oct. 1 to Dec. 31, 1983

Organism	No. of Cases
Staphylococcus aureus	2
Staphylococcus epidermidis	2
Enterococcus sp.	1
Klebsiella pneumoniae	3
Citrobacter freundii	1
Escherichia coli	1
Proteus mirabilis	1
Candida albicans	2
Candida rugosa	3
Non-candida sp. (yeast)	1
Bacillus sp.	1
Total patients cultured = 32	
Total patients positive = 7	

Mycology

The increased occurrence of nonbacterial infections in surgical patients has accentuated the need for accurate diagnosis of yeasts and true fungi recovered from surgical patients. Examinations of a Wright stain of a peripheral blood smear may reveal blastospores or pseudohyphae in patients with systemic fungal disease. In general, swabs and surface culture techniques are ineffective in the isolation of fungi and yeasts, and tissue biopsies are often necessary. In the reference mycology laboratories, an overall recovery rate of about 40% is anticipated, even using tissue biopsies, with the recovery rate from tissue specimens ranging from about 60% for yeasts to less than 30% for true fungi. It has been the experience of many mycologists that the use of tissue slivers for fungal cultures improves the yield over that from tissue homogenates. The proper handling of specimens to obtain the highest yield requires close coordination with the microbiology staff and the use of optimal media at proper incubation temperatures. Speciation of fungi usually requires coordination with a reference mycology laboratory, but generic categorization should be possible in the hospital laboratory.

As indicated in Chapter 3, Altemeier, and Pruitt and his associates, listed the yeast and fungal organisms causing infections of clinical importance in surgery as follows:

1. Candida albicans
2. Aspergillus sp.
3. Fusarium sp.
4. Histoplasma capsulatum
5. Coccidioides sp.
6. Mucor sp.

7. *Blastomyces* sp.
8. *Sporothrix schenckii*

Mycobacteriology

Every laboratory should have facilities to isolate and identify all acid-fast bacteria associated with infections. Identification should be carried out to the species level. An alternative is to use a public health or other reference laboratory to carry out such procedures.

Parasitology

Although parasite infestations are a rare cause of surgical illness in the United States, there should be a technician in the microbiology laboratory capable of carrying out the necessary procedures for the identification of such organisms. Recently, *Pneumocystis carinii* has been observed as a causative agent of pneumonitis in immunosuppressed patients. Identification of the organism requires careful examinations of the sputum of such patients with pneumonic infiltrates. *Entamoeba histolytica* is another parasite of surgical importance for which laboratory capabilities must be established. Timely collection and examination of fresh stool specimens facilitate diagnosis of amebiasis.

Virology

The incidence of opportunistic or secondary viral infection has increased recently in severely injured, debilitated, or immunosuppressed patients. Virtually all of the infections occurring in such patients have been caused by viruses in the DNA group. The viruses of varying clinical importance reported by Pruitt and his group are as follows:

Herpesviruses
    Herpes simplex, Type 1
    Herpes simplex, Type 2
    Varicella zoster
    Cytomegalovirus
Hepatitis viruses
    Hepatitis A
    Hepatitis B
    Non-A, non-B hepatitis
Paramyxovirus (mumps)
Poliovirus
Poxvirus (vaccinia)
Measles virus
Rabies virus

The most frequent cutaneous viral infections are those caused by herpes simplex virus; they commonly present as typical vesicular lesions. In the burn patient, these infections occur most commonly in healing or recently healed partial-thickness burns, and the vesicles, if ruptured, quickly become secondarily colonized by the characteristic burn wound or skin bacterial flora.

The diagnosis of viral infections may necessitate either scraping or biopsy of a suspected lesion. In the case of herpes simplex virus infections, the typical Type A Cowdry body inclusions are pathognomonic, but, if secondary infection has occurred, electron microscopy may be necessary to identify intranuclear virions. The diagnosis of cytomegalovirus infection can also be made histologically by identifying the "owl's eye" inclusion bodies in infected tissue.

Other important diagnostic maneuvers for identification of viral disease are tissue culture and animal inoculation, which permit direct isolation of the offending virus.

Serology and Immunology

The severely injured, critically ill, or immunosuppressed patient is susceptible to infection by a variety of agents, and it is necessary to assess immunological competence in such patients. Although there are numerous research tests available to identify defects of the various components of the immunological response, those commonly in clinical use today are skin tests to various antigens; absolute lymphocyte counts as rough indices of cell-mediated immunity; and serum immunoelectrophoresis, immunoglobulin quantitation, isohemagglutination, and heterophil titers as indices of the competence of the opsonic system. Chemiluminescence assays as developed by Allen permit assessment of both opsonic capacity and neutrophil oxidative activity.

For specific bacterial diseases, ASLO, rheumatoid agglutination, and acute reactive protein assays may be helpful. Other serological tests useful in diagnosis of fungal disease and their reported degree of accuracy in differentiating mucocutaneous infection from systemic infection are as follows:

Precipitin assay (90%)
Agglutinin assay (insensitive)
Fluorescent antibody (reliability uncertain)
Latex agglutination (90% and probably of prognostic value)
Counter immunoelectrophoresis (rapid, but reliability uncertain)

Additional serologic tests useful in the diagnosis of viral or mycoplasma infections are as follows:

Heterophil agglutination (infectious mononucleosis)
Cold agglutinin titer (mycoplasma pneumonia)
Hemagglutination inhibition (rubella)
Fluorescent antibodies (many viral infections; *Bacteroides fragilis; Bacteroides melaninogenicus*)
Antiherpetic IgM antibody assay (Herpes simplex virus)
HAA assay (serum hepatitis)

CHEMISTRY AND HEMATOLOGY

The chemistry and hematology laboratory support required for the high-risk or infected surgical patient is in essence that required for many other patients. For serious infection problems, it is necessary that the laboratory have 24-hour-a-day,

7-day-a-week service to provide determinations of blood gases, serum chemistries, renal function tests, blood glucose levels, and so forth. For the infected septic patient, effective treatment is vital. To this end, Clowes has emphasized that data obtained from clinical observations, physiological measurements, and laboratory determinations must be simultaneously correlated to assess the patient's condition at any particular time. This information is of value only if the nature of the local and general injury caused by sepsis is appreciated in its relationship to the impairment of metabolism and function of major organ systems. Whether the patient will survive or die depends upon the dynamic balance existing between the magnitude of the injury and the adequacy of the protective and defensive responses (Chap. 5). The ability to recognize whether or not a patient is following the normal course to recovery under these conditions of severe stress enables the physician or surgeon to institute definitive or supportive treatment directed toward correcting such deficiencies as may exist.

SURGICAL PATHOLOGY

The more frequent occurrence of newer opportunistic infections, including those caused by fungi and viruses, has increased the use of the wound biopsy as a diagnostic aid. Thus, the pathologist has become progressively involved in the management of the surgical patient. The diagnoses of bacterial burn wound infection and of surgical wound infections are often readily confirmed by histological examination of rapidly processed wound biopsies. The changes in burns and in other wounds associated with microbial infection may be focal in nature, and clinical judgment is important in selecting the site for biopsy.

The prompt reporting of biopsy histology is of obvious benefit in early confirmation of the diagnosis, and requires close coordination and frequent communication between clinician, microbiologist, and pathologist. Delays in reporting are costly in terms of morbidity and hospitalization. Review and correction of delays in reporting of surgical pathology, bacteriology, and other laboratory reporting in each hospital is recommended.

BIBLIOGRAPHY

ACCREDITATION MANUAL FOR HOSPITALS. Chicago, The Joint Commission on Accreditation of Hospitals, 1980

ALDRIDGE KE: Coagulase-negative staphylococci. Infect Control 3(2):161–165, 1982

ALLEN RC, PRUITT BA JR: Humoral–phagocyte axis of immune defense in burn patients. Arch Surg 117:113–140, 1982

ALTEMEIER WA: Bacteriology of surgical infections: Clinical and experimental considerations, pp 50–70. Presented at Vingt-quatrieme Congres de la Societe Internationale de Chirurgie, Moscow, 1971

ALTEMEIER WA, MACMILLAN BG, HILL EO: The rationale of specific antibiotic therapy in the management of major burns. Surgery 52:240, 1962

AMERICAN HOSPITAL ASSOCIATION COMMITTEE ON INFECTIONS WITHIN HOSPITALS: Statement on microbiologic sampling in the hospital. Hospitals 48:125–126, 1974

AMERICAN PUBLIC HEALTH ASSOCIATION SUBCOMMITTEE ON MICROBIAL CONTAMINATION OF SURFACES: Environmental microbiological sampling in the hospital. Health and Laboratory Sciences 12:234–235, 1975

BARTLETT RC: Making optimum use of the microbiology laboratory. III. Aids of antimicrobial therapy. JAMA 247: 1868–1871, 1982

BENNETT JV, BRACHMAN PS (eds): Hospital Infections. Boston, Little, Brown & Co, 1979

BLAIR JE, LENNETTE EH, TRUANT JP (eds): Manual of Clinical Microbiology. New York, American Society for Microbiology, 1970

COHEN S: How to get the most from your hospital microbiology laboratory. Hosp Pract 4:70, 1969

CONANT NF, SMITH DT, BAKER RD, CALLAWAY JL, MARTIN DS (eds): Manual of Clinical Mycology, 3rd ed. Philadelphia, WB Saunders, 1971

DePASS EE, FARDY PW, BOULOS, JB, ABEAR EM: Haemophilus influenzae pyosalpingitis. Can Med Assoc J 126(12):1417–1418, 1982

FAVERO MS, PETERSON NJ: Microbiologic guidelines for hemodialysis systems. Dialysis & Transplantation 6:34–36, 1977

FOLEY FD, GREEMAWALD KA, NASH G ET AL: Herpesvirus infection in burned patients. N Engl J Med 282:652, 1970

GUIDELINES FOR PREVENTION AND CONTROL OF NOSOCOMIAL INFECTIONS. Washington, DC, U.S. Department of Health & Human Services, Public Health Service, Center for Disease Control, 1983

KOLMER JA, SPAULDING EH, ROBINSON H (eds): Approved Laboratory Technique, 5th ed. New York, Appleton-Century-Crofts, 1959

LINDAN R: The role of the microbiologist in the treatment and rehabilitation of patients with spinal cord injuries. Paraplegia 16(3):237–243, 1978

MALLISON GF: Monitoring of sterility and environmental sampling in programs for control of nosocomial infections. In Cundy KR, Ball W (eds): Infection Control in Health Care Facilities, pp 23–31. Baltimore, University Park Press, 1977

MANUAL OF DIAGNOSTIC PROCEDURES FOR BACTERIAL, MYCOTIC, AND PARASITIC INFECTIONS, 6TH ED. Washington, DC, American Public Health Association, 1981

NASH G, FOLEY FD, GOODWIN MN JR ET AL: Fungal burn wound infection. JAMA 215:1664, 1971

PLATT DJ, SOMMERVILLE JS: Serratia species isolated from patients in a general hospital. Journal of Hospital Infection 2(4):341–348, 1981

PRUITT BA JR, FOLEY FD: The use of biopsies in burn patient care. Surgery 73:887, 1973

SCOTT TFM: The herpes virus group. In Rivers TM, Horsfall FL Jr (eds): Viral and Rickettsial Infections of Man, 4th ed. Philadelphia, JB Lippincott, 1965

TEPLITZ C, LINDBERG TB, SWITZER WE, MASON AD JR, MONCRIEF JA: The pathogenesis of burn death: Necropsy documentation of Pseudomonas burn wound sepsis. Annual Research Progress Report, June 30, 1963. Fort Sam Houston, Texas, U.S. Army Surgical Research Unit, Section 41, 9163.

WONG WT, BETTELHEIM KA, CHENG FC, ONG GB: Serotypes of *Escherichia coli* isolated from patients with recurrent pyogenic cholangitis. J Hyg (Lond) 88(3):513–517, 1982

16

Sterilization is the complete destruction or removal of all microbial life. Disinfection is the destruction of infectious agents (usually excluding resistant spores) by use of chemicals, germicides, boiling water, or flowing steam. Surfaces must be thoroughly cleaned prior to the use of chemical methods to ensure disinfection, since soil, especially hydrophobic soil (oil, grease), neutralizes or retards penetration by the agent used. The label *sterile* implies that the contents of the intact package are sterile. The term sterilized indicates that the package has been subjected to sterilization, but the packaging may not ensure maintenance of sterility at the point of actual use.

Sterilization and disinfection are basic components of asepsis. They deal with physical, chemical, and microbiological factors that are amenable to precise experimental definition. Such data permit management to devise systems for processing instruments and supplies for patient care expeditiously and economically. Because various combinations of cleanliness, time, temperature, concentration, and barriers achieve comparable levels of patient safety, there is no need for overkill either in methodology or control of the process. Sterilization and disinfection are but building blocks that support patterns of human behavior — the crucial element of asepsis.

Sterilization

STEAM STERILIZATION

Moist heat in the form of saturated steam under pressure is the most applicable, dependable agent for the destruction of microbial life. The microbicidal power results from two actions, both of which are essential: *wetting* and *heating*. Saturated steam possesses the following characteristics, some of which are advantages and others disadvantages.

Advantages
1. Solids are rapidly wetted and heated; textiles and porous fabrics are rapidly penetrated and moistened while being heated.
2. Dry, resistant spores are destroyed in a brief time, within 13 minutes of exposure to saturated steam at 121°C.

3. Effective temperature is easily detected and monitored.
4. There is no toxic residue.
5. It is economical.

Disadvantages
1. Residual air in the sterilizer, package, or container, or trapped in a device excludes steam, depresses temperature, and precludes sterilization.
2. Steam superheats when contacting dehydrated materials, diminishing microbicidal power to that of dry air at the same temperature.
3. Steam at customary temperature is unsuitable for sterilization of grease, anhydrous oil, and thermoplastic materials.

Gravity Air Clearance Sterilizers

Air readily escapes from a properly designed sterilizer because it is denser than steam and stratifies beneath it. A heat-activated valve at the bottom of the sterilizer vents the air by gravity, just as water flows out of a bathtub drain. When steam fills the sterilizer, the valve closes to permit pressure to rise.

In a loaded sterilizer, five factors are critical for air clearance:

1. Steam must have free access into packages. Impervious paper or plastic wrappers limit the interchange of steam and air, and retard sterilization of large packages.
2. Crowding packages of textiles results in compression of their contents and limits access by steam, hindering penetration. Sterilizers should be equipped with mesh shelves to facilitate exchange of steam for air and to preclude stacking any but small packages.
3. Sterilizers must be loaded so that there is a horizontal path for the escape of air from dry containers. Vessels trap air if placed in a steam autoclave in a position in which water could pool. Devices that trap air, such as the lumen of catheters, must be flushed with distilled water immediately prior to being packaged and put into the sterilizer to provide the moisture essential for sterilization when the device is heated.
4. Timing of exposure begins when the temperature in the exhaust line reaches 121°C.
5. Exposure is determined by the time required for penetration of the largest package plus 13 minutes thermal death time. This must be determined by experiment.

Vacuum Cycle Steam Sterilizers

Despite the complex expensive mechanics and wasteful use of energy and water, vacuum cycle steam sterilizers are being reintroduced to hospital practice. These alternately evacuate the air from the load and rapidly flood the contents with steam several times before steam pressure is ultimately built up. The intent is to shorten and standardize the penetration of steam into the load.

Depending upon the rapidity of the cycle, superheating of textiles may occur. Removal of the air trapped inside devices such as the lumen of catheters is one distinct advantage of this type of sterilizer. Extraction of moisture at the end of the sterilizing cycle is another.

No compelling microbiological advantage over the gravity air clearance sterilizer has been demonstrated. Maintenance is expensive and crucial.

Packaging

If prepackaged, presterilized single-use drapes or operating room packs are used, additional packaging and sterilizing are not necessary. Otherwise, material for use as wrappers for operating room packs must meet the following criteria:

1. It must be penetrable by steam or ethylene oxide in a period that permits sterilization of all the contents.
2. It must permit the escape of air and entry of the steam into the package.
3. It must be an effective barrier against penetration by microorganisms and dust particles.
4. It must be strong enough to resist tearing or puncture during handling.
5. It must conform easily to the shape of the contents of the pack.
6. It must lay flat when opened without the edges flipping back and contaminating the contents.
7. It should be lint free.
8. It should not attract vermin.

The contents of packages are arranged to be ready for instant sequential use when opened. The wrapper must permit ready penetration by the sterilizing gas, steam, or ethylene oxide, and it must protect its sterilized contents from the moment it is removed from the sterilizer to the point of use. It must provide a mechanical barrier to careless fingers or vermin and dust particles. Packages must be wrapped so that they can be handled by unsterile individuals and stored until needed, yet at the moment of use, the package must expose sterile contents. The wrapper also must provide a sterile protective shield or sterile field when opened by an unsterile person.

The surgical instruments, utensils, textiles, and supplies for a surgical procedure can be organized in three or four packages that can be opened after the patient has been anesthetized. The basic kit of instruments can be packaged or sterilized in an open tray (see Sterilization of Instruments). Extra or special instruments can be packaged and sterilized in small nylon or cellophane bags, ready for instant dispensing if the course of operation changes because of an unexpected finding. Supplies of sterile instruments sealed in plastic bags can be conveniently deployed in each operating room.

Effective packaging requires knowledge, studied purpose, and skill. It is important for each hospital to determine its own standards and methods of packaging and to develop written and up-to-date instructions for the assembly of operating room packs.

A convenient method of packaging drapes and utensils intended for an operation employs a trough that determines the shape and limits the size of the package to permit penetration of steam in a known period.

1. Assemble the wrapper for a surgical kit by interleafing two cotton bed sheets (180 thread count, 63 inches × 90 inches) crosswise to form four thicknesses (63 inches × 45 inches). Drape the folded sheets into the trough over a 3-yard length of venetian blind cord with a loop knot at one end that permits fastening by a library tie.
2. Deploy the supplies for use during an operation (sponges, abdominal packs, additional towels, final dressings) on the wrapper on the bottom of the trough.

3. Pleat the operative sheet (designed to cover the entire field, including the anesthetist's screen and the patient's feet) from the screen and foot ends toward the opening that demarks the operative field. Roll the pleated sheet from either end toward the opening for the operative field to form two relatively open parallel rolls that allow for easy draping.
4. Lay the pleated and rolled sheet in the center of the second layer. When properly located, the rolled sheet provides four small cross channels for ready penetration of steam throughout the bundle.
5. Place towels for draping the skin on top of the rolls and place gowns for the surgical team on either side of the central pile to fill the space in the wooden trough (Fig. 16-1). Arrange towels, sponges, and basins for disinfecting the skin on top.
6. To wrap the pack, bring the two uppermost layers of the wrapper across the top of the bundle and tuck them into the crevice between the pile of supplies and the sheet lining the trough. Lap the folded edge of the wrapper over these thicknesses. Then overlap the outer layers and tie the bundle with the prepositioned cord, using a library tie to secure it. Apply short pieces of autoclave tape to fasten the ends of the wrapper so it cannot be opened without tearing the tape.
7. Lay the package on its side for sterilizing.

After sterilization, the contents of the pack are instantly accessible in the order in which they are required during the operation.

An expiration date should be pencilled on each textile wrapped package; the Joint Commission on Hospital Accreditation recommends that hospital packs be resterilized after 1 month. Inventory should be rotated to prevent prolonged storage. Sterile packages that are sealed in plastic bags upon removal from the sterilizer can be stored indefinitely.

Sterile Pack Storage

Store sterile goods in closed cabinets rather than on open shelves if the turnover is slow. It is imperative to protect them from vermin, rodents, roaches, and silverfish that are attracted by the scent of steamed textile. Packs must be kept dry. It is important to keep free water away from sterile goods. Once any free water contacts the sterile object, it is no longer sterile. If there are cold walls, pipes, or ducts and poor humidity control in areas for storage of sterile goods, it is possible for the dew point to be exceeded, causing condensation on walls that can wet sterile supplies. Mallison has reported seeing such problems in both operating suites and central sterile storage areas in institutions. If the package is dropped on the floor, discard it or resterilize it. There should be a chemical indicator on each package of hospital sterilized goods to show that these goods have been in the sterilizer. Use a microbiological indicator routinely to give a better indication of effective operation of the sterilizers.

Date each package of stored sterile goods, preferably with an expiration date. Destroy closure tape once the package is open, so that it is not possible to reseal it with the same tape. Never reuse paper packaging. Rotate inventory to avoid prolonged storage; too long a storage period for many goods sterilized in a hospital will prove to be uneconomical.

Keep handling of sterile supplies to a minimum. Although the mechanism of

Table 16-1. Safe Storage Time for Sterile Packs

	Duration of Sterility*	
Wrapping	In Closed Cabinet	On Open Shelves
Single-wrapped muslin (two layers)†	1 week	2 days
Double-wrapped muslin (each two layers)	7 weeks	3 weeks
Single-wrapped two-way crepe paper (single layer)	At least 8 weeks	3 weeks
Tightly woven untreated pima cotton (single layer) over single-wrapped muslin (two layers)		8 weeks
Two-way crepe paper (single layer) over single-wrapped muslin (two layers)		10 weeks
Single-wrapped muslin (two layers) sealed in 3-mil polyethylene		At least 9 months
Heat-sealed, paper transparent plastic pouches		At least 1 year

* Sterility was checked daily for the first week of storage and weekly thereafter.

† Single-wrapped muslin is not recommended because it is easily penetrated by contamination, especially moist contamination.

(Simmons BP, Hooton TM, Mallison GF: Guidelines for hospital environmental control. CDC Guidelines for the Prevention and Control of Nosocomial Infections, February 1981)

contamination of sterile goods is in many cases unknown, handling appears to be a very important factor in contamination of sterile goods that are packed in porous wrappers.

Simmons, Houton, and Mallison have reported on their study of safe storage times for sterile operating room packs prepared with six combinations of wrapping materials and two methods of storage. The results of this study are summarized in Table 16-1.

Monitoring Sterilization

Verifying the efficacy of steam sterilization badgers personnel involved with asepsis anywhere in the chain of patient care. The actual process of sterilization involves two basic questions: Can a specific type of package be sterilized? Has the package at hand been sterilized? The former can be answered only by testing a typical standardized package. The latter can be answered by fastening the wrapper on each package with a paper adhesive tape imprinted with a heat-sensitive ink to indicate exposure to saturated steam. The intact tape demonstrates that the package has not been opened.

Whether a package can be penetrated readily by steam throughout must be determined experimentally. The size and shape of a package, its contents, the internal arrangement, the wrapping material, how the package is wrapped, and how

(Text continues on p 314)

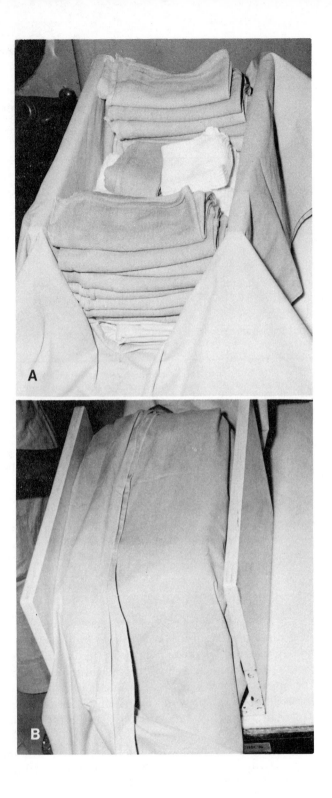

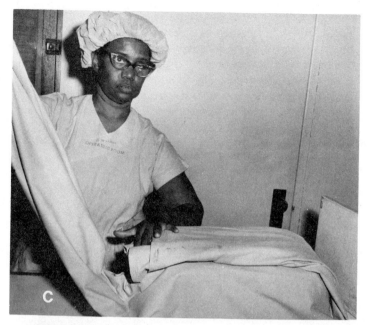

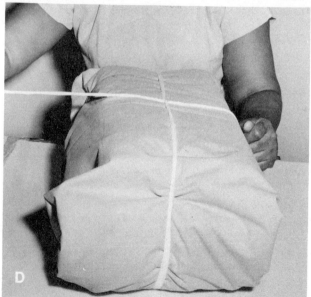

Fig. 16-1. (*A*) The placement of towels, gowns, sponges, and drapes within the wooden trough recommended by Dr. Carl Walter. (*B*) Second stage in preparation of the pack, preliminary to sterilization by autoclave. (*C* and *D*) Illustration of the technique used to complete the folding and tying of the operating room pack, which is now ready for autoclaving.

it is positioned in the sterilizer are variables that must be standardized. When this has been accomplished, it can then be determined when sterilizing conditions are reached in the densest spot. There are two ways of accomplishing this: a temperature sensor can be located in the least accessible spot, and the temperature and period of exposure recorded during a typical sterilizing cycle; alternately, a microbiological test device can be retrieved from that least accessible spot. This necessitates opening the package, since any pathway that permits easy withdrawal also invites quicker penetration by steam than does the surrounding material.

Microbiological testing is done by placing a paper strip dosed with 10^5 heat-resistant dry spores (Biological Indicator for Steam Sterilization Paperstrip USP XXI) in the test location, usually the center of a fanfolded sheet. The spore strip is packaged to permit aseptic retrieval and culturing. Because the standard incubation period for presumptive sterilization is 48 hours, and for sterility 7 days, this method is not suitable for routine monitoring of production in a Central Supply Room where prompt recycling of supplies is the key to service and economy. This test serves to correlate procedures for packaging, loading, and operation of the sterilizer, and establishes confidence in operating the sterilizer on the basis of timing the exposure when the temperature in the exhaust line reaches 121°C.

Unless packages can be segregated by size, common practice is to operate the sterilizer as if it is loaded with the most difficult packages to sterilize; hence, it is the custom to package so that sterilization is achieved by 30 minutes of exposure to steam at 121°C. The tape indicating exposure to steam attests that the package was processed through the sterilizer.

The alternate criterion is inspection of a telltale indicator. Unless that device is located in the package least accessible to steam, it is difficult to justify its use. Hence, the critical observation must be made at the point of use, and it depends upon the astuteness of a user—a method too awkward to be effective. Such monitoring is diffuse and likely to be cursory, and the marginal assurance of sterility does not justify the cost. It is more relevant to patient safety to pour a liter of water down the air and condensate drain of the gravity air clearance sterilizer each morning and see it spill through the air break, than to depend upon a telltale indicator in each pack. Failure of sterilization most often stems from a clogged chamber drain line.

The sterilizer is the crucial component of steam sterilization. It must be properly designed and installed, and the steam supply must be adequate in both quality and quantity. An inspection program must be enforced to ensure proper maintenance so that the basic physical parameters of pressure, temperature, and time can be relied upon. These parameters, plus supervision of packaging and loading, together constitute routine sterilization. Investment in competent, knowledgeable management is the crux of assuring sterile supplies.

Because sterilizers are usually remote from the source of steam, condensate and rust picked up from the iron piping are likely to be entrained. These can be separated from the steam before it is admitted to the sterilizer. Staining and spotting of packages or instruments indicate that the steam needs to be cleaned before being admitted to the chamber of the sterilizer.

The riser that supplies the steam must be dripped at the heel by a piping and trim configuration that traps condensate and debris and returns these to the boiler. In instances where oil or boiler compounds contaminate the steam, a separator can be installed just ahead of the main steam valve to the sterilizer. In most instances the jacket of the sterilizer itself serves as a separator. Under particularly adverse conditions, especially when the outer shell of the sterilizer is not corrosion resistant, a filter can be installed in the steam line from the jacket to the chamber.

Sterilization of Instruments

Three methods for steam sterilization of instruments are in use. Two use steam at either 121°C for 15 minutes or at 131°C for 3 minutes. At either temperature instruments must be unlatched, clean, and free of oil or grease. The instruments must be arranged in open perforated metal trays to afford ready access by steam. The exposure must be timed by the temperature developed in the exhaust line of the sterilizer. When instruments are packaged, additional time must be provided for penetration of steam through the wrapper in sufficient quantity to heat the instruments to sterilizing temperature.

That 8.6-kg textile absorbs one-half liter of condensate from the steam required to heat it to sterilizing temperature is readily accepted. Few people appreciate that a kit of stainless steel instruments weighing 10 kg absorbs the energy from 165 liters of steam to heat the instrument from room temperature to 121°C. Roughly 200 cc of condensate is deposited on the instruments in the process. This exchange of energy poses no problems for an exposed tray of instruments. When that tray is packaged for storage, the porosity of the wrapper becomes crucial. Not only must sufficient steam penetrate to displace the air, enough steam must penetrate to heat the instruments to sterilizing temperature. Impervious wrappers, often chosen because of the desire for prolonged storage, impede sterilization unless prolonged sterilizing periods are used. The sterilizing period must be determined by experimentation. Often, wet instruments are found when impervious wrappers are used, because the water of condensation that resulted from the transfer of heat of the instruments cannot evaporate.

The third most reliable method for the sterilization of instruments (dirty and greasy as well as clean) depends upon the use of the washer sterilizer. The method is described in the section on terminal sterilization of instruments.

Because steam sterilization depends upon physical factors, temperature, and time, which are readily and accurately determined, automation of the sterilizing cycle is the obvious control measure in an environment where professional personnel manage both sterilization and distribution. Because instruments are expensive and selection of a kit so specific for both procedure and surgeon, the processing of instruments is most efficiently done in the surgical suite. Rapid turnover permits effective use of a small inventory. Complementary supplies of special instruments or quantities that meet the idiosyncrasy of the individual surgeon can be maintained by knowledgeable personnel. Loss, damage, and theft are minimized.

Emergency Sterilization of Instruments.   The need for emergency or rapid sterilization arises daily. Every surgeon has experienced the exasperating delay caused by the omission of instruments from the kit, the inadvertent dropping of an instrument to the floor, or the unanticipated need for instruments required by a change in the operative procedure. In many clinics, "quick sterilization" (boiling for 1 or 2 minutes in a small electric sterilizer) or chemical disinfection (just wiping the instrument with a germicide) are sanctioned because of the emergency. This procedure is mentioned only to be condemned.

Emergency sterilization can be done quickly and efficiently in a small steam sterilizer equipped with large capacity controls. Steam pressure of 27 pounds/square inch is maintained in the jacket of this sterilizer during operation so that it is instantly available. Instruments must be scrubbed with soap and water and slushed in a fat solvent (*e.g.,* inhibited, 1,1,1-trichloroethane). The clean, unlocked instruments are placed in the sterilizer in a perforated metal tray and the door closed tightly. Steam is then admitted to the chamber so rapidly that a sterilizing temperature of 131°C (270°F) is attained in 40 seconds. Spores of the most heat-resistant organisms are destroyed at this temperature in 2 minutes. After a 3-minute sterilizing period, pressure in the chamber can be relieved quickly. A detachable handle is then fitted to the sterilizing tray and the sterile instruments are carried to the operative field. This technique enables the circulating nurse to return an instrument to the operating table in less than 5 minutes with no compromise of aseptic technique.

Small portable electric emergency sterilizer systems are commercially available. These liquid-phase chemical sterilizers combine ultrasonic cleaning with germicidal action. One uses 2% glutaraldehyde buffered to *p*H 7 to 8 with sodium bicarbonate; the other uses a system of sodium hypochlorite and lactic acid with triton × 100 that must be used within minutes of mixing. A third system uses nascent radicals formed by electrolysis. Microbiological documentation of these techniques is sparse.

Terminal Sterilization of Instruments and Utensils.   Transmission of viral disease, the most relevant and most common being hepatitis, the most threatening the slow viruses, is an occupational hazard for personnel processing instruments where skin penetration may occur. The hazard can be eliminated by routine terminal sterilization of instruments upon removal from the operating field. A safe, rapid technique exposes the instruments to a detergent solution in a washer–sterilizer designed to drain oil and scum from the surface. The soiled instruments are unlatched and collected in a stainless steel bucket directly from the instrument table by the gloved scrub nurse. The bucket is placed in the washer-sterilizer. A detergent, one formulated for mechanical dishwashers, is added in a quantity appropriate for the local cold water supply. The sterilizer is filled with cold water until it pours from the overflow drain. The detergent leaches the soil and debris and obviates mechanical cleaning. Steam is turned on to raise the temperature to 131°C in 7 minutes. The water is then rapidly drained, exposing the instruments to saturated steam for approximately 1 minute while the pressure is being relieved. The residual heat in the instruments flashes any adherent moisture, and the clean, dry sterile instruments are ready for immediate use upon removal from the sterilizer, or they can be safely sorted for maintenance and storage.

If the washer–sterilizer is not used, bits of tissue and congealed blood may accumulate in the serrations and joints of the instruments. The most effective method for removing this soil is by an ultrasonic cleaner. Cleaning should be routine prior to packaging and storage. Instruments cleaned in an ultrasonic cleaner must be sterilized before use, because ultrasonic energy does not sterilize.

In addition to instruments, utensils used in the operating room must also be cleaned and sterilized. Empty the contents of the basins into a kick pail and nest them into a muslin bag for sterilization in a steam autoclave, inverted, at 121°C for 30 minutes. Add sufficient chlorine hypochlorite (Chlorox) to the fluid in the kick pail to make a solution of 1:1000 free chlorine to ensure disinfection of the pail. Because plastic pail liners are likely to leak, these should not be used for discarding liquid.

Gather unsoiled dressings into a muslin bag along with the unused utensils. Sterilize them in saturated steam at 121°C for 30 minutes prior to returning them to inventory.

Gather all soiled towels, drapes, and gowns into a plastic laundry bag and send them to the laundry. Wrap wet linen in sufficient dry material to preclude bacteria-laden moisture wetting through. The laundry procedure must employ water at 82°C and hypochlorite bleach to disinfect the textiles. Bacteriological monitoring should demonstrate disinfection after such a process.

Soiled disposable supplies are gathered into a plastic bag and sealed for dispatch for incineration.

Sterilization of Solutions

Sterilization of solutions presents an apparent inconsistency in technique, because flasks are put into the sterilizer in an upright position with no provision for a horizontal path for the escape of the air from partially filled flasks. Water plays the active role in expelling the air. The temperature of the saturated steam enables it to penetrate into and condense in the bundle. The temperature of the water in a partially filled flask depends upon the heat transmitted through the flask heated by the condensing steam. In saturated steam the temperature of the liquid ultimately reaches that of the steam outside the flask, and vaporization of the water inside the flask fills it with saturated steam, which drives off the air. The air is displaced so completely from a vented flask that a high vacuum results when the flask is stoppered and cooled.

Sterilization of liquids presents a second problem not encountered with sterilization of textiles or instruments. At the end of the sterilizing cycle the liquid is as hot as the surrounding steam, and is in a stable physical state because it is subjected to the vapor pressure of the steam. When the steam pressure in the sterilizer is vented, this equilibrium is upset; the solution is too hot for the pressure exerted upon it and ebullition occurs. This results in concentration of the solution as it cools or, if the vaporization is explosive, much of the solution may be lost during the violent ebullition of steam. To prevent this, shut off the steam to the sterilizer jacket as well as to the chamber, and permit the whole sterilizer to cool to 93°C (200°F) before opening the sterilizer door. Under these circumstances, the flask of solution loses heat to the steam in the sterilizer, which in turn loses heat to the cooling walls of the sterilizer. The pressure decreases as the temperature falls and equilibrium is maintained throughout the cooling cycle.

Successful sterilization of solutions also entails detailed knowledge of the properties of the solutions themselves. It is useless to attempt to sterilize a chemical that decomposes at a temperature lower than that used for sterilization. Hydrogen ion concentration is important, since many chemicals are stable only under specific conditions. It is essential to use pyrogen-free distilled water as a diluent. Improperly rinsed glassware may add residual alkali from detergents to the solution and cause decomposition. The use of soft glass may permit the leaching of alkali at the liquid–glass interphase.

ETHYLENE OXIDE STERILIZATION

Because sterilization by ethylene oxide is more complex and less reliable than steam, it is restricted to the sterilization of articles that are damageable by heat. Ethylene oxide gas penetrates readily and has a low order of toxicity. It is easily ignited, but this hazard can be eliminated by rendering it inert with nonflammable gas such as Freon No. 11 or 12, or carbon dioxide. The process is most reliable when applied to clean, dry surfaces that do not absorb the chemical. Heavily contaminated or dessicated materials are difficult to sterilize.

During sterilization, ethylene oxide dissolves in adsorptive materials such as plastic, rubber, fabric, and leather. Chemical burns may occur when materials laden with ethylene oxide are applied to tissue. Hemolysis of blood results from contact with ethylene oxide adsorbed into plastic. The dissolved ethylene oxide escapes from materials when they are exposed to air. A minimum of 24 hours' aeration is necessary to ensure removal of the gas from sterilized articles. When the article is to be implanted, periods as long as 10 to 15 days of aeration are desirable, the bulk of the plastic being the critical factor. Vacuum and heat hasten the desorption, liberating 75% of the ethylene oxide; the remainder is dissipated by more prolonged aeration at room temperature.

An occupational hazard of exposure to ethylene oxide has been recognized. It is expressed as reproductive failure and mutagenic defects among women exposed to the gas that escapes into room air when sterilizers are opened and unloaded or aeration is done in the open. Portable ethylene oxide sterilizers are more hazardous, because exhaust gas is not disposed of through aspirators and protective ventilation is not provided. Aeration must be done in ventilated cabinets.

Ethylene oxide forms condensation products with water that damage rubber and plastic; hence, articles made of these materials must be dry when put into the ethylene oxide sterilizer. Ethylene oxide forms toxic products, such as ethylene chlorohydrin, especially when it is used to resterilize items once sterilized by radiation. Resterilization of this class of material must *not* be done in ethylene oxide.

Because ethylene oxide penetrates materials readily, certain apparently impervious materials can be used for packaging. Sealed, impervious wrappers ensure long shelf life. Conventional packaging in muslin or paper is satisfactory for short periods. Films of polyethylene, polypropylene, polyvinyl chloride, or autoclavable nylon transmit ethylene oxide readily and are completely impermeable to microorganisms. Cellophane, mylar acetate, and butyl plastics do not transmit ethylene oxide and should not be used as packaging materials.

Ethylene oxide gas destroys all forms of microorganisms; the critical factor is the amount of moisture being absorbed as the gas contacts the organism. The most resistant spores, *Bacillus subtilis* or *Clostridium sporogenes,* are only five times as resistant as *Staphylococcus aureus.* The thermochemical death time of ethylene oxide is nearly uniform for temperatures above 54°C (130°F) with a concentration of ethylene oxide at 500 mg/liter.

Relative humidity of the ambient atmosphere to which the materials are exposed prior to sterilization plays a crucial role in the action of ethylene oxide. The rate of kill decreases as the relative humidity falls below 10%; 40% relative humidity is optimal. Absorption of water and ethylene oxide at critical concentrations must occur simultaneously to be germicidal.

Heating and humidification of the material are the essential and critical time-consuming steps in the sterilizing cycle. Techniques of packaging and of loading the sterilizer influence the time required for heating and hydrating the load. A 2-hour period is allocated for a load to reach the temperature of a sterilizer heated to 54°C (130°F) by a hot jacket. A vacuum of 25 inches Hg is used to remove air. Steam is pulsed into the vacuum in quantities sufficient to hydrate the material without raising the temperature above 54°C. An additional period of 30 minutes is allotted for proper diffusion of moisture to attain equilibrium in the range of 20% to 40% relative humidity. The ethylene oxide is then admitted and a sterilizing factor accounts for the standard 4-hour sterilizing period at 54°C.

Ethylene oxide is commercially available in mixtures with an inert gas in the form of liquid under pressure. To prevent the refrigeration effect that results from the release of the gas mixture into the evacuated sterilizer chamber, a heat exchanger is used to volatilize the liquid and heat the gas as it is admitted into the chamber. This maintains the critical level of hydration established during earlier stages of the sterilizing cycle. The quantity of ethylene oxide is determined by the pressure of the gas maintained in the chamber. Adherence to the manufacturer's operating instructions for each model sterilizer and its ethylene oxide source is advisable. At the end of the cycle the sterilizing gas is evacuated, following which sterile air is admitted until ambient pressure is attained. Because the state of hydration is so critical to the thermochemical death time, table models of ethylene oxide sterilizers are suspect when sterilization, in contrast to disinfection, is required.

Because synchronization of the process and the degree of hydration are so crucial in the thermochemical death time of ethylene oxide, automation of the sterilizing cycle is not as reliable a control as in the case of steam. Frequent bacteriological monitoring is essential (*e.g.,* with Biological Indicator for Ethylene Oxide Paperstrip USP XXI). The use of packets containing 10^5 heat-resistant dry spores that have been stored in the same ambient humidity and temperature as the articles to be sterilized is critical. The incubation period for presumed sterilization is 48 hours; for sterility, 7 days. Refrigerated or moistened spores yield results that are not applicable to the load. Adhesive tape imprinted with chemicals sensitive to ethylene oxide is available to indicate that each package has been exposed to ethylene oxide.

DISPOSABLE SUPPLIES

The logistics of using commercial disposable items to complement reprocessed supplies are complex. Sterile commercial supplies follow a one-way path from the receiving dock to trash disposal. Commercial disposables are usually made of clean, new materials that are seldom contaminated with pathogens. Faults in sterilization or contamination of packages are likely to result in exotic infections. In marked contrast, the supplies and instruments that are reprocessed, recycle within the hospital. Microbiological contamination is readily fed back to personnel, the aseptic field, and patients whenever sterilization is faulty. Because heavy contamination by virulent pathogens is unavoidable when patients with infection are treated, such faults have epidemiologic significance. Therefore, processing used supplies and instruments entails full understanding of the microbiological problems involved.

Commercially, sterilization is done variously, using radioactivity, heat, or chemicals. Batches, usually identified by the sterilizer run, are quarantined until proven sterile by culture of aliquots. Standards of sterility and sterility testing procedures are specified by various authorities, including The United States Pharmacopoeia Convention, The Food and Drug Administration, The National Institutes of Health, The Joint Commission on Accreditation of Hospitals, The United States Department of Agriculture, and various state agencies. The label *sterile* implies that the contents of the intact package are sterile when opened for use. The term *sterilized* indicates that the package has been subjected to sterilization but that the packaging may not assure maintenance of sterility.

It behooves each hospital, to develop its own purchase specifications that require quality control, proper packaging, and meaningful labeling. Each hospital should also develop categories of supply usage related to the risk of cross-infection. Sterility is expensive and essential only for articles that contact tissues deep to the skin and mucous membranes. Cleanliness and freedom from pathogens suffice for supplies used on surfaces, mucous membranes, or superficial wounds of limited extent.

The initial purchase price of reusable items is high, and the use of disposable items seems to give evidence of cost savings. However, savings vanish when the initial cost is factored over the number of times an item is reused. Typical reusable systems of drapes and gowns for an operation cost 30% to 40% of comparable-use disposable supplies, depending upon the cost scale of laundry and central supply service. Also, disposable gowns and clothing may be uncomfortable since they are impervious. The advantages of properly designed disposables are that they provide a bacterial barrier that is waterproof and they reduce airborne lint particles.

Disposable supplies are ideal for free-standing surgery, for heavily contaminated procedures such as the treatment of burns, and for emergency stores. Policies that provide for efficient use of labor and storage space for disposable supplies and correct handling of the discarded material should be carefully formulated and periodically reevaluated.

OPERATING ROOM TRASH DISPOSAL

The greatly increased use of disposable operating room supplies requires a number of minor changes in details of handling. The problem of disposing of these materials and the resulting trash and pollution problems need critical examination. Few hospitals have a comprehensive disposal program that ensures asepsis for the patient, controls the occupational and public health hazards inherent in the care of patients with infections, and is compatible with institutional safety.

Few institutions recognize the extreme fire hazard embodied in the ever-increasing load of combustible supplies and their derived trash, and the loose accumulation of paper, plastic, and textiles that is characteristic of hospital trash. Perceptive fire marshals have emphasized this hazard, and incineration engineers urge that such trash not be burned on the hospital premises.

Because valuable items such as instruments and equipment are often carelessly discarded in trash, many hospitals systematically sort it, some using conveyors to facilitate scavenging. The associated danger of cross-infection is obvious. Careless disposal of sharp instruments, such as needles or blades, and the mixing of broken glass with trash creates an occupational hazard. Lacerations and needle pricks are leading occupational hazards, hepatitis being a costly complication.

Ultimate disposition of hospital trash is a mounting and an unsolved problem. Incineration is expensive and likely to pollute the air because of the dense, acrid smoke produced by burning of plastics. Dumping creates public health problems as scavengers or vermin "work over" the trash. Accidental fires add to the air pollution. Operation of a sanitary landfill must be supervised continuously on an hour-to-hour basis to ensure safety. Currently, compaction appears to be the preferable solution, since it is convenient and minimizes hazard.

STERILIZATION OF SPECIAL EQUIPMENT

Angiographic Equipment

Sterilization of apparatus used for angiography presents problems other than the microbial impact on the patient. Pyrogens and foreign bodies that accumulate in the bore of the devices are not destroyed by sterilization and can harm the patient. Worn or deteriorated items must be identified and discarded.

Residual blood in the lumens, catheters, tubing, syringes, and manifolds of the apparatus, must be flushed promptly to preclude the formation of adherent clots or the growth of pyrogen-producing bacteria. Stylets must be inspected for rough spots that abrade the walls of the bore, stripping particulates that become microemboli. Catheters and seals must be inspected critically to detect fraying or embrittlement.

Fragmentation during use, with the liberation of gross foreign body emboli, is a documented hazard.

Processing such equipment must be done by techniques developed for the preparation of parenteral fluids. The fluid pathway must be disassembled and flushed with germicidal detergent, 0.5% hydrogen peroxide or 10% household bleach containing 5.25% w/v sodium hypochlorite (Chlorox), to leach blood from the channels. Valves and plungers must be operated to expose all surfaces to both cleaning and subsequent rinsing. Other agents such as soaps, scouring powder, and tap water must be avoided. Pyrogen-free and powder-free gloves should be worn while manipulating items that will contact blood, such as stylets and catheters.

Hot, freshly distilled, pyrogen-free water must be used for thorough rinsing.

Processing must be coordinated with sterilization to reduce the interval between cleaning and sterilization, in order to preclude the growth of gram-negative bacteria in the moisture left to facilitate sterilization.

The equipment can be arranged in a metal tray and packaged in a 4-thickness, 180-count muslin wrapper. Sterilization is accomplished by exposure to steam at 121°C for 30 minutes.

Urinary Tract Equipment

Most urinary catheters in use today are disposable and come from the manufacturer in sterile packages. If reusable catheters are employed, they must be thoroughly cleansed, packaged, and sterilized by steam. The bore and the inflation channel must be flushed with distilled water shortly before sterilization to provide moisture to expel air.

Respiratory Tract Equipment

The past decade has confirmed the need for sterile apparatus intended for use on the respiratory tract and the necessity for aseptic technique. The objective is to preclude the introduction of exogenous microorganisms into a respiratory tract predisposed to infection by disease, malfunction, or invasive procedures such as intubation, suctioning, and aerosol therapy (Fig. 16-2).

The respiratory gas channels must be disassembled and washed to remove soil. The apparatus must be rinsed copiously and dried prior to packaging. Sterilization is accomplished by ethylene oxide using procedures already described. Drying before packaging is particularly important because any residual moisture will combine with the ethylene oxide to form toxic ethylene glycol residues.

Disposable segments and filters are available as an alternate method for the management of anesthesia equipment.

Aseptic Technique.   Procedures on the respiratory tract should introduce no exogenous microorganisms. For example, endotracheal tubes should be packaged and sterilized. Separate sterile catheters should be used for suctioning, and a sterile disposable glove used while accomplishing the task (see Chap. 10).

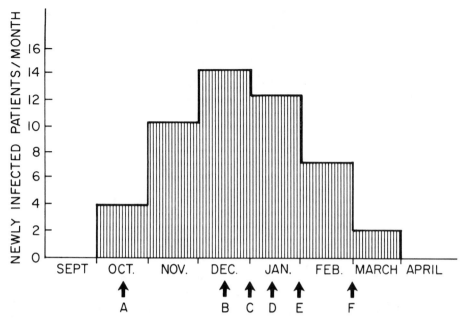

Fig. 16-2. Chronological sequence of events as they transpired during epidemic outbreak of *Serratia marcescens*. (*A*) Onset of outbreak. (*B*) *Serratia marcescens* recovered from IPPB machines. (*C*) Daily cleaning plus weekly sterilization of all machines. (*D*) Daily gas sterilization of all machines. (*E*) Daily nebulization of machines with acetic acid. (*F*) Use of sterile flex tubing, medication nebulizer, manifold, and mouth piece for each patient use. (Redrawn from Cabrera HA: An outbreak of *Serratia marcescens* and its control. Arch Intern Med 123:650–655, 1969. Copyright 1969, American Medical Association)

Medications put into nebulizers must be sterile. Too often, such medications are contaminated by bacteria that have adapted to grow in the distilled water used as the diluent. Tap water used in medication nebulizers should be sterile to avoid seeding the ventilator with bacteria common to water supplies.

Equipment Changes.   All equipment between the respirator and the patient should be changed every 48 hours (Craven and associates). The respirator should be changed every 7 to 10 days (see Chap. 10).

Anesthesia Equipment

The introduction of ethylene oxide sterilization and the development of large gas sterilizers have made possible the routine sterilizing of anesthetic equipment. Retained ethylene oxide must be eliminated from rubber, plastic tubing, or other equipment by adequate aeration.

Spinal and epidural anesthesia require essentially the same technique as that mentioned earlier for intravenous and intra-arterial procedures. The equipment used for this type of anesthesia can be sterilized in the usual manner in an autoclave. In addition, careful disinfection of the skin and a procedure similar to that used in the operating room for the surgical procedure itself is recommended for spinal anesthesia, because the skin in the lumbar area has an unusually heavy accumulation of desquamating epithelium. Scrubbing permits the disinfectant to contact the underlying skin.

Endoscopic Equipment

Because endoscopes are both complex and expensive, compromises with sterilization are tolerated to avoid damage or save time. The potential clinical effects of using contaminated endoscopes are of concern since they are often superimposed upon existing infections or delayed beyond the period of observation. The contaminated cystocope causing an acute infection of an obstructed urinary tract is one extreme; the delayed seroconversion of occult infectious hepatitis following laparoscopy is the other. With prudent management, the patient's right to a microbiologically safe endoscopy need not be violated for the sake of expediency.

Sterilization of endoscopes is a two-step process: exposing the surfaces to be sterilized and applying the microbicide. Connectors, tubes, adaptors, and nipples must be removed and moving parts operated to be certain that soil is removed and that access by microbicide is ensured. This can be accomplished while the scope is immersed in a detergent compatible with the local water supply. Channels are flushed and, when clean, the scope and detached parts are permitted to dry.

For ethylene oxide sterilization, the scope can be reassembled and packaged in a porous wrapper. Because hydration and penetration are not problems, a small cabinet-type ethylene oxide sterilizer can be used effectively. The manufacturer's instructions must be followed. Endoscopes should be sterilized in ethylene oxide after each day's use.

Because few hospitals have an inventory of endoscopes sufficient to permit ethylene oxide sterilization prior to each use, immersion in a germicidal solution is expedient. The preferred agent is 2% glutaraldehyde buffered to pH 7 to 8 with sodium bicarbonate. The exposure time is 30 minutes. Care must be taken to fill all the channels of the scope and manipulate movable parts.

When a crises makes 30 minutes an impossible burden, the clean scope can be immersed and flushed with a freshly mixed solution of equal parts of the two solutions below:

Solution A

Chlorox (5.25% sodium hypochlorite)	300 ml
Water q.s. ad.	4000 ml

Solution B

Ascorbic acid	48 gm
Triton × 100	8 ml
Water q.s. ad.	4000 ml

BIBLIOGRAPHY

ACCREDITATION MANUAL FOR HOSPITALS. Chicago, The Joint Commission on Accreditation of Hospitals, 1983

ALEXANDER EL, BURLEY W, ELLISON D, VALLARI R (eds): Care of the Patient in Surgery, Including Techniques, p 45. St. Louis, CV Mosby, 1967

ALTEMEIER WA: Surgical antiseptics. In Block SS (ed): Disinfection, Sterilization, and Preservation, 2nd ed, Chap 22. Philadelphia, Lea & Febiger, 1977

AXON AT, PHILLIPS I, COTTON PB, AVERY SA: Disinfection of gastrointestinal fibre endoscopes. Lancet 1:656–658, 1974

CABRERA HA: An outbreak of Serratia marcescens and its control. Arch Intern Med 123:650, 1969

CENTER FOR DISEASE CONTROL GUIDELINES FOR THE PREVENTION AND CONTROL OF NOSOCOMIAL INFECTIONS. Washington, DC, U.S. Department of Health & Human Services, 1981

CRAVEN DE, CONNOLLY MG JR, LICHTENBERG DA, PRIMEAU PJ, MCCABE WR: Contamination of mechanical ventilators with tubing changes every 24 or 48 hours. N Engl J Med 306:1505–1509, 1982

DECKER H et al: Air Filtration of Microbial Particles. U.S. Public Health Service Publication No. 953, p 43. Washington, DC, U.S. Government Printing Office, 1962

GINSBERG F: O.R. questions and answers. Modern Hospital 113:124, 1969

GORMAN SP, SCOTT EM, RUSSELL AD: A review: Antimicrobial activity, uses and mechanism of action of glutaraldehyde. J Appl Bacteriol 48:161–190, 1980

HARDING H: A sterility control program for the central supply service. Hosp Top 43:81 passim, 1965

ISOLATION TECHNIQUES FOR USE IN HOSPITALS. U.S. Public Health Service Publication No. (NMS) 71-8043. Washington, DC, U.S. Government Printing Office, 1973

KUNDSIN RB, WALTER CW: Asepsis for inhalation therapy. Anesthesiology 23:507, 1962

LIVINGSTON H, HEIDRICK F, HOLICKY I et al: Cross-infections from anesthetic face masks. Surgery 9:433, 1941

MALLISON GF, STANDARD PG: Safe storage times for sterile packs. Hospitals 48:77, 1974

MATHIEU A, BURKE JF: Infection and the Perioperative Area. New York, Grune & Stratton, 1982

O'CONNOR HJ, ROTHWELL J, MAXWELL S, LINCOLN C, AXON ATR: New disinfecting apparatus for gastrointestinal fibre-endoscopes. Gut 23:706–709, 1982

ORKIN FK: Herpetic whitlow—occupational hazard to the anesthesiologist. Anesthesiology 33:671, 1970

PARMLEY JB, TAHIR AH, ADRIANI J: Disposable plastic breathing bags and tubes. JAMA 217:1842, 1971

PERKINS J: Principles and Methods of Sterilization, p 340. Springfield, IL, Charles C Thomas, 1956

PERKINS J: Principles and Methods of Sterilization, 2nd ed., p 560. Springfield, IL, Charles C Thomas, 1969

REPORT AND RECOMMENDATIONS OF THE ENDOSCOPY COMMITTEE OF THE BRITISH SOCIETY OF GASTROENTEROLOGY; ENDOSCOPY AND INFECTION. Gut 24:1064–1066, 1983

RYAN P: Basics of packaging. AORN J 21(6):1091, 1975

SCHIMMELBUSCH C: The Aseptic Treatment of Wounds, p 2. London, H K Lewis, 1894

STANDARD P, MACKEL D, MALLISON G: Microbial penetration of muslin- and paper-wrapped sterile packs stored on open shelves and in closed cabinets. Appl Microbiol 22:432, 1971

STANDARD P, MALLISON G, MACHEL D: Microbial penetration through three types of double wrappers for sterile packs. Appl Microbiol 26:59, 1973

WALTER CW: Aseptic Treatment of Wounds, Chap 7, p 54; Chap 8, p 74. New York, Macmillan, 1948

WALTER WG, SCHILLINGER JE: Bacterial survival in laundered fabrics. Appl Microbiol 29:368–373, 1975

WESLEY F, ROURKE B, DARBISHIRE O: The formation of persistent toxic chlorohydrins in food stuffs by fumigation with ethylene oxide and with propylene oxide. Food Sci 30:1037, 1965

WESLEY F, CUNLIFFE AC: Hazards from plastics sterilized by ethylene oxide. Br Med J 2:575, 1967

WHITBY JL, STOREY DG: Effect of incremental doses of radiation on viability of the microbial population on synthetic operating room gowns. Appl Environ Microbiol 43:528–533, 1982

WINDING O: Foreign-body contamination at angiography. FADL's Forlag (Copenhagen), 1981

17

NECESSITY FOR AND IMPORTANCE OF ISOLATION

Isolation is an important method of preventing and controlling infections in surgical patients. Isolation plans and techniques are designed to prevent the spread of microbial disease among patients, hospital personnel, visitors, and others. The earlier that appropriate isolation procedures are instituted, the more effective will be the limitation of spread of pathogenic organisms from infected patients to other patients, to the professional staff, to the supporting hospital personnel, and to inanimate objects in the hospital.

There are two major types of isolation that can be applied in hospital practice. First, and the more frequent type, is *isolation of infected patients* in order to prevent spread of infection to other patients or hospital personnel. The second type is *reverse or protective isolation,* which is designed to protect patients with markedly reduced resistance to infection who are therefore at high risk of exposure to infection in the hospital environment. Both types of isolation are considered in detail later in this chapter.

The general and indiscriminate use of prophylactic antibiotic therapy during the 1940s and 1950s led to a widespread breakdown of isolation procedures owing to the development of a mistaken dependence on the effectiveness of the various antimicrobial agents. The effects of this trend were accentuated by the complexity of modern surgical practice, with the concentration of large numbers of infected patients in hospitals, the rapid increase in the number of high-risk patients more susceptible to infection, and the relatively common use of various diagnostic and therapeutic procedures that enhanced the possibility of cross-infection. The subsequent increase in many types of surgical infections reemphasized the importance of isolation and the necessity of a rebirth of effective isolation procedures.

Because isolation may result in a number of additional problems for physicians, nurses, and patients, there is frequently reluctance or objection to placing

Isolation for Infection Control in Surgical Patients

a patient under isolation. For the physician, for instance, additional time may be required for hospital visits. Surgical treatment and nursing care also may be more time consuming and thus increase the cost of hospitalization. If a private room is necessary for isolation, this too adds to the cost and requires space that could be used for other purposes. From the patient's standpoint, isolation results not only in increased cost but also in disorientation in time and decreased social contact. Such isolation may have psychological effects, particularly for children and the elderly confined to such an intensive care unit.

The purpose of this chapter is to provide a practical and effective guide for isolation procedures useful in the care of hospitalized patients by the surgical and nursing staffs and supporting personnel. There was a need to revise and update recommendations for isolation procedures because of various factors such as changing knowledge of the epidemiology of infectious diseases, the recognition of new syndromes such as the acquired immunodeficiency syndrome, and the emergence of new pathologies. The isolation precautions presented in this chapter are the considered opinions of the Committee on Control of Surgical Infections of the American College of Surgeons after studying the Guidelines for the Prevention and Control of Nosocomial Infections recently developed by personnel of the Center for Disease Control (CDC) and a panel of outside experts. The recommendations are based on various factors such as well-documented modes of transmission identified in epidemiologic studies, reasonable theoretical rationale, and the experience of surgical experts.

The responsibility for initiating and maintaining isolation techniques should involve everyone, including physicians, epidemiologists, nursing personnel, medical students, technicians, the housekeeping staff, and radiology and other ancillary services. All have important functions to carry out, and each must pay careful attention to details of isolation plans. The recommendations presented may be modified as necessary for individual hospitals.

In general, effective isolation depends upon the following:

1. A plan for the various types of isolation that must be formulated as appropriate and necessary for the individual case.
2. The provision of adequate and well-designed hospital facilities for the various types of isolation.
3. The availability of well-trained and competent nursing and attending personnel.
4. A method of surveillance to ensure adequacy and effectiveness of the facilities and personnel concerned with isolation.

Patients requiring isolation for specific infections in surgery are principally those with extensive draining wound infections caused by common pathogens for which Contact Isolation (Category II) and Drainage/Secretion Precautions (Category VI) should be observed. In recent years other types of infections occurring in surgical patients have required isolation considerations and practices.

Patients with impaired immunologic defenses may require what has been termed "protective isolation." These patients may include the chronically ill and debilitated, extensively burned and injured patients, very young and very old patients, patients undergoing immunosuppression therapy and cancer chemotherapy, and uremic patients. The CDC has now eliminated their former category of Protective Isolations, and this subject is discussed further in Chapter 12. Infrequently one may be called upon to provide protective isolation for a patient with a congenital immunologic defect, such as agammaglobulinemia, or an immunologic defect, such as agranulocytosis acquired during treatment for some other disease. Patients with the new acquired immunosuppressed disease syndrome also fall into this category.

"A Guideline for Isolation Precautions in Hospitals" written by Julia S. Garner and Bryan P. Simmons of the Center for Disease Control was published in July, 1983, and contains much valuable information. Copies of the article and colored cards identifying the new isolation categories now recommended can be obtained through the CDC. The CDC's data and recommendations are being used extensively in the revision of the second edition of the *Manual on Control of Infection in Surgical Patients.*

A highly recommended reference is *Control of Hospital Infection—A Practical Handbook,* edited by E.J.L. Lowbury, G.A.J. Ayliffe, A.M. Geddes, and J.D. Williams, published in 1981.

FACILITIES FOR ISOLATION

Facilities for isolation will of necessity vary from institution to institution. In some hospitals a special and separate nursing unit may be used for patients requiring various forms of isolation; in others, special rooms may be situated in different hospital areas for special isolation procedures; and in still others, a room or area may be used only as required. A busy pediatric service may require a ward for surgical patient isolation during communicable disease epidemics, and similarly there should be an area in the newborn nursery where infected infants can be effectively isolated from well infants.

Isolation Area

A private room can reduce the possibilities of transmission of infectious agents and is useful in the care of patients requiring isolation. It is indicated for those with conditions that are highly infectious or caused by highly virulent microorganisms. It should contain hand-washing, bathing, and adequate toilet facilities. There should be no cross-circulation or recirculation of air between an isolation unit and other areas of the hospital. An anteroom between an isolation room and the hall can be used as an effective airlock, provided the hall is under slightly positive pressure to prevent airborne spread of infectious agents from the isolation room. The anteroom may also provide storage space for supplies such as gowns, gloves, and masks. Ultraviolet radiation of air in the upper part of a room used for isolation of patients with active pulmonary tuberculosis has been recommended by some to reduce the density of airborne tubercle bacilli, but the effectiveness of this adjunctive measure remains essentially unconfirmed.

Hand-Washing. Hand-washing is the single most important means of preventing the spread of infection. After taking care of an infected patient or one who is colonized with microorganisms of special clinical or epidemiologic significance, personnel should always wash their hands, even when gloves are used. In addition, all personnel should wash their hands after touching excretions (feces or urine, or material soiled with them) or secretions (from wounds, skin infections, *etc.*) before touching another patient. Hands should also be washed before performing invasive procedures, touching wounds, or touching patients who are particularly susceptible to infection. Hands should be washed between all patient contacts in intensive care units and newborn nurseries.

Isolation Equipment

Sterile gowns should be used when dressing patients in isolation with extensive burns or other wounds, but clean, freshly laundered or disposable gowns may be used for all other categories of isolated patients requiring gowning of personnel. Disposable gowns should be worn only once and discarded into a designated container before the user leaves the isolation area.

Masks are recommended to protect the wearer from inhaling microbe-containing droplets or dust and to protect the patient from the transmission of some infections. When masks are required, high-efficiency, disposable filter-type masks are considered to be more effective than cotton gauze masks, and should be used only once and discarded.

Gloves reduce the possibility that personnel will become infected by or become carriers of the patients' infectious agents. They also reduce the likelihood of personnel transmitting their own microbial flora to susceptible patients. When precautions require the use of gloves, disposable single-use varieties are preferable. After direct contact with the excretions or secretions of a patient, the attending personnel should change gloves to complete the care necessary for that patient.

Needles and syringes used for patients requiring isolation precautions should be disposable, as should dishes and utensils. In general, personnel should use precautions when handling *all* used needles and syringes. After use they should be placed in a labeled, puncture proof, red-colored container designated for this purpose.

Other patient-care items, such as *stethoscopes* and *sphygmomanometers*, should be kept in the isolation area for use with the individual patient throughout his hospital course. When the patient leaves the hospital, these items should be disinfected by procedures adequate to destroy the etiologic agents involved.

All *disposable items, dressings, and tissue* actually or potentially *contaminated by excretions or secretions* of any variety should be placed in an impermeable, disposable bag within the patient-care area and enclosed in a larger disposable bag or container when removed from that area. The bag and its contents should be incinerated or sterilized by autoclaving before disposal.

PERSONNEL AND EQUIPMENT HYGIENE

It is to be reemphasized that the single most important factor in any program of isolation is *hand-washing*. It must be carried out before and after contact with each patient. A hand-washing facility should be conveniently located in each isolation area, with the water control, tissue dispenser, and soap dispenser of the type operated by the knee, foot, or arm. The soap dispenser and its contents should be cleaned and disinfected on a frequent routine basis, since they may serve as sources of bacteria such as *Pseudomonas* species.

The patient's chart should not be taken into the patient's room when strict isolation or protective isolation is being observed. Visitors should be limited to a minimum and should report to and be instructed by knowledgeable attending personnel before their visits.

Equipment used for cleaning should be disinfected at the end of each cleaning shift, and cleaning cloths laundered and autoclaved after each daily use and after terminal cleaning. For terminal cleaning, all receptacles and equipment should either be returned to central supply or cleansed with a detergent disinfectant. All disposable items should be discarded in an impervious plastic bag. All furniture, including the mattress cover, should be cleaned with a detergent disinfectant and the floors wet-vacuumed using the same solution (see Chap. 14). Disinfectant fogging is considered an ineffective procedure for decontamination, and it is not recommended.

TRANSPORTATION OF THE ISOLATED PATIENT

A patient should be moved from an isolation area for treatment or special diagnostic procedures only when essential. Notification should be given to the operating room or other area to which he is to be moved, so that appropriate isolation procedures can be observed in that area to prevent the spread of infection. The goal is to isolate the infected patient from his environment. It should be kept in mind that spread of infection may occur, theoretically at least, during transportation of the septic patient in one or more of the following ways:

1. *Contact* (most important). Infection may be passed to personnel handling septic patients and then to other patients.
2. *Airborne infection.* Infection may be spread by fine microbe-laden dust from the patient's attire, bedclothing, or dressings.
3. *Fomites.* The patient may contaminate such articles as the stretcher, operating room table, or other equipment. Syringes used on jaundiced patients may convey the virus of hepatitis. The possibility that infection may also be spread by instruments such as enema tubes, such as in the case of intestinal pathogens, should be kept in mind.

If the following technique is used for the transportation of patients in isolation, the risk of spread of infection to other patients or the staff should be greatly minimized, with the probable exception of the highly infectious exanthemata present in patients requiring anesthesia and operation.

1. The patient's operating surgical slip should indicate that he is under isolation and the type of isolation. It should give the diagnosis of the infectious condition in order that proper precautions may be planned and instituted.
2. All unnecessary personnel and equipment should be removed from the operating room.

3. The patient should be provided with a clean gown immediately before his removal to the operating room. If suppuration from a lesion has soiled a dressing, it should be replaced so that leaking of infectious material will not occur.
4. The patient should be wrapped in a freshly laundered sheet which may also be used to lift him onto the operating table.
5. The route to the operating room or other destination should be the most direct one with no unnecessary stopping at any holding areas.
6. Materials in contact with the patient should be placed in a plastic bag and carefully discarded after his arrival. Attendants must be protected from the patient or his discharges with gown, gloves, caps, masks, and boots, as indicated for the type of isolation, both during transit and after arrival.
7. The patient should be placed on the operating table, x-ray table, or examining table covered by a clean, impervious sheet with underlying rubber pad.
8. X-ray cassettes used during the operation or placed in contact with the patient's clothing should be enclosed in a plastic bag, which should be discarded after the examination.
9. All syringes and needles should be of the sterile single-use type. Care should be taken to avoid causing puncture wounds in personnel.
10. At the end of the operation the operating room table and anything with which the patient has come in contact should be cleaned with a detergent–disinfection solution (Chap. 8).
11. All persons who have come in contact with a patient in isolation should wash their hands after discarding their gowns and before further contact with other patients. *This is particularly important.*
12. The patient should be placed on and covered by clean sheets, and returned to the isolation area by the most direct route.

SPECIFIC ISOLATION TECHNIQUES

Since the publication of the first edition of this manual, there have been major changes in isolation precautions to be recommended for use in hospitals. Some of these have been defined and emphasized by the Center for Disease Control in its newly published series entitled *Guidelines for the Prevention and Control of Nosocomial Infections.* In general, two alternative systems for effective isolation procedures are now being recommended, and hospitals can choose one for their use or design one of their own. System I is based upon isolation categories and the use of seven standard color-coded, category-specific instruction cards (Figs. 17-1 to 17-7). System II is based upon the Disease-Specific System and the application of precautions which have been individualized for each patient and which have been designed to interrupt the spread of infection from him. This system will require more training and a higher level of attention by patient-care personnel for its correct application. Its use will also be guided by two color-coded cards.

System I

In System I, major changes have been made in the titles and specifications for the categories and requirements for isolation covered under each. Instead of the five categories used in the first edition of the manual, *Isolation Techniques for Use in*

Hospitals, there are now seven. Three of the original five have been retained as recommended in the new guidelines proposed by the CDC:

1. Strict Isolation (Fig. 17-1)
2. Contact Isolation (Fig. 17-2)
3. Respiratory Isolation (Fig. 17-3)

Four new categories have been created in line with the new guidelines of the CDC:

4. Tuberculosis Isolation (Fig. 17-4)
5. Enteric Precautions (Fig. 17-5)
6. Drainage/Secretion Precautions (Fig. 17-6)
7. Blood/Body Fluid Precautions (Fig. 17-7)

Category I: Strict Isolation.   Strict isolation is designed to prevent transmission of highly contagious or virulent and dangerous infections that may be spread by air and contact, such as diphtheria, viral hemorrhagic fevers, pneumonic plague, smallpox, varicella (chicken-pox), and herpes zoster localized in immunocompromised patients or disseminated (Fig. 17-1). Most diseases requiring strict isolation do not occur in surgical patients, but since they do occur under unusual circumstances, this category is included here.

Specifications for Strict Isolation
1. A private room is indicated; the door should be kept closed. Patients infected with the same organism may generally share a room.
2. Masks, gowns, and gloves should be worn by all persons entering the room. Gowns made of water-repellent material with low permeability to bacteria should give better protection.
3. Hands must be washed after touching the patient or potentially contaminated articles, and especially before taking care of another patient.
4. All equipment should be kept in the room. The room should be kept neat and uncluttered to facilitate good nursing care and cleaning procedures.
5. Articles contaminated with infective material should be discarded or bagged and labeled before being sent for decontamination and reprocessing, using a double bag technique.
6. Needles and syringes should be disposable, carefully handled, and discarded in a sealed and labeled container.
7. Charts, x-rays, laboratory reports, and so forth should be kept outside the patient's room.
8. Patients should not be transported to other departments unless necessary.
9. In case of death, special care of the body should be exercised in its removal from the room to its predetermined destination; attendants, pathologists, and morticians must be informed of possible dangers.

Category II: Contact Isolation.   Contact isolation is intended for patients with highly transmissible or epidemiologically important infections that do not require strict isolation, for example, patients infected or colonized by multiply-resistant bacteria. It is designed to prevent transmissible or epidemiologically important infections (or colonizations) that are spread primarily by close contact (Fig. 17-2).

(Front of Card)

STRICT ISOLATION

Visitors — Report to Nurses' Station Before Entering Room

1. Masks are indicated for all persons entering room.
2. Gowns are indicated for all persons entering room.
3. Gloves are indicated for all persons entering room.
4. HANDS MUST BE WASHED AFTER TOUCHING THE PATIENT OR POTENTIALLY CONTAMI-NATED ARTICLES AND BEFORE TAKING CARE OF ANOTHER PATIENT.
5. Articles contaminated with infective material should be discarded or bagged and labeled before being sent for decontamination and reprocessing.

YELLOW

(Back of Card)

Diseases Requiring Strict Isolation*

Diphtheria, pharyngeal
Lassa fever and other viral hemorrhagic fevers, such as Marburg virus disease§
Plague, pneumonic
Smallpox§
Varicella (chickenpox)
Zoster, localized in immunocompromised patient, or disseminated

YELLOW

---

* A private room is indicated for Strict Isolation; in general, however, patients infected with the same organism may share a room. See Guideline for Isolation Precautions in Hospitals for details and for how long to apply precautions.
§ A private room with special ventilation is indicated.

FIG. 17-1. A yellow card is used to give the instructions for Category I: Strict Isolation. (Garner JS, Simmons BP: CDC guidelines for isolation precautions in hospitals. Infection Control 4:284, 1983)

The more important patients in this category from a surgical point of view include the following:

1. Patients with major skin, wound, or burn infections, including those infected with *Staphylococcus aureus* or Group A *Streptococcus*.

   Isolation has been recommended for the extensively burned patient, but there are no satisfactory data confirming the effectiveness of such techniques in preventing bacterial or fungal colonization of the burn wound. The use of patient isolators has not minimized septic deaths in the patients so treated, and the gram-negative bacteria that ultimately colonized their burn wounds were often felt to originate in the patient's own gastrointestinal tract. Since the gram-negative organisms are poor air travelers, and air counts, even in busy wards, characteristically show few airborne gram-negative bacteria, the air is not considered to be a significant route of contamination of burn wounds. The transmission of bacteria from burn patient to burn patient is principally by means of personnel or fomites, so that one might anticipate a lessened patient-to-patient transmission by observing contact isolation precautions noted above. Particular attention should be given to the wearing of single-use impermeable gowns or aprons during all patient treatment procedures to prevent the front of one's clothing from becoming moist and thereby serving as a vector when attending subsequent patients.

2. Patients infected by multiple-resistant bacteria, including any of the following:
   a. Gram-negative bacilli resistant to all aminoglycosides that are tested (In general, such organisms should be resistant to gentamicin, tobramycin, and amikacin for these special precautions to be indicated.)
   b. *Staphylococcus aureus* resistant to methicillin (or to nafcillin or oxacillin if they are used instead of methicillin for testing)
   c. *Streptococcus pneumoniae* (pneumococci) resistant to penicillin
   d. *Hemophilus influenzae* resistant to ampicillin (beta-lactamase positive) and chloramphenicol

   Other resistant bacteria may be included if they are judged by the infection control team to be of special clinical and epidemiologic significance.

Other diseases are listed in Figure 17-2.

Specifications for Contact Isolation
1. Masks, gowns, and gloves are indicated for those who come close to the patient or to soiled or infective material.
2. *Hands must be washed after touching the patient or potentially contaminated articles, particularly before taking care of another patient.*
3. Articles contaminated with infective material should be discarded or bagged and labeled before being sent for decontamination and reprocessing.

Category III: Respiratory Isolation.   Respiratory isolation is designed to prevent transmission of infectious diseases, primarily over short distances through the air droplet transmission (Fig. 17-3). Patients with active tuberculosis are considered under Category IV.

(Front of Card)

CONTACT ISOLATION

Visitors — Report to Nurses' Station
Before Entering Room

1. Masks are indicated for those who come close to patient.
2. Gowns are indicated if soiling is likely.
3. Gloves are indicated for touching infective material.
4. HANDS MUST BE WASHED AFTER TOUCHING THE PATIENT OR POTENTIALLY CONTAMI-NATED ARTICLES AND BEFORE TAKING CARE OF ANOTHER PATIENT.
5. Articles contaminated with infective material should be discarded or bagged and labeled before being sent for decontamination and reprocessing.

ORANGE

FIG. 17-2. An orange card is used to give the instructions for Category II: Contact Isolation. (Garner JS, Simmons BP: CDC guidelines for isolation precautions in hospitals. Infection Control 4:285, 1983)

Diseases requiring respiratory isolation include the following: infections due to *Hemophilus influenza;* erythema infectiosum; measles; meningococcal menigitis, pneumonia, or meningococcemia; mumps; and pertussis (whooping cough). Since patients with these diseases may at times require emergency surgical operations, this category is included here.

(Back of Card)

Diseases or Conditions Requiring Contact Isolation*

Acute respiratory infections in infants and young children, including croup, colds, bronchitis, and bronchiolitis caused by respiratory syncytial virus, adenovirus, coronavirus, influenza viruses, parainfluenza viruses, and rhinovirus

Conjunctivitis, gonococcal, in newborns

Diphtheria, cutaneous

Endometritis, group A *Streptococcus*

Furunculosis, staphylococcal, in newborns

Herpes simplex, disseminated, severe primary or neonatal

Impetigo

Influenza, in infants and young children

Multiply-resistant bacteria, infection or colonization (any site) with any of the following:

1. Gram-negative bacilli resistant to all aminoglycosides that are tested. (In general, such organisms should be resistant to gentamicin, tobramycin, and amikacin for these special precautions to be indicated.)
2. *Staphylococcus aureus* resistant to methicillin (or nafcillin or oxacillin if they are used instead of methicillin for testing)
3. *Pneumococcus* resistant to penicillin

4. *Haemophilus influenzae* resistant to ampicillin (beta-lactamase positive) and chloramphenicol
5. Other resistant bacteria may be included in this isolation category if they are judged by the infection control team to be of special clinical and epidemiologic significance.

Pediculosis

Pharyngitis, infectious, in infants and young children

Pneumonia, viral, in infants and young children

Pneumonia, *Staphylococcus aureus* or group A *Streptococcus*

Rabies

Rubella, congenital and other

Scabies

Scalded skin syndrome (Ritter's disease)

Skin, wound, or burn infection, major (draining and not covered by a dressing or dressing does not adequately contain the purulent material), including those infected with *Staphylococcus aureus* or group A *Streptococcus*

Vaccinia (generalized and progressive eczema vaccinatum)

ORANGE

* A private room is indicated for Contact Isolation; in general, however, patients infected with the same organism may share a room. During outbreaks, infants and young children with the same respiratory clinical syndrome may share a room. See Guideline for Isolation Precautions in Hospitals for details and for how long to apply precautions.

FIG. 17-2 (continued)

Specifications for Respiratory Isolation

1. A private room is indicated; another patient infected with the same organism may share the room.
2. Masks are indicated for those who come close to the patient.
3. Gowns and gloves are not indicated.
4. Hands must be washed after touching the patient or potentially contaminated articles, and before taking care of another patient.
5. Articles contaminated with infective material should be discarded or bagged and labeled before being sent for decontamination and reprocessing.

(Text continues on p 340)

RESPIRATORY ISOLATION

Visitors — Report to Nurses' Station Before Entering Room

1. Masks are indicated for those who come close to patient.
2. Gowns are not indicated.
3. Gloves are not indicated.
4. HANDS MUST BE WASHED AFTER TOUCHING THE PATIENT OR POTENTIALLY CONTAMINATED ARTICLES AND BEFORE TAKING CARE OF ANOTHER PATIENT.
5. Articles contaminated with infective material should be discarded or bagged and labeled before being sent for decontamination and reprocessing.

BLUE

Diseases Requiring Respiratory Isolation*

Epiglottitis, *Hemophilus influenzae*
Erythema infectiosum
Measles
Meningitis
    Bacterial, etiology unknown
    Hemophilus influenzae, known or suspected
    Meningococcal, known or suspected
Meningococcal pneumonia
Meningococcemia
Mumps
Pertussis (whooping cough)
Pneumonia, *Hemophilus influenzae,* in children (any age)

BLUE

---

* A private room is indicated for Respiratory Isolation; in general, however, patients infected with the same organism may share a room. See Guideline for Isolation Precautions in Hospitals for details and for how long to apply precautions.

FIG. 17-3. A blue card is used to give the instructions for Category III: Respiratory Isolation. (Garner JS, Simmons BP: CDC guidelines for isolation precautions in hospitals. Infection Control 4:286, 1983)

(Front of Card)

AFB ISOLATION

Visitors — Report to Nurses' Station Before Entering Room

1. Masks are indicated only when patient is coughing and does not reliably cover mouth.
2. Gowns are indicated only if needed to prevent gross contamination of clothing.
3. Gloves are not indicated.
4. HANDS MUST BE WASHED AFTER TOUCHING THE PATIENT OR POTENTIALLY CONTAMINATED ARTICLES AND BEFORE TAKING CARE OF ANOTHER PATIENT.
5. Articles should be discarded, cleaned, or sent for decontamination and reprocessing.

GRAY

(Back of Card)

Diseases Requiring AFB Isolation*

This isolation category is for patients with current pulmonary TB who have a positive sputum smear or a chest X-ray appearance that strongly suggests current (active) TB. Laryngeal TB is also included in this category. In general, infants and young children with pulmonary TB do not require isolation precautions because they rarely cough and their bronchial secretions contain few AFB compared with adults with pulmonary TB. To protect the patient's privacy, this instruction card is labeled AFB (acid-fast bacilli) Isolation rather than Tuberculosis Isolation.

GRAY

* A private room with special ventilation is indicated for AFB Isolation. In general, patients infected with the same organism may share a room. See Guideline for Isolation Precautions in Hospitals for details and for how long to apply precautions.

FIG. 17-4. A gray card is used to give instructions for Category IV: AFB Isolation. (Garner JS, Simmons BP: CDC guidelines for isolation precautions in hospitals. Infection Control 4:287, 1983)

(Front of Card)

ENTERIC PRECAUTIONS

Visitors — Report to Nurses' Station
Before Entering Room

1. Masks are not indicated.
2. Gowns are indicated if soiling is likely.
3. Gloves are indicated for touching infective material.
4. HANDS MUST BE WASHED AFTER TOUCHING THE PATIENT OR POTENTIALLY CONTAMINATED ARTICLES AND BEFORE TAKING CARE OF ANOTHER PATIENT.
5. Articles contaminated with infective material should be discarded or bagged and labeled before being sent for decontamination and reprocessing.

WHITE

FIG. 17-5. A white card is used to give the instructions for Category V: Enteric Precautions. (Garner JS, Simmons BP: CDC guidelines for isolation precautions in hospitals. Infection Control 4:288, 1983)

Category IV: Tuberculosis isolation (AFB isolation). Category IV is an isolation category for patients with tuberculosis having a positive sputum smear or a chest roentgenogram that strongly suggests active TB (Fig. 17-4). Laryngeal TB is also included.

Specifications for Tuberculosis Isolation
1. A private room with special ventilation is indicated. The door should be kept closed. Generally, it is believed that patients infected with the same organism may share a room.
2. The wearing of masks and gown is recommended.
3. The use of gloves is not indicated.
4. *Hands must be washed after touching the patient or potentially contaminated articles, and before taking care of another patient.*
5. Inanimate articles should be thoroughly cleaned and disinfected, or discarded.

(Back of Card)

Diseases Requiring Enteric Precautions*

Amebic dysentery
Cholera
Coxsackievirus disease
Diarrhea, acute illness and suspected infectious
    etiology
Echovirus disease
Encephalitis (unless known not to be caused by
    enteroviruses)
Enterocolitis caused by *Clostridium difficile* or
    Staphylococcus aureus
Enteroviral infection
Gastroenteritis caused by
    Campylobacter species
    Cryptosporidium species
    Dientamoeba fragilis
    Escherichia coli (enterotoxic, enteropatho-
        genic, or enteroinvasive)
    Giardia lamblia
    Salmonella species

Shigella species
Vibrio parahaemolyticus
Viruses — including Norwalk agent and ro-
    tavirus
Yersinia enterocolitica
Unknown etiology but presumed to be an
    infectious agent
Hand, foot, and mouth disease
Hepatitis, viral, type A
Herpangina
Meningitis, viral (unless known not to be caused
    by enteroviruses)
Necrotizing enterocolitis
Pleurodynia
Poliomyelitis
Typhoid fever (*Salmonella typhi*)
Viral pericarditis, myocarditis, or meningitis (un-
    less known not to be caused by enterovi-
    ruses)

WHITE

---

* A private room is indicated for Enteric Precautions if patient hygiene is poor. A patient with poor hygiene does not
wash hands after touching infective material, contaminates the environment with infective material, or shares
contaminated articles with other patients. In general, patients infected with the same organism may share a room.
See Guideline for Isolation Precautions in Hospitals for details and for how long to apply precautions.

FIG. 17-5 (continued)

Category V: Enteric Precautions. On a surgical service, particularly for those patients with viral hepatitis or *Salmonella* infections, enteric isolation may also be necessary. Enteric infections are transmitted by direct contact with feces (Fig. 17-5). Hepatitis A is included in this category because it is spread through feces. Although many of these infections are not of primary surgical significance, they are included here because they may occur as complications or in association with diseases in surgical patients.

Diseases requiring enteric precautions include the following:

Amebic dysentery
Cholera
Coxsackievirus disease
Diarrhea (acute illness with suspected infectious etiology)
Echovirus disease
Enterocolitis caused by *Clostridium difficile* or *Staphylococcus aureus*
Gastroenteritis caused by
    Campylobacter species

(Front of Card)

DRAINAGE/SECRETION PRECAUTIONS

Visitors — Report to Nurses' Station
Before Entering Room

1. Masks are not indicated.
2. Gowns are indicated if soiling is likely.
3. Gloves are indicated for touching infective material.
4. HANDS MUST BE WASHED AFTER TOUCHING THE PATIENT OR POTENTIALLY CONTAMINATED ARTICLES AND BEFORE TAKING CARE OF ANOTHER PATIENT.
5. Articles contaminated with infective material should be discarded or bagged and labeled before being sent for decontamination and reprocessing.

GREEN

FIG. 17-6.   An green card is used to give the instructions for Category VI: Drainage/Secretion Precautions. (Garner JS, Simmons BP: CDC guidelines for isolation precautions in hospitals. Infection Control 4:289, 1983)

Cryptosporidium
Dientamoeba fragilis
Escherichia coli (enterotoxic, enteropathogenic, or enteroinvasive)
Giardia lamblia
Salmonella species
Shigella species
Vibrio parahaemolyticus
Viruses (including Norwalk agent and rotavirus)
Yersinia enterocolitica
An unknown agent presumed to be infectious
Hand, foot, and mouth disease
Hepatitis (viral, type A)
Herpangina
Meningitis (viral; unless known not to be caused by enteroviruses)
Necrotizing enterocolitis
Pleurodynia
Poliomyelitis
Typhoid fever *(Salmonella typhosa)*
Viral pericarditis, myocarditis, or meningitis (unless known not to be caused by enteroviruses)

(Back of Card)

Diseases Requiring Drainage/Secretion Precautions*

Infectious diseases included in this category are those that result in production of infective purulent material, drainage, or secretions, unless the disease is included in another isolation category that requires more rigorous precautions. (If you have questions about a specific disease, see the listing of infectious diseases in Guideline for Isolation Precautions in Hospitals, Table A, Disease-Specific Isolation Precautions.)

The following infections are examples of those included in this category provided they are *not* a) caused by multiply-resistant microorganisms, b) major (draining and not covered by a dressing or dressing does not adequately contain the drainage) skin, wound, or burn infections, including those caused by *Staphylococcus aureus* or group A *Streptococcus,* or c) gonococcal eye infections in newborns. See Contact Isolation if the infection is one of these 3.

Abscess, minor or limited
Burn infection, minor or limited
Conjunctivitis
Decubitus ulcer, infected, minor or limited
Skin infection, minor or limited
Wound infection, minor or limited

GREEN

* A private room is usually not indicated for Drainage/Secretion Precautions. See Guideline for Isolation Precautions in Hospitals for details and for how long to apply precautions.

FIG. 17-6 (continued)

Specifications for Enteric Precautions

1. A private room is indicated if the patient's hygiene is poor; this includes failure to wash his hands after touching infective material, causing contamination of the environment with infective material, or sharing contaminated articles with other patients. It may be possible for some patients infected with the same organism to share a room.
2. Masks are not indicated.
3. Gowns are indicated if soiling is likely.
4. Gloves are indicated when touching infective material.
5. *Hands must be washed thoroughly after touching the patient or potentially contaminated articles and before taking care of another patient.* In particular, attending personnel who handle excreta must carefully and meticulously wash their hands after contact with the bedpan, the commode, or inadvertent contact with the feces. Steam hoppers are inadequate for sterilization of bedpans and may produce dangerous aerosols. A bedpan (preferably with a disposable plastic liner) or a bedside commode for the individual patient's use should be considered.
6. Articles contaminated with infective material should be discarded or bagged and labeled before being sent for decontamination and reprocessing.

Category VI: Drainage/Secretion Precautions.   Category VI is a newly created isolation category designed to prevent infections that can be transmitted by direct or indirect contact with purulent material or drainage from an infected body site (Fig. 17-6). It was created by combining and modifying wound and skin

---

(Front of Card)

BLOOD/BODY FLUID PRECAUTIONS

1. Masks are not indicated.
2. Gowns are indicated if soiling with blood or body fluids is likely.
3. Gloves are indicated for touching blood or body fluids.
4. HANDS SHOULD BE WASHED IMMEDIATELY IF THEY ARE POTENTIALLY CONTAMINATED WITH BLOOD OR BODY FLUIDS AND BEFORE TAKING CARE OF ANOTHER PATIENT.
5. Articles contaminated with blood or body fluids should be discarded or bagged and labeled before being sent for decontamination and reprocessing.
6. Care should be taken to avoid needle-stick injuries. Used needles should not be recapped or bent; they should be placed in a prominently labeled, puncture-resistant container designated specifically for such disposal.
7. Blood spills should be cleaned up promptly with a solution of 5.25% sodium hypochlorite diluted 1 : 10 with water.

PINK

FIG. 17-7. A pink card is used to give the instructions for Category VII: Blood/Body Fluid Precautions. (Garner JS, Simmons BP: CDC guidelines for isolation precautions in hospitals. Infection Control 4:290, 1983)

precautions, discharge (lesion) precautions, and secretion (oral) precautions found in previous editions of the U.S. Public Health Manuals. Infectious diseases included are those associated with the production of infective purulent material, drainage, or secretions, except when the disease is included in another isolation category that requires more rigorous precautions. For example, minor or limited skin, wound, and burn infections are included in this category, whereas major skin, wound, or burn infections are managed under Contact Isolation (Category II).

The following infections are examples of those included in Category VI:

Abscess (minor or limited)
Burn infection (minor or limited)
Conjunctivitis
Decubitus ulcer (infected, minor or limited)
Skin infection (minor or limited)
Wound infection (minor or limited)

Specifications for Drainage/Secretion Precautions
1. A private room and masks are not indicated.
2. Gowns and gloves are indicated if soiling and touching infective material are likely.

(Back of Card)

Diseases Requiring Blood/Body Fluid Precautions*

Acquired immunodeficiency syndrome (AIDS)
Arthropodborne viral fevers (for example, dengue, yellow fever, and Colorado tick fever)
Babesiosis
Creutzfeldt-Jakob disease
Hepatitis B (including HBsAg antigen carrier)
Hepatitis, non-A, non-B
Leptospirosis
Malaria
Rat-bite fever
Relapsing fever
Syphilis, primary and secondary with skin and mucous membrane lesions

PINK

* A private room is indicated for Blood/Body Fluid Precautions if patient hygiene is poor. A patient with poor hygiene does not wash hands after touching infective material, contaminates the environment with infective material, or shares contaminated articles with other patients. In general, patients infected with the same organism may share a room. See Guideline for Isolation Precautions in Hospitals for details and for how long to apply precautions.

FIG. 17-7 (continued)

3. *Hands must be washed after touching the patient or potentially contaminated articles and before taking care of another patient.*
4. Articles contaminated with infective material should be discarded or bagged and labeled before decontamination and reprocessing.

Category VII: Blood/Body Fluid Precautions. Blood/body fluid precautions have been designed to prevent infections that can be transmitted by direct or indirect contact with infective blood or body fluids (Fig. 17-7). Included in this category are diseases that result in the production of infective blood or body fluids, unless the disease is included in another isolation category that requires more rigorous precautions, such as Strict Isolation. For some diseases included in this category, such as malaria, only blood is infective; for other diseases, such as hepatitis B (including antigen carriers), blood and body fluids (saliva, semen, *etc.*) are infective.

Diseases requiring blood/body precautions are as follows:

Acquired immunodeficiency syndrome (AIDS)
Arthropod-borne viral fevers (*e.g.,* dengue, yellow fever, and Colorado tick fever)
Babesiosis

(Front of Card)

DISEASE SPECIFIC ISOLATION PRECAUTIONS

Visitors — Report to Nurses' Station
Before Entering Room

1. **Private room indicated?**   _____ No
                                      _____ Yes

2. **Masks indicated?**   _____ No
                                     _____ Yes for those close to patient
                                     _____ Yes for all persons entering room

3. **Gowns indicated?**   _____ No
                                    _____ Yes if soiling is likely
                                    _____ Yes for all persons entering room

4. **Gloves indicated?**   _____ No
                                    _____ Yes for touching infective material
                                    _____ Yes for all persons entering room

5. Special precautions   _____ No
   indicated for handling blood?   _____ Yes

6. **Hands must be washed after touching the patient or potentially contaminated articles and before taking care of another patient.**

7. Articles contaminated with _____ should be
                                        infective material(s)
   discarded or bagged and labeled before being sent for decontamination and reprocessing.

FIG. 17-8.   Instruction card for disease-specific isolation precautions, System II. (Garner JS, Simmons BP: CDC guidelines for isolation precautions in hospitals. Infection Control 4:323, 1983)

Creutzfeldt-Jakob disease
Hepatitis B (including HB$_s$Ag antigen carrier)
Non-A, non-B hepatitis
Leptospirosis
Malaria
Rat-bite fever
Relapsing fever
Syphilis (primary and secondary with skin and mucous membrane lesions)

Specifications for Blood/Body Fluid Precautions
1.   A private room is indicated if the patient's hygiene is poor (see Categories III and VI).
2.   Masks are not indicated.
3.   Gowns are indicated if soiling of clothing with blood or body fluids is likely.
4.   Gloves are indicated for touching blood or body fluids.
5.   *Hands must be washed immediately if they are potentially contaminated with blood or body fluids, and before taking care of another patient.*

(Back of Card)

Instructions

1. On Table B, Disease-Specific Precautions, locate the disease for which isolation precautions are indicated.
2. Write disease in blank space here: _____
3. Determine if a private room is indicated. In general, patients infected with the same organism may share a room. For some diseases or conditions, a private room is indicated if patient hygiene is poor. A patient with poor hygiene does not wash hands after touching infective material (feces, purulent drainage, or secretions), contaminates the environment with infective material, or shares contaminated articles with other patients.
4. Place a check mark beside the indicated precautions on front of card.
5. Cross through precautions that are indicated.
6. Write infective material in blank space in item 7 on front of card.

FIG. 17-8 (continued)

6. Articles contaminated with blood or body fluids should be discarded or bagged and labeled before being sent for decontamination and reprocessing.
7. Care should be taken to avoid needle-stick injuries. Used needles should not be recapped or bent, but placed in a prominently labeled, impervious, puncture-resistant container labeled specifically for such disposable items.
8. Blood spills should be cleaned up promptly with a solution of 5.25% sodium hypochlorite diluted 1 : 10 with water.

System II

System II, the *Disease-Specific System of Isolation Precautions,* is a newly proposed system by the Center for Disease Control that is available as an alternative to the category-specific System I for individual hospital consideration and use. This system consists of a list of most of the common diseases and infectious agents that can be found in United States' hospitals. Listings have been made for each infectious disease by anatomical site and etiologic agent, and sometimes by a combination thereof. This listing also identifies which discharges, excretions, secretions, body fluids, and tissues are infective or potentially so. An instruction card has been designed by the CDC to give concise information about the use of these disease-specific isolation precautions (Fig. 17-8). The instruction card can be prepared for the individual use of each patient by checking off the appropriate items and filling in the blanks. When prepared, the card should be placed conspicuously near the isolated patient and attached to the front of his chart.

In presenting this system, the CDC proposes a possible saving in time and expense over the category-specific system. Such economy must be verified in actual use. Certain problems may be anticipated with its use, such as the effect of delays in specific diagnosis, possible confusion in executing indicated precautions by nurses and attendants, and potential difficulties in its administration. System II as proposed by the CDC contains much to recommend it, however, and it is worthy of the careful consideration of hospitals, particularly for nonsurgical diseases.

PRINCIPLES OF DRESSING TECHNIQUE

On a surgical service, one of the most strikingly obvious sources of contamination or of cross-contamination among hospital patients is faulty dressing technique. Improper changing and disposal of dressings or other breaches of good technique in this important area of surgical practice can result in significant morbidity and mortality. Since the equipment and dressings used have been sterilized, contamination and resultant infection usually occur through inadequate or careless technique on the part of the individual changing the dressing. Minimization of cross-contamination in infected cases is best effected by preplanned dressing changes and by the use of a technique in which clean gloves are worn to remove soiled dressings and sterile ones to apply new dressings. All dressings, tissues, and special types of apparatus are handled with sterile instruments. Upon the completion of the dressing change, thorough hand-washing is performed.

When a major dressing is to be changed, the room should be relatively quiet and free of visitors. Dressings should not be changed at a time when housekeeping personnel are carrying out or have just carried out cleaning activities in the immediate area, activities that can increase the amount of particulate matter in the air and the chances of their contained bacteria falling out onto the wound. There is probably no need for a separate dressing room in the management of the ordinary surgical patient. If, however, there are a large number of patients with severe contamination, such as is seen on a burn ward, it may be advisable to have a separate dressing room that can be thoroughly aired and repeatedly cleaned in a fashion similar to that of an operating room. Consideration should be given to changing dressings of extensive open wounds, particularly in high-risk patients, in the operating room.

Table 17-1 outlines the equipment and procedures recommended for dressing wounds. If a dressing cart is used in the routine management of the patient's wounds, it should not be taken into the patient's room. It should be left in the hallway and essential equipment moved into the room on a sterile tray or towel for the dressing change. Dressing accessories, such as suture removal sets, sponges,

Table 17-1. Equipment and Procedures Recommended in Dressing Wounds

	Infected Wound	Noninfected Wound
Hand-washing before	+	+
Gloves (2 pairs)*	+	0
Gown	+	0
Mask	+	0
Sterile equipment	+	+
Double-bag technique for soiled dressings and equipment	+	+
"No-touch" technique	+	+
Hand-washing after	+	+

*Changed between removal of soiled dressing and application of new dressing
+ = Necessary
0 = Not necessary

drains, and so forth, should be individually wrapped or put up in sets and presterilized. Extra supplies can be kept on the cart or in a supply depot in individual packages so that they may be added to any dressing change setup without the contamination of the cart. Preferably the dressing team should include two people using a technique similar to that used in the operating room: that is, one acts as a circulator to move supplies from the cart to the dressing tray, and the other actually changes the dressing. This eliminates the possibility of contaminating the cart. A plastic or impermeable bag is essential for the disposal of dressings. Contaminated dressings from infected wounds should be disposed of using the double plastic bag technique.

Other methods of management include the use of individual dressing sets sterilized in a plastic bag or linen-wrapped containers. As dressings are removed from the patient, they are carefully placed in the plastic bag which is sealed at the conclusion of the dressing change and placed in a proper receptacle for appropriate and safe disposal.

Whenever it is necessary for a single person to do the dressing, careful thought should be given to equipment and material needed for the change in order to prevent cross-contamination between the patient and the cart. As a preliminary step, the person changing the dressing should remove his rings and watch, position the patient properly, and then wash his hands. Supplies anticipated for the particular dressing should be gathered from the dressing cart or other sources and placed on the tray or dressing table next to the patient. Before opening the dressing set (if precautions are required), the nurse or physician should don a mask, gown, and gloves. Gloves need not be worn for a routine dressing if a strict "no-touch" technique is used throughout the procedure. The outer dressing is then removed, using a "no-touch" technique, and discarded into the bag. If inflammation is present or pus is seen when changing a dressing, cultures should be taken. Proper draping of the area must be carried out if manipulation of the wound is to be accomplished. The wound edges and surface may be cleansed with a mild antiseptic solution, if this is the physician's choice, or simply with saline, and a new sterile dressing applied.

Contaminated material should *never* be placed in the patient's waste can or bedside receptacle in the room. Contaminated instruments and dressing sets should be returned to the utility room and never returned to the dressing cart. The person who changed the dressing should then wash his hands prior to making appropriate notes on the patient's chart or touching other patients or equipment.

Dry occlusive dressings are preferred to wet dressings or to no dressings, although the latter choice is controversial. Most surgeons feel that skin or retention sutures should be covered by a bandage, but there has been a trend in the last decade and a half to leave the sutured wound uncovered. The wet dressing permits bacteria from the infected wound to seep upward through the dressing by capillary action, thus contaminating the bedclothing, hands, and other objects. In the same fashion, bacteria on the surface may enter through the wet dressing by capillary action and contaminate an otherwise sterile wound, particularly during the first 4 days postoperatively. Dressings that become wet with wound exudate should be changed promptly.

PROTECTIVE ISOLATION

A category of isolation achieving greater interest is that of protective isolation for patients with *immunologic impairment* and conditions associated with extreme susceptibility to infection. The isolation procedures employed with these patients vary considerably. Generally they include gown, mask, and glove precautions, assiduous hand-washing prior to contact with the patients, and the use of a private room for the patient. In some hospitals, particularly in Great Britain, experimental units with "ultra-clean" wards, rooms, or units have been set up. The Center for Disease Control, however, has recently discontinued the isolation category for protective isolation in their "Guidelines for Isolation Precautions in Hospitals."

ISOLATION IN THE OPERATING ROOM

In addition to the practice of aseptic technique, the principles of isolation must be carried out in the operating room when a patient with any of the infections listed previously requires surgery. It must be borne in mind, however, that each case in the operating room should be treated as a potentially infected one. If possible, surgery of the patient should be scheduled at the end of the operating day to avoid possible transmission of infection to subsequent surgical patients. Disposable drapes, gowns, and equipment may be used, with all instruments carefully cleansed in a detergent–disinfectant solution and handled according to standard procedure. (A terminal cleansing of the operating room should be carried out following the conclusion of the operation on an infected case; see Chap. 8.) A nonrecirculating ventilatory system in operating rooms should be used for infected cases, with the air vented 100% to the outside and changed at least 11 to 20 times per hour.

For patients who might benefit from protective isolation, airborne contamination is said to be minimized by the use of laminar flow operating rooms. This type of airflow is being used for open-heart and total hip replacement procedures in some areas. Operating room traffic, conversation, and movement should be kept at a minimum to decrease the airborne bacterial count in the operating theater. A decrease in airborne bacterial count, however, has not been shown to result in significantly decreased postoperative infection rates.

A good design for an operating room used for surgery of an infected patient ideally has a separate outside entrance so that the patient will not have to be transported through the general operating suite. If such is not available, an operating theater near the entrance to the operating suite should be designated as the operating room for septic cases.

Although a separate operating room for septic patients is considered advisable by many authorities, others believe that no special room need be set aside for "dirty" cases. The postoperative procedures for the disinfection and cleaning of operating suites following an infected case should be good enough to permit clean surgery to be performed after the cleanup routine has been completed.

Immediately prior to the patients' transfer to the surgical suite, all grossly contaminated dressings and bedding noted above should be removed from the patient and replaced by clean ones. Some authorities recommend that a septic patient being brought to the operating suite be transferred from the ward litter at a designated transfer point and placed on a "clean" litter, kept at all times in the operating suite. The patient with an infectious disease that is potentially transmissible to other patients should be returned to his previous environment and not taken to the recovery room unless an isolation area is available in the recovery suite.

Circulating and scrub nurses have specific responsibilities in the operating room where infection control is a concern. The circulator must assume responsibility for minimizing traffic into and out of the room by keeping doors closed, maintaining the sterility of the surgeons and scrub nurse(s), properly disposing of soiled and bloody sponges and linens, and the proper disposition of instruments after an operation. The scrub nurse is obligated to maintain her own sterility, as well as that of the surgeons and instruments.

Education of personnel and their constant awareness of the problem of cross-infection is of the greatest importance. Among the important points to be emphasized are the following:

1. Handle all instruments carefully to prevent danger of injury and infection of personnel, and adequately sterilize them.
2. Avoid bare-handed contact with contaminated items.
3. Be sure that the operating room air is exchanged at least 11 to 20 times per hour with high-efficiency filtration.
4. Arrange for appropriate isolation facilities in the recovery room for postoperative infected cases.

All techniques for dealing with septic cases should be clearly defined and adhered to as follows:

1. Remove all unnecessary equipment from the operating room and ask unnecessary personnel to leave.
2. Clean all surfaces after each infected case.
3. Sterilize or doubly wrap all instruments before removal from the operating room.
4. Remove gowns, caps, masks, shoe covers, and gloves before leaving the operating room and properly bag for disposal.
5. Consider the use of disposable linen when appropriate.
6. Carefully wrap all specimens leaving the room.
7. Sterilize anesthesia equipment in direct contact with the patient or use disposable equipment.

BIBLIOGRAPHY

BAGSHAWE KD, BLOWERS R, LIDWELL OM: Isolating patients in hospital to control infection. Part I — Sources and routes of infection. Br Med J 2(6137):609 – 613, 1978

BAGSHAWE KD, BLOWERS R, LIDWELL OM: Isolating patients in hospital to control infection. Part II — Who should be isolated, and where? Br Med J 2(6138):684 – 686, 1978

BAGSHAWE KD, BLOWERS R, LIDWELL OM: Isolating patients in hospital to control infection. Part III — Design and construction of isolation accommodation. Br Med J 2(6139):744 – 748, 1978

BAGSHAWE KD, BLOWERS R, LIDWELL OM: Isolating patients in hospital to control infection. Part IV — Nursing procedures. Br Med J 2(6140):808 – 811, 1978

BAGSHAWE KD, BLOWERS R, LIDWELL OM: Isolating patients in hospital to control infection. Part V — An isolation system. Br Med J 2(6141):879 – 881, 1978

BELFRAGE S, CEDERBERG A: Letter: Need hepatitis patients be isolated? Lancet 1(8170):704 – 705, 1980

BURKE JF: Identification of the sources of staphylococci contaminating the surgical wound during operation. Ann Surg 158:898, 1963

BYRNE EB: Viral hepatitis: An occupational hazard of medical personnel. Experience of the Yale – New Haven Hospital, 1952 to 1965. JAMA 195:362, 1966

CDC GUIDELINES FOR THE PREVENTION AND CONTROL OF NOSOCOMIAL INFECTIONS. Washington, DC, U.S. Department of Health and Human Services, 1981

CHARNLEY J, EFTEKAR N: Postoperative infection and total prosthetic replacement arthroplasty of the hip joint. With special reference to the bacterial content of the air of the operating room. Br J Surg 56:641, 1969

DANKERT J, GAUS W, GAYA H, KRIEGER D, LINZENMEIER G, VAN DER WAAIJ D: Protective isolation and antimicrobial decontamination in patients with high susceptibility to infection. A prospective cooperative study of gnotobiotic care in acute leukaemia patients. III. The quality of isolation and decontamination. Infection 6(4):175 – 191, 1978

DONOVAN CT: Protective isolation. Oncol Nurs Forum 9(3):50 – 53, 1982

EICKHOFF TC, BRACHMAN PS, BENNETT JV, BROWN JF: Surveillance of nosocomial infections in community hospitals. I. Surveillance methods, effectiveness, and initial results. J Infect Dis 120:305, 1969

GARNER JS, SIMMONS BP: CDC guidelines for isolation precautions in hospitals. Infect Control 4:248, 1983

JEPSEN OB: Letter: The role of an isolation unit in the control of hospital infection with methicillin-resistant staphylococci. J Hosp Infect 1(4):363 – 364, 1980

LOWBURY EJL, AYLIFFE GAJ, GEDDES AM, WILLIAMS JD: Control of Hospital Infection, 2nd ed. Philadelphia, JB Lippincott, 1981

LOWBURY EJL, BABB JR, FORD PM: Protective isolation in a burns unit: The use of plastic isolators and air curtains. J Hyg (Camb) 69:529, 1971

MAYHALL CG: Isolation techniques for hospital patients with viral hepatitis: New guidelines premature. Infect Control 1(2):71–72, 74, 1980

MOSLEY JW: The surveillance of transfusion-associated viral hepatitis. JAMA 193:1007, 1965

NAUSEEF WM, MAJI DG: A study of the value of simple protective isolation in patients with granulocytopenia. N Eng J Med 304(8):448–453, 1981

SELKON JB, STOKES ER, INGHAM HR: The role of an isolation unit in the control of hospital infection with methicillin-resistant staphylococcoi. J Hosp Infect 1(1):41–46, 1980

WILLIAMS WW: CDC guidelines for the prevention and control of nosocomial infections: Guidelines for control in hospital personnel. Am J Infect Control 12:34–63, 1984

WOODRUFF AW: Letter: Isolation to control infection. Br Med J 2(6140):831, 1978

APPENDIX 1
Contributors to Four Symposia: March 1970 – November 1972

J. Wesley Alexander, M.D., F.A.C.S.
Director, Division of Transplantation, Department of Surgery, University of Cincinnati Medical Center, Cincinnati, Ohio

J. Garrott Allen, M.D., F.A.C.S.
Professor of Surgery, Stanford University Medical Center, Stanford, California

William A. Altemeier, M.D., F.A.C.S.
Professor and Chairman, Department of Surgery, University of Cincinnati Medical Center, Cincinnati, Ohio

Betty Jane Anderson
Legal Research Department, American Medical Association, Chicago, Illinois

Curtis P. Artz, M.D., F.A.C.S.
Professor and Chairman, Department of Surgery, Medical University of South Carolina, Charleston, South Carolina

Wiley F. Barker, M.D., F.A.C.S.
Professor of Surgery, University of California Medical Center, Los Angeles, California

Folkert O. Belzer, M.D., F.A.C.S.
Professor of Surgery, University of California, San Francisco, California

John V. Bennett, M.D.
Chief, Bacterial Diseases Branch, Center for Disease Control, U.S. Public Health Service, Atlanta, Georgia

Richard P. Bergen
Director, Legal Research Department, American Medical Association, Chicago, Illinois

Harvey R. Bernard, M.D., F.A.C.S.
Professor of Surgery, Albany Medical College, Albany, New York

William F. Bernhard, M.D., F.A.C.S.
Professor of Surgery, Harvard University, Children's Hospital Medical Center, Boston, Massachusetts

William S. Blakemore, M.D., F.A.C.S.
Professor and Chairman, Department of Surgery, Medical College of Ohio, Toledo, Ohio

George H. Bornside, Ph.D.
Professor of Surgical Research & Microbiology, Department of Surgery, Louisiana State University Medical Center, New Orleans, Louisiana

Philip Brachman, M.D.
Director, Epidemiology Program, Bacterial Diseases Branch, Centers for Disease Control, U.S. Public Health Service, Atlanta, Georgia

Lloyd D. Bridenbaugh, M.D.
Department of Anesthesiology, The Virginia Mason Clinic, Seattle, Washington

Lester R. Bryant, M.D., F.A.C.S.
Professor and Chief, Division of Thoracic Surgery, Department of Surgery, Louisiana State University Medical Center, New Orleans, Louisiana

John Bunyan, M.B.
London, England

John F. Burke, M.D., F.A.C.S.
Associate Professor of Surgery, Harvard University, Boston, Massachusetts

Charles Gardner Child III, M.D., F.A.C.S.
Professor and Chairman, Department of Surgery, University of Michigan, Ann Arbor, Michigan

George H.A. Clowes, Jr., M.D., F.A.C.S.
Clinical Professor of Surgery, Harvard University, Boston, Massachusetts

William R. Cole, M.D., F.A.C.S.
Associate Clinical Professor of Surgery, University of Missouri, Sedalia, Missouri

Patricia Copenhaver, R.N.
Supervisor, Operating Rooms, Cincinnati General Hospital, Cincinnati, Ohio

Armand F. Cortese, M.D., F.A.C.S.
Assistant Professor of Surgery, New York Hospital–Cornell University, New York, New York

Peter J.E. Cruse, M.B., F.R.C.S. (C)
Assistant Professor of Surgery, University of Calgary, Foothills Provincial General Hospital, Calgary, Alberta

William R. Culbertson, M.D., F.A.C.S.
Professor of Surgery, Department of Surgery, University of Cincinnati Medical Center, Cincinnati, Ohio

John H. Davis, M.D., F.A.C.S.
Professor and Chairman, Department of Surgery, University of Vermont College of Medicine, Burlington, Vermont

Peter Dineen, M.D., F.A.C.S.
Professor of Surgery, New York Hospital–Cornell Medical Center, New York, New York

Stanley J. Dudrick, M.D., F.A.C.S.
Professor and Chairman, Department of Surgery, Baylor College of Medicine, Houston, Texas

J. Englebert Dunphy, M.D., F.A.C.S.
Professor and Chairman, Department of Surgery, University of California School of Medicine, San Francisco, California

N. Eftekhar, M.D.
Assistant Professor, Department of Orthopaedic Surgery, Columbia–Presbyterian Medical Center, New York, New York

N. Joel Ehrenkranz, M.D.
Professor of Medicine and Epidemiology, University of Miami, Jackson Memorial Hospital, Miami, Florida

Frank B. Engley, Jr., Ph.D.
Professor and Chairman, Department of Microbiology, University of Missouri, Columbia, Missouri

William F. Enneking, M.D.
Professor and Chief, Division of Orthopaedic Surgery, Department of Surgery, University of Florida, Gainesville, Florida

Maxwell Finland, M.D.
Professor Emeritus, Harvard University, Boston City Hospital, Boston, Massachusetts

William D. Fullen, M.D.
Assistant Professor of Surgery, Department of Surgery, University of Cincinnati Medical Center, Cincinnati, Ohio

Julia S. Garner, R.N., M.N.
Nurse Consultant, Hospital Infections Section, Bacterial Diseases Branch, Epidemiology Program, Centers for Disease Control, U.S. Public Health Service, Atlanta, Georgia

Elizabeth Greer
Purchasing Agent and Supervisor of Instruments, The Wilmer Institute Operating Rooms, Johns Hopkins Hospital, Baltimore, Maryland

Dieter W. Gump, M.D.
Associate Professor of Medicine, University of Vermont College of Medicine, Burlington, Vermont

Bert L. Halter, M.D., F.A.C.S.
Clinical Professor of Surgery, University of California, San Francisco, California

James D. Hardy, M.D., F.A.C.S.
Professor and Chairman, Department of Surgery, University of Mississippi Medical School, Jackson, Mississippi

Boyd W. Haynes, Jr., M.D., F.A.C.S.
Professor and Chairman, Trauma Division, Medical College of Virginia, Richmond, Virginia

Edward O. Hill, Ph.D.
Associate Professor of Research Surgery and Microbiology, Department of Surgery, University of Cincinnati Medical Center, Cincinnati, Ohio

Norman A. Hinton, M.D.
Professor and Chairman, Department of Medical Microbiology, University of Toronto, The Banting Institute, Toronto, Ontario

John M. Howard, M.D., F.A.C.S.
Professor of Surgery, Department of Surgery, Medical College of Ohio, Toledo, Ohio

Robert P. Hummel, M.D., F.A.C.S.
Associate Professor of Surgery, Department of Surgery, University of Cincinnati Medical Center, Cincinnati, Ohio

John L. Hunt, M.D.
Chief, Burn Study Branch, U.S. Army Institute of Surgical Research, Brooke Army Medical Center, Fort Sam Houston, Texas

Thomas K. Hunt, M.D., F.A.C.S.
Associate Professor of Surgery, University of California Medical Center, San Francisco, California

Saul Krugman, M.D.
Professor and Chairman, Department of Pediatrics, New York University Medical Center, New York, New York

Ruth B. Kundsin, D.Sc.
Surgical Bacteriology Laboratory, Peter Bent Brigham Hospital, Boston, Massachusetts

Calvin M. Kunin, M.D.
Veterans Administration Hospital, Madison, Wisconsin

Thomas J. Krizek, M.D.
Professor of Surgery, Chief, Section of Plastic and Reconstructive Surgery, Department of Surgery, Yale University, New Haven, Connecticut

Norman K. Kurtz, M.M.E.
Consulting Engineer, New York, New York

Harold Laufman, M.D., F.A.C.S.
Chairman, Committee on Control of Operating Room Environment, American College of Surgeons, Montefiore Hospital and Medical Center, Bronx, New York

William J. Ledger, M.D.
Professor of Obstetrics/Gynecology, University of Southern California Medical Center, Women's Hospital, Los Angeles, California

E. Stanley Lennard, M.D.
Department of Surgery, University of Washington School of Medicine, Seattle, Washington

James Lindsey, M.D.
Centers for Disease Control, U.S. Public Health Service, Atlanta, Georgia

Bertha Yanis Litsky, M.P.A.
Consultant Bacteriologist, Echo Hill, Amherst, Massachusetts

Warren Litsky, Ph.D.
Department of Environmental Sciences, Marshall Hall, University of Massachusetts, Amherst, Massachusetts

E.J.L. Lowbury, D.M.
Medical Research Council, Industrial Injuries & Burns Research Unit, Birmingham Accident Hospital, Birmingham, England

Lloyd D. MacLean, M.D., F.R.C.S.(C)
Professor of Surgery and Chairman, Department of Surgery, McGill University, Montreal, Quebec

Bruce G. MacMillan, M.D., F.A.C.S.
Professor of Surgery, University of Cincinnati Medical Center; Director, Shriners Burns Institute, Cincinnati, Ohio

George F. Mallison, M.P.H.
Chief, Microbiological Control Section, Bacterial Diseases Branch, Epidemiology Program, Centers for Disease Control, U.S. Public Health Service, Atlanta, Georgia

A.E. Maumenee, M.D.
Director, The Wilmer Institute, Johns Hopkins Hospital, Baltimore, Maryland

Brian F. McCabe, M.D., F.A.C.S.
Professor and Chairman, Department of Otolaryngology, University of Iowa Hospital, Iowa City, Iowa

John J. McDonough, M.D.
Chief Surgical Resident, Department of Surgery, University of Cincinnati Medical Center, Cincinnati, Ohio

John E. McGowan, M.D.
Boston City Hospital, Boston, Massachusetts

A.P.H. McLean, M.D., F.A.C.S.
Associate Professor of Surgery, McGill University, Royal Victoria Hospital, Montreal, Quebec

Jonathan L. Meakins, M.D.
Surgical Resident, McGill University, Montreal, Quebec

Don R. Miller, M.D., F.A.C.S.
Professor of Surgery, University of California College of Medicine at Irvine, Irvine, California

George E. Miller, M.D.
Assistant Professor of Surgery, University of Cincinnati Medical Center, Cincinnati, Ohio

Ronald Lee Nichols, M.D.
Department of Surgery, West Side Veterans Administration Hospital, Chicago, Illinois

Michael J. Patzakis, M.D.
Assistant Professor, Section of Orthopedic Surgery, Los Angeles County – University of Southern California Medical Center, Los Angeles, California

Fernando Paulino, M.D., F.A.C.S.
Rua Joao Berges, Rio de Janeiro, Brazil

Jerry G. Peers, R.N.
Executive Director, Association of Operating Room Nurses, Inc., Englewood, Colorado

Hiram Polk, M.D., F.A.C.S.
Professor and Chairman, Department of Surgery, University of Louisville School of Medicine, Louisville, Kentucky

Basil A. Pruitt, Jr., M.D., F.A.C.S.
Colonel, M.C., U.S. Army; Commander and Director, U.S. Army Institute of Surgical Research, Brooke Army Medical Center, Fort Sam Houston, Texas

Frank Rhame, M.D.
Acting Chief, Comprehensive Hospital Infections Project, Bacterial Diseases Branch, Epidemiology Program, Centers for Disease Control, U.S. Public Health Service, Atlanta, Georgia

Jonathan E. Rhoads, M.D., F.A.C.S.
Professor of Surgery, University of Pennsylvania, Department of Surgery, Philadelphia, Pennsylvania

Jonathan E. Rhoads, Jr., M.D.
Assistant Professor of Surgery, Medical College of Pennsylvania, Philadelphia, Pennsylvania

Robert E. Richie, M.D.
Assistant Professor of Thoracic Surgery, Vanderbilt University, V.A. Hospital, Nashville, Tennessee

Brooke Roberts, M.D.
Hospital of the University of Pennsylvania, Philadelphia, Pennsylvania

Leon D. Sabath, M.D.
Associate Professor, Department of Medicine, Harvard University, Boston, Massachusetts

William R. Sandusky, M.D., F.A.C.S.
C. Bruce Morton Professor of Surgery, University of Virginia Medical Center, Charlottesville, Virginia

Jay Sanford, M.D.
Professor of Internal Medicine, and Chief, Infectious Disease Section, University of Texas Southwestern, Dallas, Texas

Paul E. Shorb, M.D., F.A.C.S.
Associate Professor of Surgery, George Washington University, Washington, D.C.

David Smith, M.D.
Children's Hospital, Boston, Massachusetts

Gordon T. Stewart, M.D.
Professor and Chairman, Department of Epidemiology, School of Public Health and Tropical Medicine, Tulane University, New Orleans, Louisiana

Frank E. Stinchfield, M.D., F.A.C.S.
Professor of Surgery, Director of Orthopaedic Service, Columbia–Presbyterian Medical Center, New York, New York

Lawrence Swartz, Ph.D.
Assistant Professor of Economics, University of North Dakota, Grand Forks, North Dakota

Malcolm C. Todd, M.D., F.A.C.S.
Associate Clinical Professor of Surgery, University of California College of Medicine at Irvine, Irvine, California

Jeremiah Turcotte, M.D., F.A.C.S.
Professor of Surgery, University of Michigan, Ann Arbor, Michigan

Carl W. Walter, M.D., F.A.C.S.
Clinical Professor of Surgery, Harvard Medical School, Boston, Massachusetts

Norton G. Waterman, M.D.
Associate Professor of Surgery and Microbiology, University of Louisville, Louisville, Kentucky

Henry T. Winkelman, A.I.A.
Caudill Rowlett Scott Design, Inc., Houston, Texas

Lillian Wittmeyer, R.N.
Surgical Nursing Supervisor, Cincinnati General Hospital, Cincinnati, Ohio

R. Lewis Wright, M.D., F.A.C.S.
Department of Neurosurgery, Medical College of Virginia, Richmond, Virginia

Stephen Wysocki, M.D.
Chirurgische Universitätsklinik, University of Heidelberg, Heidelberg, Germany

Jack Zimmerman, M.D., F.A.C.S.
Associate Professor of Surgery, Johns Hopkins University School of Medicine, Baltimore, Maryland

APPENDIX 2
Agenda of Symposia

First Symposium on Control of Surgical Infections
Fort Lauderdale, Florida
March 5–7, 1970

I   Opening Remarks
      Jonathan E. Rhoads, M.D.
      and James D. Hardy, M.D.

II   The Nature and Scope of the Problem of Surgical Infections
      Introduction
      William A. Altemeier, M.D., Chairman
      Changing National Patterns of Hospital Infections
      Philip Brachman, M.D.
      Morbidity and Mortality from Surgical Infections
      William R. Sandusky, M.D.

III   Economic Problems
      The Cost of Hospital Infections
      Lawrence Swartz, Ph.D.
      Malpractice and Professional Liability Insurance Problems
      Bert L. Halter, M.D.
      Legal Issues Involved
      Betty Jane Anderson

IV   Surgical Infections
      Development of a Working Classification of Surgical Infections
      William R. Cole, M.D.
      Incidence of Wound Infections and Relationship to Types of Operation
      John H. Davis, M.D.
      Types of Bacteria Causing Infections
      John V. Bennett, M.D.
      Surveillance of Hepatitis in Hospitals
      N. Joel Ehrenkranz, M.D.
      Types of Bacteria Causing Infections and Emerging New Pathogens
      Edward O. Hill, Ph.D.
      Epidemiology of Hospital-Based Infections
      Gordon T. Stewart, M.D.
      The Hospital Reservoir
      Jay Sanford, M.D.
      The Host Factors
      John F. Burke, M.D.
      Immunologic Factors
      J. Wesley Alexander, M.D.

The Biology of Response to Infection, Including Normal and Altered Patterns of Recovery
George H. A. Clowes, Jr., M.D.

V   The Prevention and Control of Surgical Infections
The Sources and Relative Significance of Contamination of Surgical Wounds
William R. Culbertson, M.D.

Sterilization Procedures and Control
Carl W. Walter, M.D.

Preparation and Regulations for Operating Room Team
Robert P. Hummel, M.D.

Preparation of the Patient and His Operative Area
William R. Cole, M.D.

VI   Summary Reports of Discussion Groups
Chairman of Each Group

VII   Concluding Remarks
W.A. Altemeier, M.D., Chairman

Second Symposium on Control of Surgical Infections
Washington, D.C.
March 8–9, 1971

I   Purpose and Plan of the Symposium
W.A. Altemeier, M.D., Chairman

II   Development of a Working Classification of Surgical Infections
The Problem of Classifying Surgical Infections
W.A. Altemeier, M.D.

Operating Room-Based Surgical Infections
William R. Sandusky, M.D.

Hospital-Based Surgical Infections
Hiram Polk, M.D.

Preoperative and Community-Based Surgical Infections
William R. Culbertson, M.D.

Viral and Non-Bacterial Infections
Basil A. Pruitt, Jr., M.D.

III   Control of Microbial Contamination in the Operating Room
Definition and Significance
W.A. Altemeier, M.D.

Recommended Sterilization Technics for the Modern Operating Room, Including Removal, Control and Decontamination of Soiled Linen, Instruments, and Equipment
Carl W. Walter, M.D.

Disinfection Technics and Agents in the Modern Operating Room
Ruth B. Kundsin, Sc.D.

Control of Microbial Contamination of Surfaces in the Modern Operating Room, and Pitfalls in Sterilization Procedures Currently Used in the Operating Room.
Frank B. Engley, Jr., Ph.D.
Environmental Air
William S. Blakemore, M.D.
Monitoring Technics
E.J.L. Lowbury, D.M.
Special Considerations in Control of Microbial Contact Contamination
William R. Cole, M.D.

IV Review of the First Symposium
W.A. Altemeier, M.D., Chairman

V Special Problems in the Control of Microbial Contamination in the Operating Room
Personnel as a Special Problem in Cross Contamination in the Operating Room
John H. Davis, M.D.
Carriers
Carl W. Walter, M.D.
Regulations for Control of Operating Room Activities of Consultants, X-ray and Laboratory Personnel
John F. Burke, M.D.
Architectural Designs for Control of Bacterial Contamination in the Operating Room
Harold Laufman, M.D.
Traffic Control
Wiley F. Barker, M.D.
Effect of Design in Architectural Patterns of Operating Rooms to Control Traffic and Air Circulation
Henry T. Winkelman, A.I.A.
Environmental Control
John F. Burke, M.D.
Housecleaning
George F. Mallison, M.P.H.
Air Circulation
Norman K. Kurtz, Consulting Engineer
Report of the Collaborative Study on Ultraviolet Irradiation in Operating Room Practice
John M. Howard, M.D.
Tracheostomy Care
Don R. Miller, M.D.
Surveillance and Reporting of Surgical Infections
John V. Bennett, M.D.

VI Summary Reports of Discussion Groups
Chairman of Each Group

VII Concluding Remarks
          W.A. Altemeier, M.D., Chairman

**Third Symposium on Control of Surgical Infections
Washington, D.C.
January 10–11, 1972**

  I Welcome and Orientation
          Opening Remarks
            James D. Hardy, M.D.
          Purpose and Plan of Symposium
            W.A. Altemeier, M.D., Chairman
 II Iatrogenic Infections in Surgical Patients
          The Problem
            W.A. Altemeier, M.D.
          Operating Room-Based Iatrogenic Infections — Types, Sources and
            Treatment
            Hiram C. Polk, M.D.
          Iatrogenic Infections of the Urinary Tract
            Calvin M. Kunin, M.D.
          Iatrogenic Respiratory Tract Infections
            Jay Sanford, M.D.
          Recent Studies of Nosocomial Infections from Intravenous Infusions
            Frank Rhame, M.D.
          Antibiotic Related Infections
            Maxwell Finland, M.D.
          Drug Related Infections
            J. Wesley Alexander, M.D.
III Environmental Control and the "Clean Room"
          Definition and Significance of the Problem
            W.A. Altemeier, M.D.
          Bacteriologic Studies of Alteration in O.R. Environmental Contami-
            nation with "Clean Room"
            William F. Enneking, M.D.
          The Birmingham Experience
            E.J.L. Lowbury, D.M.
          The Use of the Clean Air Room — Is It Essential or Not?
            N. Eftekhar, M.D.
          Report of the American College of Surgeons' Committee on Control
            of Operating Room Environment
            Harold Laufman, M.D.
          Report on Legal and Malpractice Liabilities Relative to Non-Use of the
            "Clean Room"
            Malcolm C. Todd, M.D.

VIII   Laboratory Support and Special Planning for Prevention and Control of
         Infections in the Operating Room
            Recommended General Procedures
               Bruce G. MacMillan, M.D.
            Special Considerations for the Septic Case
               George H.A. Clowes, M.D.
            Recent Experiences in Quality Control of Clinical Microbiological
               Testing
               John V. Bennett, M.D.
            Pharmacokinetics and Dynamics of Antibiotics
               Stephen Wysocki, M.D.
            Special Considerations for Burn Patients
               Basil A. Pruitt, Jr., M.D.
  IX   Summary Reports of Discussion Groups
            Chairman of Each Group
   X   Closing Remarks and Discussion
            W.A. Altemeier, M.D., Chairman

Fourth Symposium on Control of Surgical Infections
Washington, D.C.
November 10–11, 1972

    I   Welcome and Orientation
            Opening Remarks
               Jonathan E. Rhoads, M.D. and
               James D. Hardy, M.D.
            Purpose and Plan of the Fourth Symposium
               W.A. Altemeier, M.D., Chairman
   II   Assessment of Patient Risk to Infection
            General Factors
               William R. Culbertson, M.D.
            Immunologic Factors
               J. Wesley Alexander, M.D.
            Pathophysiologic State of Wounds
               John H. Davis, M.D.
            Surgical Procedures
               Paul E. Shorb, Jr., M.D.
            Anesthesia Procedures
               Lloyd D. Bridenbaugh, M.D.
            Respiratory Assistance Procedures and Antibiotic-Induced Changes in
               the Endogenous Flora
               Jay Sanford, M.D.

Hospital Differences in Mortality
Charles Gardner Child III, M.D.

Computerized Current Patterns of Surgical Use of Antimicrobial Agents in Community Hospitals
James Lindsey, M.D.
Julia S. Garner, R.N.
John V. Bennett, M.D.

Prospective Study of 20,105 Surgical Wounds with Emphasis on Use of Topical Antibiotics and Prophylactic Antibiotics
Peter J.E. Cruse, M.B.

III   Principles and Technics of Prophylactic Antibiotic Therapy

Definition and Significance of the Problem
W.A. Altemeier, M.D.

Modes of Action of Antibiotic Agents
Leon D. Sabath, M.D.

Time and Routes of Administration
John F. Burke, M.D.

Influence of Antibiotic Therapy on Changing Patterns of Infecting Microorganisms
Stephen Wysocki, M.D.

Bacterial Acquired Antibiotic Resistance (Transfer of R-Factors)
David Smith, M.D.

Host – Pathogen – Drug Relationships
Maxwell Finland, M.D.
John E. McGowan, M.D.

Studies on the Decisive Period of Prophylactic Antibiotic Therapy
Hiram C. Polk, M.D.

Relationship of Antibiotic Treatment to Super- and Opportunistic Infections
N. Joel Ehrenkranz, M.D.

IV   Symposium on Controversial Issues

Antibiotic Prophylaxis in Preoperative Preparations for Colon Operations
Hiram C. Polk, M.D.
Robert P. Hummel, M.D.
Jeremiah Turcotte, M.D.
George Bornside, Ph.D.
Jay Sanford, M.D.
Ronald Lee Nichols, M.D.
W.A. Altemeier, M.D.

Special Considerations of Prophylactic Antibiotic Therapy
John H. Davis, M.D.
Maxwell Finland, M.D.
J. Wesley Alexander, M.D.
William S. Blakemore, M.D.

VI   Summary Recommendations for Use of Prophylactic Antibiotic Therapy
        Chairman of Each Discussion Group
VII   Development of Tables and Charts for Reference and Clinical Use
VIII   Closing Remarks
        W.A. Altemeier, M.D., Chairman

Index

An *f* following a page number indicates a figure; a *t* indicates tabular material.